The Double-Edged Helix

The Double-Edged Helix

Social Implications of Genetics in a Diverse Society

Edited by

Joseph S. Alper, Catherine Ard,
Adrienne Asch, Jon Beckwith,
Peter Conrad, and Lisa N. Geller

The Johns Hopkins University Press
Baltimore and London

The Johns Hopkins University Press
2715 North Charles Street
Baltimore, Maryland 21218-4363
www.press.jhu.edu

Library of Congress Cataloging-in-Publication Data

The double-edged helix : social implications of genetics in a diverse society
/ edited by Joseph S. Alper . . . [et al.].
    p.   ; cm.
Includes bibliographical references and index.
ISBN 0-8018-6964-1 (alk. paper)
    1. Human genetics—Social aspects.
[DNLM: 1. Bioethics. 2. Genetic Techniques. 3. Genetics, Medical. QH 438.7
D727 2002] I. Alper, Joseph S., 1946–
QH438.7 .D68 2002
599.93'5—dc21   2001006618

A catalog record for this book is available from the British Library.

Contents

Contributors

Joseph S. Alper, Ph.D., is a professor of chemistry at the University of Massachusetts–Boston. He is one of the original members of the Genetic Screening Study Group.

Catherine Ard, M.H.H.S., is a Ph.D. candidate at Brandeis University specializing in the diffusion of emerging genetic technologies. She has been a member of the Genetic Screening Study Group since 1992.

Adrienne Asch, Ph.D., M.S., is Henry R. Luce Professor in Biology, Ethics, and the Politics of Human Reproduction at Wellesley College. She has written many articles and books on genetics and assisted reproduction and has been a member of the Genetic Screening Study Group since 1995.

Carol I. Barash, Ph.D., a trained philosopher, is founder and principal consultant at Genetics, Ethics and Policy Consulting, which optimizes the integration of genomics into twenty-first-century health care.

Jon Beckwith, Ph.D., is American Cancer Society Research Professor of Microbiology and Molecular Genetics at Harvard Medical School. He is one of the original members of the Genetic Screening Study Group.

Diane Beeson, Ph.D., is a professor of sociology and chair of the Department of Sociology and Social Services at California State University, Hayward. She was one of the first social scientists to study prenatal genetic testing.

Paul R. Billings, M.D., Ph.D., is cofounder and chief medical/scientific officer of GeneSage, Inc., in San Francisco.

William Byne, M.D., Ph.D., is director of the Laboratory of Neuroanatomy and Morphometrics in the Department of Psychiatry at the Mount Sinai School of Medicine in New York and has examined the human brain for anatomical correlates of sexual orientation.

Peter Conrad, Ph.D., is Harry Coplan Professor of Social Sciences at Brandeis University and studies the public discourse of genetics and behavior and the meanings of biomedical enhancement. He has been a member of the Genetic Screening Study Group since 1993.

Jack Drescher, M.D., is a training and supervising analyst at the William Alanson White Psychoanalytic Institute and author of *Psychoanalytic Therapy and the Gay Man.*

Troy Duster, Ph.D., is a professor of Sociology at New York University and served as a member of the National Advisory Council of the National Center for Human Genome Research.

Lisa N. Geller, Ph.D., J.D., is a technology specialist at Fish & Richardson. She is one of the original members of the Genetic Screening Study Group.

Mitchell Lasco, Ph.D., teaches at Lehman College, Bronx, New York. His research interests include the role of the hypothalamus in sexuality and brain reward systems.

C. Phoebe Lostroh, Ph.D., is a postdoctoral fellow in the Department of Microbiology at the University of Iowa. She has been a member of the Genetic Screening Study Group.

Susan Markens, Ph.D., is an assistant professor of sociology at Temple University. Her current research concerns the rise of new genetic and reproductive technologies, with a particular focus on the medicalization of pregnancy and the impact of prenatal genetic screening of women's reproductive autonomy.

Udo Schuklenk, Ph.D., is associate professor of bioethics and human rights in the Faculty of Health Sciences at the University of the Witwatersrand, Johannesburg, South Africa, and head of the division of bioethics.

Alan Stockdale, Ph.D., is a senior research and development associate at the Center for Applied Ethics and Professional Practice at Education Development Center in Newton, Massachusetts.

Sharon F. Terry is the founding executive director of PXE International and Vice President of Consumers for the Genetic Alliance.

Amanda Udis-Kessler, Ph.D., is assistant professor of sociology at Ripon College and has written extensively about sexuality, feminism, and social justice.

Deborah R. Zucker, Ph.D., M.D., an internist and molecular geneticist, is currently a faculty clinician and health services researcher at New England Medical Center and Tufts University School of Medicine.

Acknowledgments

More than most books, this volume is a collective effort. Not only did we have a larger than usual editorial team, but many other people also contributed useful comments, constructive criticism, and various kinds of support to this book. The editors are particularly grateful to the current and past members of the Genetic Screening Study Group (GSSG) who lived with this project from its inception. Many of the chapters were discussed during the biweekly GSSG meetings. The group provided a continuity, an intellectual camaraderie, and an exchange that sharpened our thinking and clarified complex issues. GSSG members whose contributions are of special note are Joseph Chen, C. Phoebe Lostroh, Susan Markens, Joel Roselin, Daniel Goldstein, Amanda Udis-Kessler, and Deborah Zucker.

The editors appreciate the hospitality of the Geller-Rauch household for hosting most of our meetings: Lisa for cheese and wine; Steve and Jay for the spontaneous entertainment. This book would not, of course, have been possible without the authors who generously contributed their efforts to this volume and who tolerated our group process and requests for revisions with considerable fortitude.

We owe much to the reviewers and editors of the Johns Hopkins University Press, whose comments stimulated lively discussion. Tom Murray especially encouraged us to pursue this project and provided support, notably in the initial stages. Celestia Ward, our copyeditor, suggested numerous revisions that resulted in a much clearer and more readable book. Finally, we laud Wendy Harris, our editor at the Johns Hopkins University Press, for her patience, persistence, and ability to understand the processes of six editors.

The Double-Edged Helix

Perspectives on Perspectives

Joseph S. Alper, Catherine Ard, Adrienne Asch,
Jon Beckwith, Peter Conrad, and Lisa N. Geller

In February 2001, two competing research groups announced the near-completion of the primary goal of the Human Genome Project: the DNA sequence of the entire set of human chromosomes (International Genome Sequencing Consortium, 2001; Venter et al., 2001). This analysis allowed the identification of approximately thirty thousand genes carried by the forty-six human chromosomes. Since its inception, leaders of the project have used such metaphors as the "book of life," the "holy grail," and the "blueprint for life" to describe the importance of the human genome sequence (Beckwith, 1999). Its first director, James Watson, stated that we now know, by and large, that "our fate is in our genes" (Jaroff, 1989). Genome scientists suggested, and the media eagerly reported, that the information from the Genome Project would revolutionize the diagnosis of disease and would lead to the cures, or at least treatments, of many of our most feared illnesses (see Chapter 2 of this volume).

Historical Background

Not everyone was so sanguine about the consequences of a tremendous increase in the availability of genetic information. Historically, the use of genetic information (usually misinformation) has been detrimental and some-times catastrophic to countless people's lives (Marks, 1995). Psychologists in the early twentieth century devised IQ tests that purportedly measured the inherited portion of intelligence (Kamin, 1974). They studied thousands of people, especially army recruits, and concluded not only that intelligence was inherited but also that racial and ethnic groups differed in their inborn intel-ligence. In the 1920s, these claims were used to justify the restrictive immigra-tion laws that were enacted in the United States (Chase, 1980). During the first third of the twentieth century, German researchers used these ideas to argue that the racial purity of the German people (which they called the Aryan race) was being corrupted by mixing with the blood of inferior peoples (Muller-Hill, ˌ1988). The importance of these ideas from the scientific community as causal factors of the Holocaust is still a matter of debate. Nevertheless, justification for the Holocaust was frequently couched in the language of eugenics.

After millions of people were murdered simply because they were not Aryan, many researchers around the world came to believe that studying the genetics of race, and, more generally, genetic differences among people, was unacceptable. However, by the late 1960s, these strong feelings had dissipated. In a widely reported paper published in 1969, psychologist Arthur Jensen, of the University of California–Berkeley, maintained that black people had a lower intelligence than white people and that efforts such as the Head Start program, designed to overcome the substandard educational environment of many black students and poor children of other races, were doomed to failure (Jensen, 1969). A few years later, psychologist Richard Herrnstein of Harvard University argued that because intelligence was inherited and because an indi-vidual's financial success in the United States depended on intelligence, finan-cial success was inherited. Furthermore, he argued, inequality in the United States will increase, since people tend to marry people of their own intelligence level (Herrnstein, 1973).

In 1975 E. O. Wilson published *Sociobiology: The New Synthesis* (Wilson, 1975a). The final chapter of this book applies sociobiology to the human species. In it, Wilson attempted to show that most human behavior can be explained in terms of evolutionary processes. Since evolution is driven by genetic variation, Wilson argued that human social behavior must be largely genetic. It may sound quaint today, but in a 1975 *New York Sunday Times* magazine article, Wilson stated that because of genetic differences, "even with identical education and equal access to all professions, men are more likely to play a disproportionate role in politics, business, and science" (Wilson, 1975b).

In response to these interpretations of human genetics, a group of Boston academics who were part of a radical science organization called Science for the People began meeting to discuss these issues. We called ourselves the Sociobiology Study Group. In a series of papers, talks delivered at scientific conferences, and organized public meetings, the group critiqued the extension of sociobiology to contemporary human social behavior. Of special concern were the evolutionary explanations, typified by Wilson's *New York Times* pronouncement, of the continued and pervasive sexism in American society.

The Genetic Screening Study Group

By the mid-1980s, the "sociobiology debate" had run its course. At the same time, the science of human molecular genetics was on the verge of becoming mature. Within a few years, funding provided by the Human Genome Project would further accelerate progress in the field. We realized that the social and political consequences of genetics would no longer be restricted to theoretical descriptions of human behavior, such as those given by sociobiology. The new applied genetics, which focused on finding the actual chemical entities responsible for diseases and traits, could have serious social side effects in addition to the obvious benefits, such as early diagnosis and treatment of diseases. We decided that it was important first to study and then to address the potential consequences of the advances in human genetics, and we renamed ourselves the Genetic Screening Study Group. Three of the coeditors of this book (Joseph S. Alper, Jon Beckwith, and Lisa N. Geller) were among the original members of this group.

As our first project, we endeavored to determine the effect of the increasing availability of DNA-based genetic tests. How does genetic testing, especially predictive genetic testing, affect the lives of people who are found to carry mutations conferring increased susceptibility to genetic diseases? We were particularly interested in determining whether any of these people suffered discrimination and, if so, the form that the discrimination took. Our preliminary study suggested that what has been termed genetic discrimination was indeed a problem (Billings et al., 1992). A grant from the ELSI (Ethical, Legal, and Social Implications) program funded by the Department of Energy enabled us to conduct an extensive survey designed to study the forms and prevalence of genetic discrimination. We found that genetic discrimination did in fact exist and manifested itself in many forms. Some people were denied insurance and employment. Others were subjected to discrimination by the army and by educational institutions. The article reporting our results (Geller et al., 1996) is reprinted as Chapter 12 of this book.

Since the publication of our study, concerns about this type of discrimination have increased dramatically. As of August 2001, approximately forty states and the federal government had passed a variety of laws and regulations banning genetic discrimination. In June 2001, President George W. Bush decried the use of genetic discrimination by health insurance companies and called for legislation to remedy the problem.

The Genesis and Purpose of This Book

This book expands our explorations of the impact of genetic research on contemporary social life. When genetic researchers urged the U.S. Congress to allocate $3 billion for the project to study the human genome, they argued that genomic information would help society in treating and curing disease, would aid in the birth of healthy children, would reveal the origins of many traits linked to positive and negative attributes, and would ameliorate social problems of poverty, substance abuse, crime, and violence. Since then, in numerous books and articles, philosophers, ethicists, sociologists, lawyers, and geneticists have examined the ethical, legal, political, and other social implications of the Human Genome Project.

By the late 1990s, the efforts of these scholars had resulted in an extensive and important body of work that sought to clarify the issues and to suggest answers to troubling ethical and social questions raised by the new genetic research. Four examples of such issues are: the privacy and confidentiality of an individual's genetic information (Rothstein, 1997); the morality of genetic therapy and enhancement (Walters and Palmer, 1997; Parens, 1998); the implications of genetics for access to health care (Murray, Rothstein, and Murray, 1996); and the economic and legal questions concerning ownership of genetic information (Guenin, 2000).

Despite this vast literature, our group felt that an important aspect was missing from the analysis of the new genetics. Nearly all of the existing books and articles dealt with the issues from the point of view of "society." All too often, this point of view had been interpreted to mean the point of view of those with the greatest economic and political power. For example, much had been written about the science and economics of developing new pharmaceuticals for rare genetic diseases and about the possibilities of population screening for genetic conditions. However, little was written about how such developments would affect the lives of people with these conditions.

Our approach in this book supplements the existing bioethical and social science literature. We have attempted to highlight how those members of society who do not always make their way into policy deliberations understand and are affected by genetic technology. In our opinion, previous literature did not pay adequate attention to the full range of values, voices, and interests that should be included in any discussion of the social and ethical impact of the new genetics. To remedy this deficit, we decided to focus on a few illustrative problems and allow voices of nondominant groups, which are not normally heard, to speak.

Like a growing number of observers, we believe that science itself incorporates values. Values are reflected in the choices made about what problems to study, what research to fund, and even what approaches to take in solving scientific problems. These choices can both directly and indirectly affect the various communities represented in this book.

Consider the following example illustrating the choices involved regarding a disabling but nonlethal disease that is believed to be caused in part by mutated genes. Should researchers focus their attention on discovering the underlying genetics of the disease with the goal of preventing it, or should they study the disease itself with the goal of improving treatment? (Assume, for the sake of simplicity, that these approaches do not overlap.) What criteria should be used for deciding how much effort should be devoted to each approach?

Scholars seeking such criteria must choose a perspective. A successful perspective would enable them to evaluate on a single scale the merits of each of the conflicting sets of values underlying the two approaches. If such a scale can be found, the values can be reconciled.

In the biweekly meetings of the Genetic Screening Study Group, we did not feel constrained to find the best single set of criteria, to continue our example. Instead, we felt free to explore in detail the potentially irreconcilable values held by different groups. Prospective parents might urge that every effort be made to prevent their baby from being affected by the disease; people with disabilities might be more concerned with treating people already affected by the disease.

In discussing conflicts like these, we realized that it would be useful to present to the general public an exposition of such issues and conflicts from the perspectives of the groups involved. Since our group was itself composed of people representing quite varied disciplines and experiences, we believed that we were well situated to engage in a study of groups. During the course of preparing this book, the Genetic Screening Study Group has included scientists, physicians, a lawyer, sociologists, ethicists, a high school biology teacher, journalists, and students in various fields. The skills we developed for talking and interacting across disciplines were essential to the construction of this book.

The Focus on Perspectives and Communities

We decided to prepare a book whose chapters would each focus on a different "community" in society, discussing how that community was materially affected by genetic discoveries and how members of that community experienced and responded to these discoveries. We use the term *community* to refer to an identifiable group of people who have similar social situations and similar perspectives and interests: for example, geneticists, people with genetic diseases or disabilities, or African Americans. This definition of community is, of course, an oversimplification. First, individuals and groups within a single community often differ in their views and concerns. Second, a single individual may be a member of more than one community. A woman, as a member of the community of research geneticists, might participate in the development of genetic reproductive technology. As a geneticist, she experiences the advances in her field differently from a woman who, belonging to the community of consumers, must decide what type of assistive reproductive technology, if any, is best for her. Of course, the same woman may be both a geneticist and a prospective user of reproductive technology. She might find that her assessment of the products of genetic reproductive research may differ depending on whether she is working in her lab or is at home with her family.

In soliciting chapters for this book, we first prepared a list of those communities, and in some cases subcommunities, for whom genetic issues are especially relevant. A book of thirteen chapters cannot hope to provide the full range of the diversity of perspectives on genetics held by all the subcultures within our society. Nevertheless, the range of views and the complex social dynamics that are presented in the various chapters encompass many of the problems faced by other groups and subcultures not specifically included in this volume. For each of the chosen communities or subcommunities, we sought contributors who would explore the impact of genetic discoveries and technologies. Some of the contributors are academic researchers who present the results of their research on various communities; other contributors are themselves members of a target community.

The differing perspectives among the communities presented in our book have led to conflicts among these communities over many issues arising from applications of genetics. In recent years, controversies have arisen over the marketing of new genetic tests for such diseases as cystic fibrosis and breast cancer, the search for genes contributing to homosexual behavior, and research programs to study the genes of certain ethnic groups.

These controversies occur because professional communities, religious organizations, governmental agencies, business interests, and different segments within the public can perceive genetics in very different ways. It is evident from the stridency of some of the debates that clashes arising from differing perspectives are becoming crucial in an increasing number of people's lives. Several chapters of this book explore these irreconcilable conflicts. We, the editors, have made no effort at reconciliation. Instead, by presenting the voices of groups that are typically not heard, we hope that those debating public policy will begin to take the interests of these groups more seriously.

Because this book is about genetics, we start with the community of geneticists who have developed the new technology. Geneticists advance our knowledge about genetic diseases and potentially about treatments of these diseases. However, the community of people with these genetic diseases, their families, and their advocates have a different perspective from the researcher on what it means to live with these diseases. Many members of this community prefer to use the term *conditions* instead of *genetic diseases* to emphasize this difference in perspective.

The community of people with disabilities is also extremely troubled by the increasing prevalence of selective abortion. Selective abortion and other forms of genetic reproductive technologies raise other issues that primarily affect women. Reports of the existence of a "gay gene" have provoked such a diversity of responses that we solicited two chapters: the first is by male psychiatrists and genetic researchers, and the second, by two women who identify themselves as belonging to the gay/lesbian/bisexual/transsexual community.

No book about communities can avoid the subject of race. In the United States, genetic screening programs for sickle cell disease have had a major impact on African American communities. The racial history and current racial environment in the United States inevitably affects the reception of new genetic technologies into these communities. On the global scale, geneticists have been carrying out population genetic studies on various ethnic groups throughout the world. These studies went largely unnoticed until geneticists proposed that their efforts be organized into what is now called the Human Genome Diversity Project. This project, designed to systematize the search for genetic differences among ethnic groups, has been attacked because of its potentially racist implications. We have devoted separate chapters to each of these two very different types of genetic programs.

As a result of our focus on the perspectives of communities, several important social issues arising from advances in molecular genetics were omitted. The authors were instructed to focus on those problems that they believed to be most important to their respective communities. Some omitted issues, such as gene therapy and gene enhancement, are in their infancy and have not yet had any significant effect on the communities discussed in this book. Others, such as privacy and the confidentiality of genetic records, can be analyzed under the rubric of genetic discrimination, which is discussed in the last two chapters of this book.

As a result of advances in genetic technology, the controversies over certain other issues, such as DNA fingerprinting, have faded. In just a few years the debate over DNA fingerprinting has been transformed from concern with its validity and the possibility of convicting innocent suspects to the demand that all convicted criminals be granted the right to DNA fingerprinting so they can use that information in attempts to exonerate themselves. This development suggests that the impact of genetics on communities can change over time. It is quite conceivable that the perspectives of many of the communities discussed in this book will change significantly as a result of future advances in genetic technology and as a result an increasing familiarity with and understanding of these advances.

A Tour through the Book

The title of this book, *The Double-Edged Helix: Social Implications of Genetics in a Diverse Society,* reflects the messages we wished to convey. "The double-edged helix" suggests that each group in society, even those groups who traditionally receive much less of their share of social benefits, experience both the pluses and the minuses of genetic technology. Perhaps the greatest challenge in preparing this book was striking the proper balance between irrational enthusiasm for the new technology and Luddite rejection of any change from the way things always have been. "Social implications of genetics in a diverse society" emphasizes the idea that in a society like ours, much of the story is lost if it is told exclusively from a monolithic "top-down" point of view.

Until recently, the assumption that most human traits are controlled by genes and, in particular, that there is one gene primarily responsible for each trait, appeared to inform most analyses of the social implications of genetics. In Chapter 1, "Genetic Complexity in Human Disease and Behavior," Joseph S. Alper, a theoretical chemist with a longstanding interest in the social implications of human genetics, introduces some fundamental concepts of genetics to show that traits are a result of complex interactions among genes and the environment. The complexity of these interactions explains why it is so difficult to develop accurate diagnostic genetic tests, why there have been no confirmed reports of genes for mental illnesses such as schizophrenia and bipolar disorder that seem to be strongly inherited, and why the genetics of human behavior is so poorly understood. Alper concludes that only after we appreciate genetic complexity can we hope to discuss intelligently any of the contentious societal issues arising from the new genetics.

The people who actually do the research and produce the technological and conceptual advances in genetics can significantly affect the impact their work has on society. Historically, the presence or absence of geneticists in public discussions may have played a critical role in the applications of their discoveries. Jon Beckwith, a geneticist, reviews this history in Chapter 2, "Geneticists in Society, Society in Genetics," and analyzes the factors that influence the stance geneticists take on such issues as genetic determinism and the implementation of genetic screening. While geneticists as a group may be quite diverse in their views, statements by leaders of the genetics community do not always mirror this diversity. Beckwith describes some of the factors that determine the public positions taken by geneticists. He also offers explanations for the failure of many geneticists to express their opposition in the face of misuses and misrepresentation of genetics.

In Chapter 3, "Genetics and Behavior in the News: Dilemmas of a Rising Paradigm," Peter Conrad, a sociologist, examines the public discourse surrounding genes and behavior. He investigates how the news media cover stories involving human genetics and shows that the media, as a professional community, create the lens (or lenses) through which the public views genetics. Consequently, the media play an important role in shaping public discourse on genetics. In view of this role, it is unfortunate that the media have often exaggerated the influence of genes on human behavior. In many cases, it propagated the inaccurate "one gene–one disease" model of genetic causality and downplayed retractions of previously reported discoveries of these genes. This flawed coverage of genetics not only results in the overemphasis of the role of genes in human problems but also raises unrealistic expectations about the fruits of genetic research.

The next several chapters explore one of the most important promises of the new genetics: improved human health. Genetic knowledge may yield the information that will be required to treat and cure chronic illnesses or disabilities that arise at birth or later in life. It will also allow the testing of individuals or screening of populations to prevent the birth of children who are likely to be affected by one or another such condition. People with disabilities, their families and friends, women of childbearing age, and members of ethnic groups that carry genes for particular conditions have all been concerned that genetic information may affect their freedom, equality, and well-being. Chapters 4 through 7 deal with aspects of these concerns.

Genetic self-help groups are organizations composed primarily of individuals with genetic disabilities and their families and friends. These groups provide information and support to their members and lobby for increased funds for developing treatments. The two authors of Chapter 4, "Advocacy Groups and the New Genetics," present different perspectives on these groups. Alan Stockdale, an anthropologist, offers a historical and critical analysis of the Cystic Fibrosis Foundation from the point of view of an outside observer. Sharon F. Terry, an activist mother whose two children have PXE, a rare genetic disease, founded PXE International. She writes about her experiences as an activist and advocate trying to shape the organization to meet the needs of the affected individuals.

In Chapter 5, "Invisible Women: Gender, Genetics, and Reproduction," Susan Markens, a sociologist, contends that women are often neglected in debates about the uses of genetic knowledge and technologies. Markens draws on recent feminist scholarship that highlights the gendered nature of much genetic decision making. Using data derived from her own collaborative research on women offered prenatal testing, she shows that despite common involvement of couples, women maintained a significant autonomy over decision making. However, although prenatal testing creates more "choice" and gives women more control, it also engenders new anxieties and familial and social pressures. While women generally view genetic technologies favorably, Markens suggests that access to genetic information is not always desirable.

In Chapter 6, "Prenatal Diagnosis and Selective Abortion: A Challenge to Practice and Policy," Adrienne Asch, who teaches and does research in reproductive ethics, women's studies, and disability, discusses the impact of the growing practice of selective abortion on the community of people with disabilities. She also examines society's quest to alter its understanding of life with disease and disability. In contrast to Stockdale and Terry, who focus on science and medicine to solve the problems of disease and disability, Asch believes that many of the difficulties faced by people with disabilities can be ameliorated by means of societal change. And in contrast with Markens's empirical approach based on her own research, Asch focuses on a theoretical analysis of the empirical studies reported in the literature. The contrasting approaches of Chapters 4, 5, and 6 complement one another in presenting a more complete picture of the implications of reproductive technologies.

Chapters 7 and 8 deal with issues involving racial and ethnic groups. The understanding of genetics and its uses can be mediated by culture and ethnicity. Chapter 7, "African American Perspectives on Genetic Testing," by sociologists Diane Beeson and Troy Duster, continues the discussion of the application of genetic technology to health care, but it does so from the perspective of African Americans. Beeson and Duster focus on African Americans' response to the genetic test for the sickle cell trait. When comparing African Americans who have a relatively high likelihood of developing sickle cell disease with white Americans who are similarly at risk for cystic fibrosis, the authors found that the concerns and actions of the two groups were in many ways remarkably similar in their ambivalence about the new genetic medicine. But among African Americans, they observed a higher level of what the authors call "narratives of resistance." African Americans tended to distrust the motives of those promoting genetic medicine. They were concerned about the risk and stigma associated with genetic testing in the context of racism. And they tended to regard the threat of genetic disease as comparatively minor alongside the more immediate threats to their well-being, such as poverty, disease, and the stresses of everyday life. Beeson and Duster echo themes from Asch's critique and from Stockdale and Terry's analysis of the role played by genetic information in the lives of individuals and families affected by characteristics considered abnormal and negative.

An overwhelming majority of geneticists who study human genes and anthropologists who study human societies agrees that there is no scientific concept of race. However, the social concept of race remains exceedingly important in our divided society. In Chapter 8, "Genetics, Race, and Ethnicity:

Searching for Differences," Alper and Beckwith examine how genetics has historically played and still plays a role in discussions about racial differences. Certain diseases are more prevalent in certain racial and ethnic groups than in others. Can and should therapies be targeted to specific groups? A variety of research projects have been proposed or implemented to conduct a systematic analysis of genetic differences among a wide variety of ethnic groups throughout the world. Could the genetic differences that will undoubtedly be found be used to justify racial discrimination? Alper and Beckwith discuss these problems and provide a framework for their analysis.

In contrast to the concept of race, which has been stripped of its scientific validity, the concept of "sexual orientation" has, in recent years, been situated by some scientists in the realm of biology. In 1993, a group of National Institutes of Health (NIH) researchers announced they had found a region of the human X chromosome that they said was associated with male homosexuality. The publicity engendered by this report stimulated heated debates in the gay community and elsewhere. Would this finding lead to abortion of male fetuses who carried the "gay gene," or would a genetic explanation for homosexuality result in greater acceptance of gays by the population at large?

In Chapter 9, "The Origins of Homosexuality: No Genetic Link to Social Change," psychiatrist and researcher William Byne and his colleagues review the history of research into the origins of homosexuality, with a particular focus on the NIH study. They outline the variety of models, biological and social, that have been proffered to explain why some people are gay, and they raise the broader questions of scientific and medical definitions of normal and defective. Byne and his coauthors argue that supposed discoveries of biological bases for homosexuality present more dangers than benefits to the gay community. Therefore, they suggest that researchers who investigate this area have a serious responsibility to prevent such harm.

Many communities that are generally characterized by outsiders as being homogenous, are, in reality, quite diverse. For example, nonheterosexual people are often labeled as "gay" or "gay and lesbian." In Chapter 10, "Diversity and Complexity in Gay/Lesbian/Bisexual/Transsexual Responses to the 'Gay-Gene' Debate," C. Phoebe Lostroh, a geneticist, and Amanda Udis-Kessler, a sociologist, examine the diversity among nonheterosexuals in their views about genetics and homosexuality. In particular, they discuss how they, and respondents to a questionnaire they distributed, react to the possibility that the "gay gene" actually exists. Lostroh and Udis-Kessler conclude that nonheterosexuals show a wide variety of views about the genetics of homosexuality and its implications. These views are often at variance with those of the researchers conducting the search for the "gay gene."

Various groups and individuals are directly affected by the new genetics when scientific advances are developed into consumer products. In Chapter 11, "The Commercialization of Genetic Technologies: Raising Public Awareness," Catherine Ard, a researcher on social policy, and Deborah Zucker, a physician and biomedical researcher, examine the interests of the groups involved in and affected by technological development. Using four cases, the authors explore how academic scientists, universities, corporations, government, and consumers sometimes cooperate and at other times compete with each other to bring research into the marketplace. These collaborations promote development, yet raise concern regarding corporate influence on the direction of basic research, the possibility that a company could limit access to scientific findings, and possible conflicts of interest for researchers with a stake in a company's success. Ard and Zucker consider the risks to public trust in academia and science as biomedical research and private profit mix in the genetic era. In the view of the authors, the arrangements between academic science and the corporate world may have serious implications for consumers who rely on the products and services produced by these collaborations.

Chapter 12, "Individual, Family, and Societal Dimensions of Genetic Discrimination: A Case Study Analysis," reprints the article that reported the results of the original study of genetic discrimination carried out by members of the Genetic Screening Study Group. The study not only demonstrated the existence of genetic discrimination but also provided insight into its many manifestations. In Chapter 13, "Postscript: Current Developments in Genetic Discrimination," Lisa Geller, the lead author of the genetic discrimination article and now an attorney specializing in intellectual property and issues related to genetic technology, updates the article and discusses the current state of genetic discrimination legislation. She notes that there is still reason to be concerned both about maintaining the privacy of an individual's genetic information and about the unfairness of discrimination based on medical and, in particular, genetic information.

Conclusion

As the book developed, genetic complexity—the idea that most human behaviors and illnesses result from a complex interdependence among genetic and environmental influences—emerged as a central theme. This was not surprising. The Genetic Screening Study Group and its predecessor, the Socio-biology Study Group, had been emphasizing the importance of genetic complexity and the errors of biological determinist beliefs for twenty-five years.

We were also aware of other types of complexity. The moral, philosophical, social, political, legal, and even personal issues involved in the implications of the new molecular genetics have been extensively discussed. Nevertheless, we were not prepared for the degree of complexity we found. The complexity in the perspectives of the various communities discussed in this book strengthened our initial belief that resolving disputes over the appropriate uses of genetic information requires recognizing the differing needs, histories, and social situations of different groups within contemporary society. Rather than offering a bioethical analysis ourselves, we have let voices from many communities speak about their own concerns and conclusions. In so doing, we hope to enable a greatly expanded public policy debate.

Problems in the "real world" arise because different individuals and groups in society have different interests which are often competing. With the advancement of genetic knowledge and its applications, we need to consider the interests of scientists, who produce the knowledge; the media, who disseminate it; the corporations, who commercialize it; and, finally, the consumers, who use this knowledge and its applications.

The use of genetic technology in medicine introduces additional participants, namely, a wide range of health care providers. When this technology is applied to reproduction, subcommunities of the consumer group using this technology become important. Within the consumer group, conflicts may arise between husband and wife, genetic and gestational parent, and parent and fetus.

The issues affecting communities defined by race or ethnicity, gender, and disability are especially important because prejudice and discrimination and the resulting economic and political inequalities are still major problems in our society. Unfortunately, as the chapters of this book reveal, genetic information is currently divisive; people see themselves, even more than they might have otherwise, as members of distinct communities with different needs and interests. On the other hand, the finding that *all* people carry genes that may predispose them to a wide variety of health problems may help alleviate the problems caused by discrimination on the basis of genotype. The recognition that we all carry within us the potential for a genetic disability may lead to policies and practices that help people flourish irrespective of their genomes.

As editors who value biological and social diversity, we hope that our book will be of help in reaching this goal.

Although genetic advances resulting in increased predictive power and increased control over reproduction have raised some new dilemmas, the basic ethical and social issues and the conflicts arising over these issues are not new. It is our belief that these longstanding issues and conflicts cannot be resolved by ignoring the different contexts in which people make decisions and conduct their lives. Psychological, social, and economic factors must always be taken into account. In our present society, these factors include, but are not limited to, economic inequality, racial prejudice, and differences in cultural traditions, educational attainment, and even professional ambitions. Understanding these aspects of the social dynamics of early twenty-first century American society is necessary to help us deal with our burgeoning genetic knowledge.

If we are to cope with the social implications of the new genetics, we must learn to understand and appreciate the complexity and diversity of perspectives. Society is not monolithic. The views and interests of each of the diverse and overlapping groups of society must be heard, respected, and, to whatever extent possible, served. It is the responsibility of groups with more power, such as health care professionals, scientists, and corporations, to be aware of and respond to the needs of the less powerful, such as women, minorities, the economically disadvantaged, and people with disabilities.

Each conflict among these groups raises its own issues, and in attempting to resolve the conflict we must consider all perspectives. There are no easy answers. Resolving the twenty-first-century questions that genetics raises requires many of the same ideas that have characterized the best aspects of American democracy, primarily the recognition of the moral equality and worthiness of individuals and communities, regardless of their differing attributes. If our book contributes to such recognition and to a renewed commitment to such goals, we will be gratified indeed.

REFERENCES

Beckwith, J. 1999. "Genes and Human Behavior: Scientific and Ethical Implications of the Human Genome Project," in *Handbook of Molecular-Genetic Techniques for Brain and Behavioral Research*, Crusio, W., and Gerlai, R., eds. Amsterdam: Elsevier, pp. 917–26.

16   *Joseph S. Alper and Others*

Billings, P. R., M. A. Kohn, M. de Cuevas, J. Beckwith, J. S. Alper, and M. R. Natowicz. 1992. "Discrimination as a Consequence of Genetic Testing," *American Journal of Human Genetics* 50:476–82.

Chase, A. 1980. *The Legacy of Malthus: The Social Costs of the New Scientific Racism.* Urbana: University of Illinois Press.

Geller, L. N., J. S. Alper, P. R. Billings, C. J. Barash, J. Beckwith, and M. R. Natowicz. 1996. "Individual, Family and Societal Dimensions of Genetic Discrimination: A Case Study Analysis." *Science and Engineering Ethics* 2:71–88.

Guenin, L. M. 2000. "Patents, Ethics, Human Life Forms," in *Encyclopedia of Ethical, Legal and Policy Issues in Biotechnology,* eds. T. H. Murray and M. J. Mehlman. New York: J. Wiley and Sons, pp. 866–80.

Herrnstein, R. J. 1973. *I.Q. in the Meritocracy.* Boston: Atlantic Monthly Press.

International Human Genome Sequencing Consortium. 2001. "Initial Sequencing and Analysis of the Human Genome," *Nature* 409:860–921.

Jaroff, L. 1989. "The Gene Hunt," *Time,* March 20, p. 67.

Jensen, A. R. 1969. "How Much Can We Boost IQ in Scholastic Achievement?," *Harvard Educational Review* 33:1–123.

Kamin, L. J. 1974. *The Science and Politics of I.Q.* Potomac, Md.: Lawrence Erlbaum Associates.

Marks, J. 1995. *Human Biodiversity: Genes, Race, and History.* Hawthorne, N.Y.: Aldine de Gruyter.

Muller-Hill, B. 1988. *Murderous Science: Elimination by Scientific Selection of Jews, Gypsies, and Others, Germany, 1933–1945.* Oxford: Oxford University Press.

Murray, T. H., M. A. Rothstein, and R. Murray, Jr., eds. 1996. *The Human Genome Project and the Future of Health Care.* Indianapolis: Indiana University Press.

Parens, E., ed.. 1998. *Enhancing Human Traits: Ethical and Social Implications.* Washington, D.C.: Georgetown University Press.

Rothstein, M. A., ed. 1997. *Genetic Secrets: Protecting Privacy and Confidentiality in a Genetic Era.* New Haven: Yale University Press.

Venter, J. C., M. D. Adams, E. W. Myers, P. W. Li, R. J. Mural, et al. 2001. "The Sequence of the Human Genome," *Science* 291:1304–51.

Walters, L., and J. G. Palmer. 1997. *The Ethics of Human Gene Therapy.* New York: Oxford University Press.

Wilson, E. O. 1975a. *Sociobiology: The New Synthesis.* Cambridge: Harvard University Press.

———. 1975b. "Human Decency Is Animal," *New York Times Magazine,* October 12, 38–50.

CHAPTER ONE

Genetic Complexity in Human Disease and Behavior

Joseph S. Alper

The knowledge that certain diseases run in families is thousands of years old. But only in the past twenty-five years or so has it become practicable to link individual genes, the units of heredity, with particular diseases. For some single-gene diseases, the particular alleles (the possible structural forms of a gene) of the single gene responsible for the disease have been identified. In complex diseases like breast cancer, alleles have been found that are associated with increased likelihood of developing the disease, especially in women with a strong family history of breast and ovarian cancer (Sack, 1999).

Once an allele has been associated with a disease, it is a relatively simple matter to develop a genetic test that will determine whether or not a person carries that allele. The test results are simple to state: allele "X" has been found in patient "A." However, the interpretation of the test result is not simple. Because of genetic complexity, the subject of this chapter, a positive test indicating the presence of the allele does not necessarily mean that the patient will, or is even highly likely to, develop the disease. Consequently, in many cases the positive result may not be of much use to a physician in planning a course of prevention or to a patient in planning her or his life. Moreover, although a positive test result may not be useful to either physician or patient, it might be used by an insurance company or an employer to deny a policy or a job.

In addition to discovering genes associated with somatic diseases, researchers are now finding genes they believe to be associated with mental illnesses and with various aspects of human personality (Hamer and Copeland, 1998). These human traits include schizophrenia and manic depression among the mental illnesses, and intelligence, novelty seeking, sexual orientation, aggression, and addictive behavior among the personality traits. Behavioral geneticists have long believed that these traits and behaviors are influenced by genes (Plomin et al., 1997). However, their beliefs had been based on studies of family resemblances and differences. Such familial studies can at best provide clues about genetic influences, but they cannot identify the individual genes responsible for the illnesses and behaviors.

The evidence for genes associated with mental illnesses and behaviors is much weaker than the evidence for genes associated with somatic diseases like cystic fibrosis and breast cancer (Risch, 2000). Furthermore, differences in any given single gene from one person to another will probably account for only a small percentage of the wide variation in the manifestations of a corresponding illness or behavior (Tobin, 1999). These conditions and behaviors are the result of many genes operating in the context of a complex environment. No single gene is likely to explain an illness or behavior.

Despite the limitations of these genetic studies, people remain fascinated by genetic accounts of their behavior (Nelkin and Lindee, 1995). How much of our personalities, abilities, and accomplishments are inborn, and how much do we control? How can we understand the similarities (and differences) between parents and children and the differences (and similarities) between siblings? Beliefs about the role of genes have influenced, sometimes in contradictory fashion, how people think about themselves and others. On the one hand, claims about the genetic influences on differences in IQ scores among racial groups have been used to explain and rationalize social inequality and discrimination (Herrnstein and Murray, 1994). On the other hand, some members of the gay community believe that an understanding of the genetic basis of sexual orientation will lead to more acceptance of and less discrimination against homosexuals (Halley, 1994).

In their enthusiasm for the remarkable discoveries in the genetics of disease and behavior, some researchers and commentators have even suggested that genes play the dominant role in determining the course of our lives. James

Watson, the codiscoverer of the structure of the DNA, stated that "in large measure, our fate is in our genes" (Watson, 1997). In this view, genes are the blueprint for our lives. They determine who we are and what we are like. Free will is a myth because our minds and will are simply consequences of biochemical processes determined by our genes.

How is the layperson to make sense of these grandiose claims? Do our genes determine the course of our lives? How important is the sequencing of the human genome, the detailed listing of the approximately 3 billion bases that encode the genetic information carried by our DNA? The discussion of complexity in this chapter is designed to enable the reader to interpret these new genetic findings and to make informed decisions about the implications of these findings both for society and for their own lives.

Genetics 101 in Seven Paragraphs

To understand the genetic complexity involved in human disease and behavior, we first need to become familiar with the rudiments of human genetics (Griffiths et al., 1993). Genes are units of heredity. The dramatic progress in our understanding of human genetics stems from the discovery that genes are chemicals and that the operation of these chemicals can be understood in terms of their structure.

The genetic material in each cell consists of DNA (the abbreviation for the formal chemical name deoxyribonucleic acid), a long stringlike molecule. A string of DNA is composed of two strands that look like the two banisters of a freestanding spiral staircase. Since the mathematical name for a spiral is a helix, DNA is said to have the form of a double helix. For the understanding of genetics, the most important structural components of DNA are groups of atoms called bases, which are arrayed along the length of each strand of the string. There are four different bases: adenine, guanine, cytosine, and thymine, with the obvious abbreviations A, G, C, and T. The bases at corresponding positions along each strand of the string, in other words, at the two ends of the same step of the staircase, are always complementary. This means that if A appears at one end of a step, T appears at the other, and vice versa. Similarly, G and C are always paired. This pairing occurs because A-T pair and the G-T pair fit together like two pieces of a jigsaw puzzle. As Watson and Crick immediately realized upon their discovery of the structure of DNA, this complementarity enables the DNA to reproduce itself.

A gene is a section of DNA that has some particular function. This function is determined by the order of the bases in the gene, just as a word is determined by a particular sequence of letters. Most genes direct the synthesis of proteins. In humans, some of these proteins are structural (muscles), while others regulate the chemical reactions (for example, those required for digestion, vision, and thought) that are continually occurring within us.

Each chromosome contains one double-stranded string of DNA. With the exception of the sperm and egg cells, each cell of our bodies contains 23 pairs of chromosomes. The two chromosomes in each pair are related. The two genes in corresponding positions on the two paired chromosomes are associated with the same function. However, these genes need not be identical; the sequence of bases in the two genes may be somewhat different. The various possible forms of a gene found at a particular position on a particular chromosome are called alleles.

Each sperm or egg cell contains just one chromosome (selected at random) from each pair of related chromosomes. In reproduction, when a sperm and egg merge, the paired nature of each chromosome is restored. As a result of this mechanism, we inherit one chromosome of a pair from our father and the other chromosome from our mother. I am genetically different from each of my parents because one-half of my genes were inherited from the other parent. I am genetically different from my brother because each pair of our genes derives from one gene from our mother and one gene from our father. For each gene, the chances that both of us received the same allele from our mother's pair is one-half, and similarly the chances that both of us received the same allele from our father's pair is also one-half.

As I have noted, in different individuals, corresponding genes (those in the same location, or locus, on the chromosome) can differ chemically. In many cases, these different alleles of the same gene perform their prescribed function equally well. In some cases, the different alleles result in the normal genetic variation in such traits as eye color that we see from one person to the next. In other cases, an allele may differ sufficiently from the typical allele so as not to function properly.

A singe-gene disease is a disease caused by a single malfunctioning allele. Such diseases typically can develop in practically all usual environments. These single-gene diseases are termed *simple* because changes in only a single gene can result in drastically different phenotypes (manifestations of a trait). In addition, because only one gene is involved, these diseases usually exhibit simple inheritance patterns. Single-gene diseases are called Mendelian because they recall Mendel's original experiments in which differences in what we now call single genes resulted in clear differences in, for example, the color and texture of his peas. The simple inheritance patterns of these characteristics led Mendel to formulate his laws. But, as we shall see, most diseases and behaviors are non-Mendelian because no single gene is the star of the show; instead, each gene contributing to the trait seems to play a supporting role. It is the combined effect of these supporting actors, in interaction with the environment, that results in the disease.

Genetic Complexity

I have emphasized the point that only a small minority of genetic diseases and behaviors are controlled by the actions of the alleles of a single gene. Most traits are *polygenic;* they involve several or even large numbers of genes. Sometimes the genes act independently of one another. More commonly, however, the genes interact, a phenomenon called *gene-gene interaction* or *epistasis.* In gene-gene interaction, the action of each individual gene depends on which other genes are present and on what these other genes are doing. Consider the following hypothetical example. Suppose gene *A* (in the absence of gene *B*) contributes five units to some trait while gene *B* (in the absence of *A*) contributes three units to the same trait. If *A* and *B* act independently of each other, when both are present they would contribute 5+3=8 units to the trait. However, if there is an interaction, the combined effect of two genes might be either more or less than eight units.

We are all familiar with the fact that the environment has an effect on some traits and little or no effect on others. A typical person, irrespective of his genes, brought up on a substandard diet will invariably be shorter, lighter, and more prone to disease than someone brought up on a normal diet. But, irrespective of the environment, a person who was conceived with genes for blue eyes will be born with blue eyes and will remain blue-eyed. However, it is less appreciated that genetic and environmental influences do not always act independently of each other.

The interdependence of genetic and environmental influence takes two forms. First, certain forms of genes may be more likely to be present in certain environments. This effect is called *gene-environment covariance.* For example, in the United States, genes responsible for dark skin are associated with (on average) lower income than genes for light skin. This statistic could be interpreted to mean that the genes of people with dark skin render them less capable of making money than light-skinned people. However, the statistic could also reflect an environment shaped by the continuing racism in the United States. Aspects of this environment (e.g., inferior schooling and less adequate health care) could result in fewer economic and social opportunities for dark-skinned people than for light-skinned people. Consequently, the relatively low income of people with dark skin compared with that of people with light skin would not be explained by the direct action of their genes. Instead, we would invoke an explanation based on gene-environment covariance: dark-skinned genes are more likely to be found in less advantageous environments than light-skinned genes.

Second, as a result of *gene-environment interactions*, gene *A* might result in a more favorable trait in environment *1* than would gene *B* in environment *2*, but *A* in environment *2* might be less favorable than *B* in environment *1*. For example, it may be the case that because of genetic differences, there is no single best method of teaching reading. Pupils with one genotype (the genetic makeup of an organism) will learn to read more easily using one pedagogic method, while pupils with a different genotype may do better with a different method.

The term *genetic complexity* encompasses all these phenomena: polygenic traits, gene-gene interactions, complex environmental influences, gene-environment covariances, and gene-environment interactions. Geneticists are now studying these complexities. Several of their studies are showing that the task of separating genetic from environmental influences is even more daunting than previously thought. In part, this complexity can be ascribed to the fact that, in contrast to the central dogma of molecular biology (as described above in "Genetics 101"), information does not flow unidirectionally from genes to proteins. In fact, signals from the internal and external environment can both activate DNA to produce the appropriate proteins (Gottlieb, 1998).

Somewhat paradoxically, the study that most dramatically highlighted the difficulties in unraveling genetic complexity in human behavior involved the study of genetically identical mice. Researchers in three geographically separated laboratories gave the same behavioral tests to mice that had been carefully bred to be genetically identical (Crabbe, Wahlsten, and Dudek, 1999). Within each laboratory, the mice behaved similarly in repeated experiments. However, despite the researchers' best efforts to create identical experimental conditions, the behavior of the mice in each laboratory differed significantly from the behavior of the mice in the other two laboratories. The researchers note in their published report that they were unable to account for these differences. This result suggests that when researchers think that they have shown that some genetic difference is responsible for a behavioral difference, they cannot be sure that the difference was not really caused by subtle environmental differences.

In February 2001, scientists announced the near-completion of the sequencing of the human genome and the identification of all the human genes. The sequence of the genome refers to the order of the bases, A, G, C, and T (defined in the second paragraph of "Genetics 101"), that constitute each chromosome. The most spectacular of the reported results was the finding that we humans possess approximately 30,000 genes. Previously, nearly all geneticists had thought that the number of genes was closer to 100,000. This result suggests that the relationship between genes and proteins and, consequently, the relationship between genes and traits is even more complicated than previously thought. With fewer genes, it seems likely that an individual protein or trait arises from complex interactions among at least several genes. Some scientists have hypothesized that different parts of the same gene may work together in various combinations to produce a wide variety of different proteins. Although the exact nature of this genetic complexity is not yet known, it is becoming increasingly evident that genetic complexity is the rule. We should not be surprised that geneticists have been finding it so difficult to identify single genes responsible for (as opposed to associated with) illnesses like schizophrenia and personality traits like intelligence (Morange, 2001).

Genetic Diseases

The simplest examples of genetic complexity involve genetic diseases that are caused by alterations in a single gene. Yet even these single-gene diseases display a remarkable degree of complexity. A recent review of the thalassemias, a group of inherited, single-gene disorders characterized by abnormal forms of hemoglobin, discussed the "remarkable phenotypic diversity of the ß-thalassaemias." The author attributes this diversity to a variety of forms of genetic complexity as well as to the influence of a wide range of environmental factors (Weatherall, 2001). This complexity has practical consequences. Most importantly, it affects decisions about whether one should undergo prenatal genetic testing or genetic predictive testing for a serious or potentially fatal disease. In many cases, breast cancer being a prime example, the information provided by the genetic tests is ambiguous. Moreover, even if the results of the test were definitive, the best course of medical intervention may not always be clear.

Cystic Fibrosis and Other Single-Gene Diseases

Cystic fibrosis is the most common recessive (defined in the following paragraph) disease affecting Caucasians, occurring in approximately 1 in twenty-five hundred newborns. The disease is characterized clinically by sticky viscous secretions of the pancreas and lungs. Improvements in treatment have enabled people with this disease to survive into adulthood. Nevertheless, at present, there is no cure (Sack, 1999).

Cystic fibrosis results from the malfunctioning of a single gene. Recall that there are two copies of each gene and that the particular form a gene takes is called an allele. For the disease to be present, both of the alleles must be malfunctioning. A person with one malfunctioning allele is not affected by the cystic fibrosis but is a *carrier*. There is a 25 percent probability that a child of two carriers of cystic fibrosis will inherit two malfunctioning alleles, one from each parent, and thus be affected by the disease. This probability is a consequence of the paired nature of chromosomes described above: each child has a 50 percent chance of receiving the malfunctioning allele from her father and a 50 percent chance of receiving one from her mother. Diseases of this type in which both alleles must be malfunctioning are called *recessive*.

It was long believed that the genetics of cystic fibrosis was simple: a person has cystic fibrosis if and only if he or she has two malfunctioning alleles of the single gene associated with the disease. In recent years we have learned that the genetics of cystic fibrosis is much more complex (Sack, 1999). Different alleles have slightly different sequences of their bases. Cystic fibrosis is complex because there are hundreds of different alleles of the cystic fibrosis gene, and different alterations can affect normal function in different ways.

In the majority of cases of cystic fibrosis (CF), especially in people of Caucasian descent, one particular allele (called deltaF508) is present on both chromosomes. However, many people with the disease have various combinations of different alleles. Other people with still different alleles have symptoms that seem to have nothing to do with cystic fibrosis, and still others have no symptoms at all (Desgeorges et al., 1994; Parad, 1996; Donat et al., 1997).

These observations show that individual genes do not perform specific functions independent of the presence or absence of other genes. As a result of gene-gene interactions, the expression of different alleles of the CF gene may vary substantially because the expression of each allele may depend on the expression of a particular set of other genes. The lesson from these phenomena is that information about the effects of mutations in a gene sometimes provides little or no information about the normal functioning of that gene.

Because of the large number of different alleles of the CF gene, it has been very difficult to develop a complete prenatal screening test for cystic fibrosis. For such a test to yield meaningful results for each person who is tested, all the types of altered genes that cause cystic fibrosis must be detected. It is both technically and financially impractical to test for all these alleles. The currently available tests are designed to detect only the most commonly occurring alleles. Consequently, a negative test result does not mean that the fetus will not develop cystic fibrosis but only that it is unlikely. In view of this ambiguity in the test, there is still considerable debate concerning the advisability of using genetic tests for screening individuals who do not have a family history of cystic fibrosis (Andrews et al., 1994). Of course, for a couple with a history of cystic fibrosis caused by mutations included in the genetic test, the test result, whether positive or negative, provides significant information.

Huntington disease and fragile X syndrome are other single-gene diseases that show additional levels of complexity (Sack, 1999). Huntington disease is a fatal neurological disease whose symptoms typically begin to appear between the ages of thirty and fifty. It is a dominant disease. Unlike a recessive disease like cystic fibrosis, only one malfunctioning allele of the gene is sufficient to result in Huntington disease. Fragile X syndrome, meanwhile, is the most common cause of inherited mental retardation. Fragile X disease results from an allele on the X chromosome, one of the sex chromosomes, that seems to weaken the chromosome. Women have two X chromosomes; men have an X and a Y sex chromosome. Since the presence of one functioning X chromosome is sufficient to protect against the disease, fragile X disease is much more common in boys than in girls.

The complexity in both Huntington and fragile X diseases arises from a segment of the gene called a triplet repeat. A triplet repeat consists of repetitions of a sequence of three bases. In recent years, researchers have discovered that the number of repetitions affects the age of onset of these diseases, the severity of symptoms, and even whether the disease will appear at all. However, although the gene is inherited from the parent, the precise number of repeats is not inherited. In some cases, the number of repeats will increase from one generation to the next. In the case of fragile X, the degree of increase also depends on the sex of the parent. As a result of this type of complexity, a person in a family with a history of one of these triplet-repeat diseases may be healthy but have a child affected by the disease. The parent carried the altered gene, but the number of repeats in parent's gene was small while the number of repeats in the child's gene was large (Warren and Nelson, 1994). If, on the other hand, the number of repeats in one of the mother's genes is large, then a boy inheriting that gene would have at least that number of repeats and would almost certainly develop the disease.

Cancer Genetics and Genetic Testing

Cystic fibrosis, Huntington disease, and fragile X syndrome are rare diseases. In contrast, breast, colorectal, and prostate cancers are common. For example, approximately 10 to 15 percent of women develop breast cancer in the course of their lifetimes. Scientists regard cancer as a collection of genetic diseases. By this they mean that cancers arise when mutations occurring in normal genes interfere with the orderly growth of cells and allow the uncontrollable growth of cells into tumors. It is generally believed that at least two mutations are required in a cell before its normal functioning breaks down and a cancer develops (Thompson, McInnes, and Willard, 1991). Some mutations are caused by environmental insults (e.g., smoking and exposure to asbestos); others are inherited. In studying the causes and mechanisms involved in cancer, it is natural that geneticists would focus on the heritable aspects of the disease.

Genes have been found that are associated with cancer. Most famously, in 1994 and 1995, researchers found two genes, named BRCA1 and BRCA2, associated with susceptibility to breast cancer (Sack, 1999). Scientists believe that the normal forms of these genes act to suppress the growth of tumors. DNA mismatch-repair genes have been found to be associated with hereditary nonpolyposis colorectal cancer (Sack, 1999), and a candidate gene, HPC1, has been linked to prostate cancer (Fearon, 1997).

In view of these genetic discoveries, how important are genetic as opposed to environmental factors in the causation of cancer? This question is exactly the topic of a recent study of almost forty-five thousand pairs of twins listed in the Swedish, Danish, and Finnish twin registries (Lichtenstein et al., 2000).

The researchers calculated the probability that if one twin had a particular type of cancer, that person's co-twin would also have the same type of cancer. They then compared the probabilities for identical twins, who are genetically the same, with the probability for fraternal twins, who on average are 50 percent genetically identical. Assuming that each twin pair experienced a similar environment, a statistical analysis of this data would quantify the amount of genetic variation responsible for a particular type of cancer.

In summarizing the results of the Scandinavian study, we first note that, according to the statistical analysis of the data, most of the cancers studied did not seem to be heritable at all. Three common forms of cancer were found to be heritable: breast, colorectal, and prostate cancers. The researchers found that the proportion of the susceptibilities to each of the three diseases that was due to heritable genetic variation was 27, 35, and 42 percent, respectively. However, it should be noted that the statistical uncertainties in these percentages were very high. For example, the figure of 27 percent for the breast cancer susceptibility is more precisely expressed as the range 4 to 41 percent.

Based on their data, Lichtenstein and colleagues concluded that most cancers are sporadic (nonfamilial) and are caused predominantly by environmental factors and somatic events. However, in a recent paper, Neil Risch argues that these authors used an incorrect statistical model to analyze their data (Risch, 2001). Reanalyzing the same data, Risch concluded that genetic factors play a significant role in the great majority of cancers. Of course, even if correct, this conclusion does not mean that there are "cancer genes," genes that if present will result in cancer. Rather, as Risch stated (Holden, 2001), "we should be looking for susceptibility genes for all cancers."

Risch's paper indicates that not only is the genetics of cancer complex, but the analysis of that complexity is complex as well. Both Lichtenstein's team and Risch emphasize that there are probably several or many genes associated with each type of cancer. Each of these genes may be fairly common and carry only moderate risk. Some of these genes may not even be expressed in all individuals who carry them. These characteristics all contribute to the difficulty of finding the genes involved in cancer etiology.

In addition to the presence of several genes acting independently, there are very likely to be complex interactions among these genes, and complex interactions between genes and the environment. For example, even though much of prostate cancer is attributable to heredity (42%), the risk among migrant groups tends to approach the level of risk in their adopted country within a few generations (Hoover, 2000). Despite this strong evidence for environmental factors, few such risk factors have been identified. This example suggests that both genetic and environmental factors are important but that interactions between the genetic and environmental effects make it difficult to attribute a causal role to any specific gene or environmental factor.

What are the implications of this and other studies of cancer etiology? It is evident that reports in the press announcing predictive genetic tests for various cancers and highlighting advances in pharmacogenetics that promise a tailor-made drug for each individual may be overly optimistic. Cancer genetics is so complicated that a test for a specific gene or even group of genes is unlikely to be relevant in more than a small percentage of individuals and will probably have limited predictive value.

For the sake of concreteness, consider genetic testing for BRCA1 and BRCA2. If a woman is a member of a high-risk family, those with several cases of both breast and ovarian cancer among first-degree relatives in successive generations, and she has a positive genetic test, the probability that she will develop breast cancer may be as high as 90 percent. Because these probabilities are so high, many physicians recommend testing for women in these groups. There is now evidence that for women in these groups with a positive genetic test, prophylactic surgery to remove breasts and ovaries greatly increases the chances of avoiding the disease (Eisen and Weber, 1999).

However, for most women, genetic testing for breast cancer will not be very informative (Holtzman and Marteau, 2000). Women who test positive for the BRCA1 or BRCA2 susceptibility genes will account for less than 5 percent of all those women who develop breast cancer. Moreover, a negative test does not mean that the woman will never develop breast cancer (Ponder, 1997). Assuming the test is accurate, the negative result simply means that the woman does not have the particular mutations tested for; it does not mean that she will never get cancer and need not get periodic mammograms. In fact, her risk of cancer has decreased very little from that of a woman in the general population who has never been tested. This is because so little breast cancer is caused by the BRCA1 and BRCA2 genes.

Genetic testing may even be harmful (Ponder, 1997). The results of a positive test may fall into the hands of an insurance company, which may then deny a policy to an applicant. There is already strong evidence that insurers have discriminated against people who may have genes for a particular disease but who are presently free from any symptoms (Chapter 13 in this volume).

Because of the complex genetics of most such diseases, even though they carry the altered gene many of these people will never develop the corresponding disease.

Genes Affecting Mental Illness and Personality

Scientists attempting to understand the genetic influences on mental illness and human behavior face additional complexity. In the case of breast cancer, for example, there is no question that alterations in BRCA1 and BRCA2 are associated with the disease. But when dealing with mental illnesses like schizophrenia or behavioral traits like shyness, finding genes associated with these behaviors has presented monumental problems. Many of the reports of the discovery of genes for both mental illnesses and behavioral traits have either been retracted or have failed to be confirmed by other researchers.

Single-Gene Diseases Affecting Behavior

Genes do affect behavior. In a variety of diseases, the alteration of a single gene has severe effects on mental function (Sack, 1999). Phenylketonuria (PKU), caused by the mutation of a gene involved in the metabolism of the amino acid phenylalanine, results in severe mental retardation. Fortunately, this disease, unlike most genetic diseases, can be treated. All babies are tested for PKU at birth. If they are found to have the disease, they are placed on a phenylalanine-free diet, which enables them to develop normally. Individuals with Lesch-Nyhan disease, another single-gene disorder, engage in uncontrollable self-mutilating behavior. In Wilson disease, the mutation in a single gene affects the metabolism of copper. Some of the symptoms of this disease mimic those of schizophrenia.

In 1993, a Dutch research team studying one particular family discovered a mutation in a gene called MAOA that was immediately labeled by the press as "the criminal gene" (Brunner et al., 1993; Cowley and Hall, 1993). Men in the family who had this allele were reported to engage in violent behavior. This mutation has a severe impact on many of the biochemical reactions required for the normal functioning of the nervous system. Consequently, it is not surprising that this mutation affects mental functioning and might even cause antisocial behavior. Nevertheless, these findings do not imply that the MAOA gene is a "criminal gene."

The MAOA gene should not be called a criminal gene for the same reason that the gene whose mutation causes PKU should not be called an intelligence gene, even though people with untreated PKU have lower than average intelligence. The purpose of the PKU gene is not to regulate intelligence but rather to regulate a chemical reaction involved in digestion. In addition, PKU is a rare disease; very few instances of mental retardation are caused by PKU. Consequently, very little of the variation in intelligence among people is due to variations in this gene. Studying the PKU gene is unlikely to lead to a greater understanding of human intelligence.

Analogously, the mutation in MAOA results in a disease. However, the MAOA gene is designed to regulate not violent tendencies but rather the metabolism of certain neurochemicals involved in a wide variety of neurological functions that are not specific to the brain. This mutation is extremely rare, much rarer than PKU, and, as a result, is responsible for at most a tiny fraction of violent antisocial activity. Thus, studying MAOA mutations is unlikely to increase our understanding of criminal behavior. It is important to note that Brunner himself has written two articles emphasizing these points and criticizing the overinterpretation of his results (Brunner, 1995, 1996).

People who commit violent crimes such as robbery and murder are clearly more aggressive than the average person, and it may even be true that their aggressive behavior is influenced by their genes. However, it does not follow that differences in aggression among people can be explained by the presence or absence of mutations in a few identifiable genes. In view of what we know about the genetic complexity of human behavior, it is quite unlikely that there are such simple, singly acting "criminal genes" (Alper, 1998).

The Genetics of Mental Illness

Mental illnesses such as schizophrenia and manic depression are complex conditions. Often, these illnesses run in families; if several of a person's close relatives have the illness, that person is more likely than the average person to also develop it. However, *familial* does not necessarily mean *genetic*. It is possible, but by no means proven, that some mental illness may arise as a result of a "dysfunctional" family environment and that children of these families may recreate the dysfunction when they marry and have children of their own.

To determine whether mental illnesses are genetic, researchers have studied the patterns of these illnesses in families (Plomin et al., 1997). Some researchers study separated identical twins who have been brought up in different households. Suppose that in most cases, such cotwins either both have or both do not have the illness. Assuming the environments in the two households are no more similar than any two randomly selected households, then the illness is likely to be genetic. Other researchers compare identical twins with fraternal twins. If the illness is genetic, the siblings of an identical twin pair are much more likely to be either both well or both ill than are the siblings from a fraternal twin pair.

Although most researchers in the field believe that these and other family studies show convincingly that schizophrenia and manic depression are inherited to at least some extent, other scientists are not so sure (Beckwith and Alper, 1998). They note that for the studies involved, the households in which the separated twins were raised are often quite similar to each other. Adoption agencies usually attempt to chose adoptive homes that match the biological home with regard to such environmental influences as socioeconomic status and religion. If the separated homes are similar, then the similarity between the separated twins could be due to environmental factors as well as to genetic factors. Critics also note that the environments experienced by identical twins are much more similar than the environments experienced by fraternal twins or by ordinary siblings (Joseph, 1998). Although these arguments have been challenged by behavioral geneticists (Rowe and Jacobson, 1999), I believe that they have not made a convincing case that their methods are able to separate environmental influences from genetic influences on behavior.

Since the Lichtenstein et al. (2000) study of cancer etiology depended exclusively on data concerning twins, some of the criticisms discussed above also apply to their study. However, there are several factors that mitigate these criticisms. First, the study involved such a large number of subjects that the statistical analysis is much more reliable than that of the typical twin study of intelligence. Second, it seems reasonable to believe that the aspects of the environment that are relevant to cancer etiology are more similar for the cotwins than are those aspects that are involved in psychosocial development.

In an effort to obtain a more detailed understanding of mental illness, molecular geneticists have spent more than ten years searching for the individual genes associated with schizophrenia and manic depression. The results of their searches have been disappointing (Risch and Botstein, 1996). There have been many articles reporting that a gene on one chromosome or another is associated with one of the two illnesses. For example, a recent report argues that a major susceptibility locus for familial schizophrenia is on chromosome 1 (Brzustowicz et al., 2000). Nevertheless, at the time of this writing (December,

2001), none of these reports has both (1) passed the statistical tests required for the demonstration of an association between a gene and the illness and (2) been replicated by other researchers. Replication is important, because in several cases the researchers who reported positive findings of an association later retracted their work.

If there are genes associated with schizophrenia and manic depression, an assumption that most scientists find reasonable, why has it been so hard to find them? We may recall that for all the genetic complexity in a disease like breast cancer, at least there is no doubt that the presence of mutated forms of the genes BRCA1 and BRCA2 increase the likelihood that a woman will develop breast cancer.

There are several reasons for the difficulty in finding genes associated with mental illness, all of which illustrate the additional complexity inherent in the genetics of these conditions. First, in view of the weaknesses in the classical family studies, we cannot rely on them to be sure that there actually are genes responsible for mental illness. Second, a mental illness might arise as the effect of many malfunctioning alleles working together. If this situation is true, it would be very difficult to detect the effect of any one of these so-called minor genes. Third, the set of symptoms grouped together and labeled as a particular illness may actually represent several illness, each resulting from a different specific cause. Thus even if all cases of, for example, manic depression resulted from altered genes, it is possible some cases of manic depression might be caused by mutations in one particular gene on one chromosome and other cases might be caused by mutations on a completely different gene in a different chromosome. If this is the case, a researcher who studied one set of patients might report the finding of a gene associated with manic depression, but a second researcher whose patients had mutations on a different gene would find no evidence that the gene reported by the first researcher had anything to do with the disease.

Fourth, just as is the case in breast cancer, even if a gene is found to be associated with a mental illness, many individuals with the illness may not carry that particular mutated gene. And conversely, some people who carry that mutated gene may not develop the illness. In the language of logic, the mutated gene is neither a necessary nor a sufficient cause of the condition. As a result of these complexities, researchers need large numbers of subjects, they must be extremely careful in the types of controls they use (controls are people who are similar in all respects to the subjects except they do not have the mental illnesses), and they must use very stringent statistical criteria in assessing whether their data show an association between a gene and the mental illness. In recent years, several articles explaining these difficulties and suggesting procedures for overcoming them have appeared in the technical literature (Uhl, Gold, and Risch, 1997). We would expect that as more researchers adopt the proposed recommendations, future reports of genes associated with mental illnesses will be more reliable than those of the past.

Genes for Human Personality Traits

All of the complexities described above also apply to the study of the genetics of traits such as shyness and risk-taking that are part of what we call personality. In addition, the genetics of these personality traits present difficulties of their own. With regard to a diseases like breast cancer, there is usually no dispute about whether a woman does or does not have the disease. Similarly, in most cases, clinicians would agree on a diagnosis of such mental illnesses as schizophrenia and manic depression.

The situation with respect to the normal variation in personality traits is quite different. For these traits we have the additional problem of defining the trait or type of behavior. Consider the case of intelligence. Books have been written about what intelligence means and about whether intelligence is one property or whether there are really many different types of intelligences (Mackinstosh, 1998). In addition, unlike a disease, intelligence is not an either-or trait. Behavioral geneticists are interested in quantifying degrees of intelligence. To achieve their aims, they simply define the degree of intelligence of a person to be that person's score on an intelligence (IQ) test. Yet many psychologists would deny that an IQ score measures intelligence in any meaningful way (Harrington, 1997). If they are correct, finding a gene that is associated with scores on an IQ test would not provide any information about the genetics of intelligence.

Traits like shyness, novelty-seeking, aggressiveness, and homosexuality are equally difficult to define and quantify. For example, the degree of homosexuality versus heterosexuality in a person is often measured by means of the Kinsey scale. Even if we assume that this scale is valid (i.e., it measures accurately what it is supposed to measure), behavioral geneticists looking for a "homosexuality gene" have a problem. Which point on the Kinsey scale is the correct dividing point separating nonhomosexuals from homosexuals? If the point is chosen on the middle of the scale, the genetic analysis is difficult. People near the middle of the scale show both types of behavior; however, they either have the presumed "homosexuality gene" or they don't. If the dividing point is chosen so that only those at one extreme end of the scale are considered homosexuals, then a gene that is discovered to be associated with this type of homosexual behavior may be associated only with the sexual orientation of this relatively small group of people. This ambiguity in definitions may explain why two studies reach opposite conclusions about the existence of an association between male homosexuality and a gene on the X chromosome (Wickelgren, 1999).

Because behavioral genes are so difficult to identify, behavioral geneticists studying the genetics of behavior still rely on the nonmolecular, traditional types of familial studies already described in the section on mental illness. As is the case with mental illness, there is considerable debate about whether these familial studies do indeed prove that genes are responsible for the normal variation in behaviors. In addition, we should emphasize again that these studies do not identify individual genes that are responsible for the behavior. Instead, they use statistical methods to support their contention that genetic differences are more important than environmental differences in causing the variation in the behavioral trait between one individual and another. These results have been used by molecular geneticists as guides for suggesting which traits should be examined in the search for the individual genes that may influence behavior. These molecular genetics studies have resulted in reports of genes associated with intelligence, addictive behavior, homosexuality, and novelty-seeking.

The Genetics of Novelty-Seeking

The genetics of novelty-seeking can serve as a textbook example of genetic complexity. It illustrates the difficulties in establishing the existence of a gene for a personality trait. The studies themselves also indicate that even if such a gene did exist, it would most likely be of little importance.

In early 1996, two groups of researchers found an association between the degree of a trait they called novelty-seeking and the length of a particular portion of a particular gene (the D4 dopamine receptor gene on chromosome 11) (Cloninger, Adolfsson, and Svakic, 1996). Novelty-seeking involves exploratory, thrill-seeking, and excitable behavior. This behavior, which shows continuous variation, was measured by means of a psychological test. Despite the questions concerning the possibility of defining any complex behavioral trait using such a test, we will assume that the test does in fact measure a real trait called "novelty-seeking."

When first published, these studies seemed very convincing. After all, two independent groups had found the same gene for novelty-seeking. Unfortunately, soon after, other researchers reported that they were unable to find the same gene. In addition, one of the original two groups could not, in a follow-up study, replicate the clear-cut results they had obtained previously. In fact, to obtain a positive result at all, they were forced to redefine novelty-seeking, restricting it to an extreme type of thrill-seeking behavior (Baron, 1998).

How could two independent studies reaching the same conclusion both be wrong? As is the case in the search for genes for mental illness, the answer lies in the statistics of gene searches. There are probably thousands of genes involved in the functioning of the human brain, any of which could conceivably be associated with a trait like novelty-seeking. Because of this large number of genes, it is more likely than not that an association due solely to coincidence would be found between one of these genes and *any* trait whatsoever. The statistical methodology used by the researchers did not take this fact into account. As a result, they vastly overestimated the likelihood that the association between the gene they studied and the trait of novelty-seeking was a real association rather than a coincidence.

Even if the two groups of researchers had been correct in their claim that they had found a "novelty-seeking gene," the existence of this gene, taken in isolation, would not explain novelty-seeking behavior. Novelty-seeking is only a moderately heritable trait (Cloninger, Adolfsson, and Svakic, 1996). This means that roughly 50 percent of the variation in novelty-seeking behavior from one person to another is due to genetic influences, and the remainder is due to environmental influences. Furthermore, the gene reported in these studies accounts for only approximately 10 percent of the heritability of novelty-seeking. Finally, individuals with novelty-seeking gene segments of the same length may behave very differently. For example, an extrovert with a mature creative character, a bulimic, an antisocial alcoholic, and a schizotypal individual all may be novelty-seekers. This variability is presumably the result of interactions among various hypothesized temperament genes and interactions of these genes with the environment. It seems evident that the identification of individual temperament genes will be of little help in explaining or predicting the behavior of a person.

Conclusion

This chapter has examined the various aspects of complexity that arise in the genetic analysis of human traits. We have seen that, in the progression from single-gene diseases to multifactorial diseases to mental illnesses and then to normal behavior, the types and degree of complexity increase dramatically. As a result, although the genetics of some single-gene diseases is quite well established, little progress has been made in our understanding of the genetics of any type of normal human behavior. In practical terms, this complexity means that we cannot expect simple solutions to genetic problems. Because the interpretation of genetic medical tests is so difficult, presymptomatic testing for diseases like cancer, as well as prenatal testing, presents difficult medical problems in addition to the more obvious psychological and ethical ones. And with regard to human behavior, the simple notion that there is a single gene or several genes "for" a particular trait like intelligence or homosexuality is clearly erroneous.

Despite the reality of genetic complexity, we cannot ignore either the genetics or the complexity. Many of us, at some time or another, will need to make medical decisions about the risks and benefits of some genetic test. It seems quite likely that genetic tests for Alzheimer disease will become available within a few years. We are all concerned about such societal issues as privacy, genetic discrimination, and the implications of genetic differences among races and between sexes. We are also interested in the genetic and environmental influences that were important in shaping the individuals we are today. All these difficult issues involve complex genetic questions. In dealing with them, we must first realize that the genetics involved in these issues is indeed immensely complicated. We will not make much progress if the focus is on a "gene for X." Once we appreciate this complexity, we can then approach the task of understanding and interpreting reports of genetic advances.

REFERENCES

Alper, J. S. 1998. "Genes, Free Will, and Criminal Responsibility." *Social Science and Medicine* 46:1599–1611.
Andrews, L. B., J. E. Fullarton, N. A. Holtzman, and A. G. Motulsky, eds. 1994. *Assessing*

Genetic Risks: Implications for Health and Social Policy. Washington, D.C.: National Academy Press.

Baron, M. 1998. "Mapping Genes for Personality: Is the Saga Sagging?" *Molecular Psychiatry* 3:106–8.

Beckwith, J., and Alper, J. S. 1998. "L'Apport Reel des Etudes sur les Jumeaux." *La Recherche* 311 (July–August): 72–76.

Brunner, H. G. 1995. "Monoamine Oxidase and Behaviour." *Annals of Medicine* 27:431–32.

———. 1996. "MAOA Deficiency and Abnormal Behavior: Perspectives on an Association." In *Genetics of Criminal and Antisocial Behaviour*, ed. M. Rutter, pp. 155–64. Chicester: Wiley.

———, M. Nelen, X. O. Breakefield, H. H. Ropers, and B. A. van Oost. 1993. "Abnormal Behavior Associated with a Point Mutation in the Structural Gene for Monoamine Oxidase A." *Science* 262:578–83.

Brzustowicz, L. M., K. A. Hodgkinson, E. W. C. Chow, W. G. Honer, and A. S. Bassett. 2000. "Location of a Major Susceptibility Locus for Familial Schizophrenia on Chromosome 1q21-q22." *Science* 288:678–82.

Cloninger, C. R., R. Adolfsson, and N. M. Svakic. 1996. "Mapping Genes for Human Personality." *Nature Genetics* 12:3–4.

Cowley, G., and C. Hall. 1993. "The Genetics of Bad Behavior." *Newsweek*, April 30: 59.

Crabbe, J. C., D. Wahlsten, and B. C. Dudek. 1999. "Genetics of Mouse Behavior: Interactions with Laboratory Environment." *Science* 284:1670–72.

Desgeorges, M., P. Kjellberg, J. Demaille, and M. Claustres. 1994. "A Healthy Male with Compound and Double Heterozygosities for DeltaF508, F508C, and M470V in Exon 10 of the Cystic Fibrosis Gene." *American Journal of Human Genetics* 54:384–85.

Donat, R., A. S. McNeil, D. R. Fitzpatrick, and T. B. Hargreave. 1997. "The Incidence of Cystic Fibrosis Gene Mutations in Patients with Congenital Bilateral Absence of the Vas Deferens in Scotland." *British Journal of Urology* 79:74–77.

Eisen, A., and B. L. Weber. 1999. "Prophylactic Mastectomy: The Price of Fear." *New England Journal of Medicine* 340:137–38.

Fearon, E. R. 1997. "Human Cancer Syndromes: Clues to the Origin and Nature of Cancer." *Science* 278:1043–50.

Gottlieb, G. 1998. "Naturally Occurring Environmental and Behavioral Influences on Gene Activity: From Central Dogma to Probabalisitic Epigenesis." *Psychological Review* 105:792–802.

Griffiths, A. J. F., J. H. Miller, D. T. Suzuki, R. C. Lewontin, and W. M. Gelbart. 1993. *An Introduction to Genetic Analysis*, 5th ed. New York: Freeman.

Halley, J. 1994. "Sexual Orientation and the Politics of Biology: A Critique of the Argument from Immutability." *Standford Law Review* 46:503–68.

Hamer, D., and P. Copeland. 1998. *Living with Our Genes: Why They Matter More Than You Think.* New York: Doubleday.

Harrington, G. M. 1997. "Psychological Testing, IQ, and Evolutionary Fitness." *Genetica* 99:113–23.

Herrnstein, R. J., and C. Murray. 1994. *The Bell Curve: Intelligence and Class Structure in American Life.* New York: Free Press.

Holden, C. 2001. "Genes Come to the Fore in New Cancer Analysis." *Science* 293:601.

Holtzman, N. A., and T. M. Marteau. 2000. "Will Genetics Revolutionize Medicine?" *New England Journal of Medicine* 343:141–44.

Hoover, R. N. 2000. "Cancer—Nature, Nurture, or Both." *New England Journal of Medicine* 343:135–36.

Joseph, J. 1998. "The Equal Environment Assumption of the Classical Twin Method: A Critical Analysis." *Journal of Mind and Behavior* 19:325–58.

Lichtenstein, P., N. V. Holm, P. K. Verkasalo, A. Iliadou, J. Kaprio, M. Koskenvuo, E. Pukkala, A. Skytthe, and K. Hemminki. 2000. "Environmental and Heritable Factors in the Causation of Cancer." *New England Journal of Medicine* 343:78–85.

Mackintosh, N. J. 1998. *IQ and Human Intelligence.* New York: Oxford University Press.

Morange, M. 2001. *The Misunderstood Gene.* Cambridge: Harvard University Press.

Nelkin, D., and M. S. Lindee. 1995. *The DNA Mystique: The Gene as a Cultural Icon.* New York: W. H. Freeman.

Parad, R. B. 1996. "Heterogeneity of Phenotype in Two Cystic Fibrosis Patients Homozygous for the CFTR Exon 11 Mutation G551D." *Journal of Medical Genetics* 33:711–13.

Plomin, R., J. C. DeFries, G. E. McClearn, and M. Rutter. 1997. *Behavioral Genetics,* 3d ed. New York: W. H. Freeman.

Ponder, B. 1997. "Genetic Testing for Cancer Risk." *Science* 278:1050–54.

Risch, N. 2000. "Searching for Genetic Determinants in the New Millennium." *Science* 405:847–56.

———. 2001. "The Genetic Epidemiology of Cancer: Interpretation of Family and Twin Studies and Their Implications for Molecular Genetic Approaches." *Cancer Epidemiology Biomarkers & Prevention* 10:733–41.

———, and D. Botstein. 1996. "A Manic Depressive History." *Nature Genetics* 12:351–53.

Rowe, D. C., and K. C. Jacobson. 1999. "In the Mainstream: Research in Behavioral Genetics." In *Behavioral Genetics: The Clash of Culture and Biology,* ed. R. A. Carson and M. A. Rothstein, pp. 12–34. Baltimore: Johns Hopkins University Press.

Sack, G. H., Jr. 1999. *Medical Genetics.* New York: McGraw-Hill.

Thompson, M. W., R. R. McInnes, and H. F. Willard. 1991. *Genetics in Medicine,* 5th ed. Philadelphia: W. B. Saunders.

Tobin, A. J. 1999. "Amazing Grace: Sources of Phenotypic Variation in Genetic Boosterism." In *Behavioral Genetics: The Clash of Culture and Biology,* ed. R. A. Carson and M. A. Rothstein, pp. 1–11. Baltimore: Johns Hopkins University Press.

Uhl, G. R., L. H. Gold, and N. Risch. 1997. "Genetic Analyses of Complex Behavioral Disorders." *Proceedings of the National Academy of Sciences, USA* 94:2785–86.

Warren, S. T., and D. L. Nelson. 1994. "Advances in Molecular Analysis of Fragile X Syndrome." *Journal of the American Medical Society* 271:536–42.

Watson, J. D. 1997. "President's Essay: Genes and Politics." *Cold Spring Harbor Laboratory Annual Report,* 1–20.

Weatherall, D. J. 2001. "Phenotype-Genotype Relationships in Monogenic Disease: Lessons from the Thalassaemias." *Nature Reviews/Genetics* 2:245–55.

Wickelgren, I. 1999. "Discovery of 'Gay Gene' Questioned." *Science* 284:571.

CHAPTER TWO

Geneticists in Society, Society in Genetics

Jon Beckwith

Some scientists sit down daily at the laboratory bench to carry out experiments; others spend most of their time in front of computers; still others travel to exotic countries to study flora or fauna; and there are those who may simply think, formulate new theories, and write. For many, their work may gain attention within their scientific community but never attract the public's interest. For others, the subject they study may be so connected with people's concerns that it is the constant subject of news reports. In biology and biomedical science, the subjects that attract the most public attention include those that promise practical social benefits, such as medical treatments or cures, or those that attempt to explain human origins, human behavior, and human health. Because genetics plays a prominent role in each of these endeavors, it is often in the media spotlight.

Since the founding of modern genetics, at the beginning of the twentieth century, geneticists have participated in public discussions of genetics' relevance to social concerns. These discussions have influenced social policy and molded public attitudes. From the heyday of the eugenics movement to the ongoing Human Genome Project, geneticists have spoken out, disagreed, and even directly involved themselves in the formulation of policy. What stances have geneticists taken on these policy issues? Do geneticists largely agree on the relevance of their science to social concerns? What factors have influenced the positions that geneticists have taken on these issues?

In this chapter, I focus largely on issues surrounding human behavior genetics, where the interface between science and social concerns has been most prominent, and discuss the role geneticists have played in these discussions. While, for the purposes of my analysis, I refer to "geneticists" as though they represent a single community within science, one should remember that the field of genetics is, in fact, extraordinarily diverse. It includes scientists involved in clinical genetics, molecular biology, animal and human behavior genetics, evolutionary biology, and population genetics.

Human Genetics and Society: A Brief History

The birth of genetics led to a remarkable series of insights into genes, their function, and their mode of inheritance. A number of traits in plants, fruit flies, humans, and other organisms were shown to be traceable to single Mendelian units—genes. Among these traits were several human genetic diseases. The enormous success of this newborn field led geneticists, perhaps understandably, to generalize from their actual scientific results. They argued that not only the traits they studied but also many human health problems and much of human social behavior could be attributed to variations in human genes. Mendelian explanations were extended to explain complex human traits such as intelligence and criminal behavior.

It is the nature of science that when a successful new theory or paradigm appears, it is often invoked to explain a wide range of phenomena well beyond the scope of the studies that led to it. The very acceptance of such theories depends, in part, on their explanatory power (Kuhn, 1970; Boyd, 1995). Moreover, the establishment of a paradigm can be a prerequisite for the expansion of a field. Although attempts to extend the scope of a paradigm eventually confront limits, without those attempts scientific progress might be hindered. Indeed, most scientists hope that their findings will be applicable to a much larger set of phenomena than the particular problem they are studying. Thus, it is not surprising that geneticists would speculate about the implication of their results. Such speculation can take different forms depending on the social and cultural environment in which it evolves.

I will use the term *reductionist* to describe this focus on genes providing the ultimate explanation for many aspects of human health, social arrangements, and life activities (Levins and Lewontin, 1985; Longino, 1990). This reductionist position is valid in genetics at least in the trivial sense that most human diseases and much of human social behavior and aptitudes are species-specific and, therefore, must reflect our genetic inheritance. But the genetic reductionist stance, at its extreme, proposes much more than that. It argues that the best approach for studying these phenomena is a genetic one and that other approaches will not be successful. Thus, it posits that genes are the fundamental elements to which human phenomena can be reduced. This approach has its attractions, since genetics appears to provide much more solid quantitative and often verifiable results than other approaches—epidemiological, sociological, psychological.

This extreme version of the genetic paradigm has had serious social consequences. One example concerns the human disease pellagra (Chase, 1977). Pellagra, now known to be due to a vitamin deficiency, is a condition that begins with a severe skin disease and progresses to cause diarrhea, lassitude, dizziness, and mental illness. The physician Joseph Goldberger demonstrated in 1915 that the disease was due to poor diet. However, the U.S. government's Pellagra Commission, established to deal with a condition very common among poor people, concluded that the disease was due to a genetic susceptibility of the lower classes. The commission was dominated by people such as geneticist Charles Davenport, a leader of the eugenics movement. As a result, Goldberger's arguments for improved diet were ignored for the next fifteen years. It was not until the depression, when the U.S. government instituted programs to feed the large number of hungry people in the country, that pellagra essentially disappeared as a significant disease. In the meantime, many people suffered and died due to the ruling of the Pellagra Commission, following the genetic paradigm.

Many scientists who promoted the genetic reductionist position also were genetic determinists. Genetic determinism refers to the belief that any human trait influenced by genes is a relatively fixed trait, one that is little affected by changes in the physical and social environment. In the early eugenics movement, the reductionist perspective was invariably accompanied by the conclusion that traits ascribed to genes were unchangeable.

The reductionist and genetic determinist positions came together early in the twentieth century in the attitudes toward the genetics of human behavior.

Human behavior genetics has historically covered topics ranging from the genetics of mental illness to those of antisocial traits such as criminality to those of everyday human activities such as novelty-seeking, sexual behavior, and shyness (Beckwith and Alper, 1997). This science has attracted particular social attention and has informed social policies ranging from destructive eugenics movements in the United States, Germany, and elsewhere to the more recent screening of youth for the XYY chromosome makeup, the supposed "criminal chromosome" (Katz, 1972). In the nineteenth century Sir Francis Galton's writings, including the book *Hereditary Genius* (Galton, 1884), provided impressive support for the role of heredity in the development of intelligence. In the early twentieth century, many leading geneticists publicly proclaimed the genetic basis of a variety of behavioral traits. Most prominent among them was Charles Davenport, a Harvard-trained geneticist and head of the Eugenics Record Office at Cold Spring Harbor, Long Island, in the early part of the century. Davenport proffered that criminality, poverty, intelligence, and even seafaring affinity could be attributed to single genes (Ludmerer, 1972).

Attitudes toward reductionism, determinism, and genetic theories of human behavior provided the base of eugenic attitudes. Eugenics refers to practices intended to improve the human gene pool either through reduction of gene variants in the population that are considered deleterious or through increasing those genes considered beneficial or superior. Inherent in eugenic theory and in its historical practice are both the reductionist assumption that many human traits can be traced to genes and the determinist assumption that gene-based traits are so fixed that eliminating the particular gene is the preferred way to prevent the "deleterious" consequences of harmful mutations. These assumptions are valid for some well-characterized genetic diseases. That is, certain diseases (e.g., Tay-Sachs) can be traced to an altered form of a gene, which invariably leads to the disease condition, and the diseases are not treatable even today. However, therapies exist for other genetic diseases, and certain treatments are being continuously improved (e.g., those for sickle cell and cystic fibrosis).

Historically, eugenics-influenced social policy has gone beyond the focus on diseases that are clearly physical to assume that human social behaviors such as criminality, mental illness, and homosexuality, as well as human aptitudes such as intelligence, can be traced to the genetic makeup of individuals or groups (Allen, 1975; Kevles, 1985; Beckwith, 1993). While the genetic basis of a large number of physical diseases is well-established, the same cannot be said for the genetic basis of social behaviors and aptitudes. In this case, the genetic reductionist view of human traits has far outrun the scientific evidence.

The Role of Geneticists in Discussions of Eugenics

Eugenics theory and practice had disastrous social consequences, especially in the United States and Germany. What role did geneticists play in the public debates over the issues outlined above? Did geneticists stay in the lab doing what they know how to do best, or did they participate in public discussions of social questions that involve arguments from genetics?

During the first two decades of the twentieth century, the heyday of the eugenics movement in the United States, many leading geneticists expressed genetic reductionist views about human behavior and supported eugenic policies such as sterilization programs. Most members of the first editorial board of the journal *Genetics*, which included the leading geneticists of the day, supported eugenics policies (Ludmerer, 1972). In one of the most widely used human genetics texts of the day, German geneticists Erwin Baur, Eugen Fischer, and Fritz Lenz argued that stereotypes such as fraud among Jews, the laziness of Negroes, the Russians' tendency to "excel in suffering," and the superior mental gifts of the Nordic race were all real traits, ones that were genetically based (Baur, Fischer, and Lenz, 1931).

Many of the leading geneticists in the United States eventually dissociated themselves from the eugenics movement, either because they became more sophisticated about the limitations of the available genetic approaches or because of their distaste for the actual implementation of eugenics practice (Ludmerer, 1972; Allen, 1975). This defection occurred at the same time (late in the second decade of the twentieth century through the early 1920s) that those promoting eugenics were achieving enormous successes. Laws were passed in many states allowing sterilization of those considered to carry bad genes for such traits as low intelligence or criminality. Despite their increasing disdain for the scientific arguments of eugenics, geneticists generally failed to speak out publicly. For instance, Thomas Hunt Morgan, one of the most prominent geneticists of the day, was very critical privately of the genetic arguments underlying eugenics. Yet he never confronted the social consequences of these arguments, saying in a 1915 private letter: "If they [eugenicists] want to do this sort of thing, well and good . . . but, I think it is just as well for some of us to set a better standard, and not appear as participators in the show. I have no desire to make any fuss" (Allen, 1975).

Only in the late 1920s, after much of the damage had been done, did geneti-cists begin to express their opinions (Kevles, 1985). The first concerted effort by geneticists to deal with the consequences of eugenics programs did not come until 1939, when a leading international group of geneticists issued a manifesto as a response to the increasingly appalling extension of eugenics ideas in Germany (Crew et al., 1939).

Recent History

The Human Genome Project (HGP) was established in 1989, with the major goal of determining the complete DNA sequence of all human chromosomes by sometime early in the twenty-first century (Cook-Deegan, 1994). Supported by the National Institutes of Health and the Department of Energy, this project not only has provided substantial new funds for research in genetics but also has become a catalyst for public discussion of the significance of genetics and the social implications of genetic research (Beckwith, 1991). During the early stages of the project, there was considerable debate over the value of undertaking such an effort. Those scientists who have played a major role in the proposal and in the evolution of the HGP have sometimes argued for the importance of this project in terms that suggest a genetic reductionist point of view. James Watson, the first director of the HGP, stated, "We used to think our fate was in our stars. Now we know, in large measure, our fate is in our genes" (Jaroff, 1989). Harvard biologist Walter Gilbert suggested that, from the human genome sequence, "we can have the ultimate explanation of a human being" (DelGuercio, 1987). University of California biologist Daniel Koshland argued that the HGP will ultimately lead to a cure for homelessness (Koshland, 1991).

There is no genetic evidence to support these claims. Rather, they may reflect a belief in the power of genes—a belief derived from the successes of genetics in illuminating numerous biological phenomena. This perspective appears to conflate the dramatic achievements of contemporary genetics with a view of genetics as promising "universal reducibility" (Longino, 1990). Particularly today, the technologies of genetics allow a degree of precision in gene mapping, measurement of gene expression, and defining development pathways of organisms, which ensures replicability of findings. But the old cautionary saw that one looks for lost objects where the light is brightest may be as relevant for these perspectives as for others. That is, much would be missed by focusing on genetics alone.

While no consequences of this reductionism have arisen with regard to the treatment of human disease on a scale comparable to that seen with pellagra in an earlier era, a rather minor recent incident shows striking parallels. A number of babies die each year from what has been termed sudden infant death syndrome (SIDS). Some researchers have argued that SIDS in some cases may be caused by a heritable defect. One piece of evidence came from Dr. Alfred Steinschneider, who reported on a family in which five children had died from SIDS. However, subsequent investigations revealed that the mother had murdered all of the children (Steinschneider, 1972; Pinholster, 1994, 1995). Here, the prevailing genetic paradigm had so directed the interpretation of the family's misfortune that alternative "environmental" factors were ignored. When leading geneticists such as Paul Berg argue that "many if not most human diseases are clearly the result of inherited mutations" (Berg, 1991), the danger of failing to explore other sources of disease can become very real.

Geneticists and Genetic Determinism

In 1993, geneticist Dean Hamer and his coworkers from the United States National Institutes of Health reported that they had found a region of the human X chromosome that was associated with male homosexual behavior in some families (Hamer et al., 1993,. and see Chapters 9 and 10 of this volume). In a press release and elsewhere, Hamer took care to point out the limitations of the study and the likelihood that environment factors as well as genes play a role in homosexuality (Hamer et al., 1993; Hamer and Copeland, 1998). Dr. Hamer was subsequently called to testify in the Colorado Supreme Court, where plaintiffs were asking that an anti–gay rights amendment to the state constitution be declared unconstitutional. There, after summarizing the evidence for a genetic "component" of sexual orientation, he admitted that "sexual orientation is not completely genetic." Despite Hamer's cautions, the plaintiffs used the science and other arguments to "argue that homosexuality is inborn"(Bayliss, 1993), contending that the "fact" that homosexuality was not a choice supported their request for a revocation of the amendment. A *U.S. News and World Report* writer referred to the "strange twist" in which "liberals found themselves arguing the deterministic position" (Herbert, 1997). Later,

Hamer himself took a more deterministic position in a *Washington Post* interview: "On the one hand, having a gene is practically useful because you can argue that it's an immutable trait" (Weiss, 1994).

Owing to the array of disciplines subsumed under the term *genetics*, it is impossible to speak of the attitude among geneticists toward the power of genes in determining human traits. Nevertheless, many of the geneticists who act as spokespeople for the HGP or for genetics in general tend to speak in determinist terms. Most of these geneticists do not make extreme determinist statements such as those attributed to James Watson, as essentially all geneticists agree that our behavior and our health are a mix of nature and nurture. However, the oft-claimed end of the nature-nurture debate has not really materialized. There are still those at one end of the spectrum who will ignore the role of genes in a range of human traits; and there are those who, while admitting the importance of nurture, will argue that the genetic contributions are so strong as to place severe limitations on changes in those traits.

The determinist view is perhaps most explicit in the field of behavior genetics. While the term *determinism* implies "immutability," this is not generally the way the concept is elaborated by behavior geneticists. Rather, some geneticists present a moderated view of determinism that speaks of *limits* to changing traits imposed by genetics. This is certainly a more accurate way of speaking of the role genes play in shaping human traits. Depending on the nature of a gene or a mutation of a gene, interactions with the environment or with other genes in the individual may either yield wide variations or a very limited variation in the degree to which a trait is expressed. The problem is we simply don't know what the degree of this variation is for most traits. We don't know, in most cases, what environments will allow the greatest changes in manifestation of a disease or a behavior. So, when geneticists or the media speak of limits to change, they rarely have a basis for the specificity of such claims.

For example, it has been suggested, on quite weak evidence, that genetics may play an important role in the difference between boys and girls in performance on tests of mathematics ability. Two scientists who published a study on this subject also made statements in interviews that reflected the "limits" perspective on genetically influenced traits or abilities. According to one of them, Dr. Camilla Benbow, women would be "better off accepting their differences" (Kolata, 1980). Such statements are not innocuous when uttered publicly. After this study, there were some instances of negative impacts on public attitudes toward the potential of girls in math (Beckwith, 1983).

One of the largest projects designed to assess the genetic contributions to human behavior and aptitudes is the study of identical twins led by Dr. Thomas Bouchard at the University of Minnesota (Bouchard et al., 1990). Published reports from this group have suggested that a wide range of such traits are substantially influenced by genetics, with heritability estimates hovering around the 50 percent range. These findings have led some of the researchers associated with the project to express the "limits" view of genetic influences and even to make prescriptive statements. For instance, referring to their claim that "fearlessness" is subject to strong genetic determinants, team member Dr. Nancy Segal states, "Parents can work to make a child less fearful, but they can't make that child brave" (Leo, 1987). Segal's colleague, Dr. David Lykken, speaking of the supposed genetic limits in some individuals that establish a "set point" of happiness, recommends, "Find the small things that you know give you a little high. . . . In the long run, that will leave you happier than some grand achievement that gives you a big lift for a while" (Goleman, 1996).

Both of these prescriptions recognize that genetics does not imply a fixed limit to the expression of a trait, but, by suggesting how people should behave, their authors implicitly claim knowledge of just how flexible the impact of genes is.

It has to be said that even the reported heritability estimates from research projects such as the Bouchard group's have been subject to criticism (Billings, Beckwith, and Alper, 1992; Feldman et al., 1997; Joseph, 2001). Furthermore, tested heritabilities of a trait tell us only about the variability in that trait under the existing set of conditions to which the population being tested is subject (Feldman and Lewontin, 1975; Lewontin, 1976; Stoltenberg, 1997). So, even if we accepted these heritability estimates, they simply do not tell us how much change in a genetically influenced behavior is possible, nor do they indicate what changes in the familial, social, or cultural environment would foster such change. It is possible that someday genetics might help us to determine what some of those changes might be. In the absence of such information today, the "limits" approach appears more like a fallback position that essentially retains the deterministic attitude toward genetics.

Are There Eugenic Attitudes Today?

In the first half of this century, many prominent geneticists openly expressed eugenicist points of view. Even during the Nazi period in Germany, those geneticists in other countries who publicly opposed Nazi eugenics programs still favored the principles of eugenics if they could be implemented in the future, in a more egalitarian society. As opposed to the German goal of purifying the race, these geneticists viewed programs to alter the gene pool as reducing suffering and enhancing life experiences for humans as a whole (Crew et al., 1939). Despite these different outlooks on the role of eugenics, both points of view became largely suppressed after World War II; the horror that Nazi atrocities inspired made it difficult to express the strong eugenic position and may even have influenced people to change their views. For instance, a statement issued by UNESCO argued that the role of environment in the development of human behavior and capabilities was more important than had been realized, making the use of eugenics in such cases questionable (Montagu, 1963). This statement was signed by some of the same geneticists who had earlier expressed their support for the principles of eugenics.

Today, any eugenics perspectives comparable to those of the earlier era are expressed only by fringe groups, some of them with links to or enthusiasm for aspects of the Nazi regime. And, overall, the revulsion at the Nazi experience and the awareness of the poor science that underlay eugenics programs has resulted in a genetics community that shies away from eugenic proposals (Kevles, 1985; Kitcher, 1996; Paul, 1998). What little debate there is on these issues revolves around the role of genetic counselors, doctors, and clinical geneticists in reproductive decision making. There are no laws or proposals for laws in the United States that would dictate reproductive decisions based on eugenics. Rather, discussions concern whether genetic professionals should encourage prospective parents who have the probability or certainty of bearing children with known genetic conditions to terminate pregnancies or forego conception (see Chapter 6). Some geneticists believe that it doesn't make sense to bring a child into the world who would suffer from a genetic condition and would impose an additional financial health care burden on society, but they rarely express this point of view openly. James Watson, because of his out-spokenness on any issue, expresses a point of view perhaps more common than we realize. In discussing the pros and cons of families deciding whether or not to bear a child with a predictable handicap, Watson wrote: "Is it more likely for such children to fall behind in society or will they through such affliction develop the strengths of character and fortitude that lead, like Jeffrey Tate, the noted British conductor, to the head of their packs? Here I'm afraid that the word handicap cannot escape its true definition-being placed at a disadvantage. From this perspective, seeing the bright side of being handi-capped is like praising the virtues of extreme poverty" (Watson, 1997).

Another even stronger expression of these thoughts has been presented by Margery Shaw, past president of the American Society of Human Genetics, who argued that "parental rights to reproduce will diminish as parental responsibilities to unborn offspring increase" (Shaw, 1984). Robert Edwards, the British embryologist who created the first test-tube baby, stated: "Soon it will be a sin of parents to have a child that carries the heavy burden of genetic disease" (Rogers, 1999).

Ethicists and other scientists who disagree with Watson, Shaw, and Edwards have been quite open about their opposition to these positions. But many geneticists who share the conceptions of parental responsibility stated by Shaw and Edwards dare not speak out publicly on these issues, owing to the dark history of eugenics and the bitter abortion debate. Even with little public debate over these questions, such eugenic points of view may be influencing daily decisions in clinical genetics practice.

Perhaps the most mainstream contemporary example of the classic eugenics point of view is found in the book *The Bell Curve*, written by psychologist Richard Herrnstein and political scientist Charles Murray (Herrnstein and Murray, 1994). Here, the authors suggest that "dysgenic" trends are the root cause of a number of social problems in the United States. That is, people with genes for lower intelligence and for antisocial traits are outbreeding those with better genes. To remedy these problems, Murray and Herrnstein propose that women from the upper classes be encouraged by new social programs to bear more children and that welfare and remedial education programs be ended.

Yet a widely accepted antieugenic tenet of genetic counseling today is that the interaction between genetic professional and parents should be nondirective (Wertz and Fletcher, 1998). That is, in cases where a genetic condition can be predicted as a result of genetic testing, the counselor should only present options and likely consequences of various actions and not direct the individuals to a decision that he or she might favor. A recent survey reports that, in the United States, between 65 and 80 percent of medical geneticists stated they would be nondirective in counseling parents about several different genetic conditions (Wertz, 1997). The same survey, conducted in a wide range of other countries, reported that 35–40 percent of respondents stated that they would be nondirective for the same conditions.

While the nondirective stance reflects a belief in patient autonomy, such counseling can never be truly neutral (Bernhardt, 1997; Michie et al., 1997). The choice of which information to give prospective parents will reflect the beliefs of the counselor as to which information is important. These beliefs will vary from one genetic counselor or geneticist to another. For instance, a counselor informing parents could show, on the one hand, a recently made film about the joys of family life with a Down syndrome child or an episode of a TV show starring an individual with Down syndrome. Another counselor might discuss the range of outcomes but emphasize those children who suffer severe ailments, are subject to recurrent operations, and die at an early age. A third might emphasize both outcomes equally. These are all valid stances and simply represent differing perspectives on what is important information. Nevertheless, the current emphasis on nondirectiveness probably reflects concerns that eugenic decisions not be imposed on families by anyone from government officials to genetic professionals.

Another position expressed by geneticists that may influence the future course of genetic reproductive decision making is economic cost-benefit analysis (Lauria et al., 1993). These analyses are often placed in the context of the costs to society of caring for an individual with a chronic illness or a physical or mental disability versus the costs of genetic testing and abortion. In Cyprus, the program to encourage abortions of fetuses with ß-thalassemia was based on the costs to the government of providing health care for the relatively large number of individuals with that condition (Angastiniotis, Kyriakidou, and Hadjiminas, 1988; Angastiniotis and Middleton, 1997). Directive counseling was justified by its practitioners based on potentially severe economic consequences to society. As health care costs grow, particularly with more modern technological innovations becoming available, this reason for jettisoning nondirective counseling may increase. Nevertheless, the cost-benefit analyses usually do not include ethical and social concerns related to autonomy, family relations, attitudes toward disability, and other nonquantifiable factors.

Public Stances of Geneticists

I have mentioned the failure of geneticists to speak out against the misuse of genetics during the eugenics movement in the early part of the twentieth century. Such misuses continue to this day, providing new opportunities for geneticists to participate in public discussion of genetic issues with significant social import. In *The Bell Curve*, the authors argue that many of our social problems and social inequalities are the inevitable result of differences in genetic background between the different racial groups. Aside from a small number of researchers such as Luca Cavalli-Sforza (1997) and Steven Jay Gould

(1994), geneticists have remained silent (see Chapter 8 in this volume). One leading scientist active in the Human Genome Project, Dr. David Botstein, offers a possible explanation for why the silence has persisted: "People keep asking me why I do not rebut *The Bell Curve*. The answer is because it is so stupid it is not rebuttable" (Botstein, 1997).

This answer appears to ignore the potential social consequences of theories such as those found in *The Bell Curve*, when they remain unchallenged. Oddly enough, in the next sentence, Botstein speaks of the fact that most of his immediate family was murdered by the Nazis. Whether the theories are stupid or not seems beside the point when the stakes may be so high. Perhaps Botstein's attitude really derives from the conception of science as a neutral pursuit where scientists have no role in entering into discussions of social issues, even when there is a scientific component to the discussions. Such an attitude would hark back to Morgan's suggestion in an earlier era that scientists should "not appear as participators in the show." Or perhaps Botstein simply believes that the truth will win out.

While responses specifically to *The Bell Curve* from geneticists have been limited, a handful, including Richard Lewontin, David Suzuki, Neil Holtzman, and Paul Billings, have spoken out in the past on such issues (Lewontin, 1976; Suzuki and Knudson, 1988; Holtzman, 1989; Billings, Beckwith, and Alper, 1992). The broader community of geneticists has not participated in these debates, even while academics from other fields such as psychology, statistics, sociology, and anthropology have been considerably more outspoken (Beckwith, 1997; Devlin et al., 1997).

Cultural Values and Social Factors in the Attitudes of Geneticists

My attempts to outline modes of thought among geneticists concerning issues of reductionism, determinism, and human behavioral genetics have relied largely on the experience in the United States. One can ask whether these attitudes are inherent in the nature of the discipline. If this were the case, we would expect cross-cultural analysis to reveal similar attitudes among geneticists in different countries. After all, paralleling the strong eugenics movement in the United States in the early part of the century, England and Germany, among others, were also fonts of eugenic thought and practice. Yet we have seen in the case of directiveness of genetic counseling that there is substantial variation between the positions of medical geneticists in the United States and those in other countries. To examine some of these differences, I will focus on France, where, in addition to the Gaullist tradition of demonstrating independence from U.S. policies, geneticists have taken very different stances.

Differences in geneticists' attitudes in the two countries show up perhaps most clearly in the importance of human behavioral genetics studies and in the role of scientists in public debate on these topics. Scientists in France have played a large role in the evolution of contemporary genetics, including pioneering studies on the genetics of human disease. This tradition continues with the substantial effort put into the Human Genome Project through CEPH (Centre d'Etudes des Polymorphismes Humaines), a center for collecting genetic information on human polymorphisms, and Genethon, a consortium that is directly involved in the genome projects (Rabinow, 1999). Yet there is strikingly little effort to extend these research efforts into the realm of the genetics of human behavior.

Furthermore, clear lines of conflict between French and some other European behavior geneticists (many of whom work in animal behavior), on the one hand, and those from the United States, on the other, were recently exposed as controversy engulfed the Behavior Genetics Association (BGA), based in the United States (Holden, 1995a, 1995b; Carlier, 1999). At the annual meeting of this organization in 1995, the outgoing president, Glayde Whitney, devoted a portion of his speech to the likelihood that genetic factors contribute to the difference in violent behavior between African Americans and whites in the United States. A number of members of the association, including the incoming president, French scientist Pierre Roubertoux, walked out of the talk in protest, stating that this was not science but politics. This walkout represented the culmination of concerns among many behavior geneticists that the organization was placing too much emphasis on human studies that were seriously flawed in their conception and paying less attention to more carefully controlled animal experiments. Roubertoux subsequently resigned the presidency of the association. These concerns have led many of the European members of the BGA and a significant number from the United States to participate instead in the newly established International Behavioral and Neural Genetics Society, which holds its annual meetings in Europe.

French geneticists have also gone beyond the walls of academia to speak out publicly against determinism and arguments for the genetic basis of intelligence, aggression, and other complex human social traits or aptitudes. Nobel laureate François Jacob has given interviews and published articles in French newspapers arguing against faulty genetic arguments about racial differences and proposals for eugenics (Jacob, 1979, 1980; Todd, 1973). Daniel Cohen, who has played a major role in genome projects in France, raises many questions about the behavioral genetics research that is attracting so much media attention and of possible eugenic consequences in his 1993 book *Les genes de l'espoir* (Cohen, 1993) and in interviews (Charles and Harrois-Monin, 1993). Geneticist Albert Jacquard has published numerous books that warn against the misuse of human behavior genetics to inform social policy (Jacquard, 1994). Behavior geneticists Pierre Roubertoux and Michele Carlier published a book and an article in the popular science magazine, *La Recherche*, critiquing studies that purport to show the genetic basis of intelligence (Roubertoux and Carlier, 1996a, 1996b).

Some of the French scientists' activism around these issues may come from the fact that issues of genetics and race are rather prominent in the French political scene. French geneticists have confronted racist genetics-based statements made by members of the right-wing National Front political party. After the mayor of Vitrolles, Catherine Mégret, was fined by a French court for stating in an interview that "there are differences between the races . . . in the genes" (Associated Press, 1997) and statements about genetic inequality between the races were made by Jean-Marie Le Pen, the leader of the National Front (Anonymous, 1996a), more than six hundred scientists and historians signed a statement criticizing Le Pen from a scientific point of view (Anonymous, 1996b; Butler, 1996). No comparable array of prominent scientists in the United States have spoken out on such issues.

These differences between the United States and France have prompted French historian of science Jean-Paul Gaudillière to ask: "Why is behavior genetics practiced mainly in the Anglo-Saxon world? Why are French researchers so little represented in a domain which, in terms of scientific publications, seems to be in full bloom?" He points out that "there is only a handful of researchers [in France] officially concerned with genetic factors predisposing to autism or schizophrenia. There is nothing comparable to the many American projects to model and discover the genes implicated in diverse psychiatric syndromes, alcoholism, drug addiction and violent behavior" (Gaudillière, 1998).

Gaudillière traces these differing traditions back in history and raises a number of explanations, none of which is completely satisfactory. These in-

clude differing religious histories (Catholic and Protestant), contrasting political traditions, and the Pasteurian focus on environmental sources of human
disease. Another possible explanation is the resistance to accepting Mendelian
genetics that lasted in France from 1910 to 1940 (Burian and Gayon, 1999).

Conclusion

It is clear from the public role that geneticists have played and from the
contrasting attitudes in different cultures that being a geneticist does not imply
a commitment to the more extreme forms of reductionism or determinism.
Nor can one ascribe any particular stance on eugenic practices to those doing
genetic research. Among geneticists, the critics of these modes of thought have
themselves used genetic arguments to offer a more holistic, complex view of
human disease and human aptitudes and behavior (Wolf, 1995; Strohman,
1993).

Nevertheless, the view of geneticists most often heard by the public tends to
overestimate the role of genes in human affairs. There have been periods in
history when certain geneticists have taken an active role in promoting such
views, resulting in destructive social impact. Depending on the society, the
response of critics from the field of genetics has usually been limited to a small
minority. I would suggest that the lessons of history mandate a greater participation in public debates over the importance of genes and a greater involvement in public education by scientists.

REFERENCES

Allen, G. 1975. "Genetics, Eugenics and Class Struggle." *Genetics* 79:29–45.
Angastiniotis, M., S. Kyriakidou, and M. Hadjiminas. 1988. "The Cyprus Thalassemia
Control Program." *Birth Defects: Original Article Series* 23:417–32.
———, and L. Middleton. 1997. "Genetic Services in Cyprus." *European Journal of
Human Genetics* 5, suppl. 2:51–57.
Anonymous. 1996a. "Inégalité des races: 600 scientifiques répondent a Le Pen." *L'Hu-
manité*, September 27.
Anonymous. 1996b. "M. Le Pen demande à ses militants de se préparer à une 'révolu-
tion.'" *Le Monde*, September 17, 1.
Associated Press. 1997. "French Mayor Fined for Racism." *Boston Globe*, September 9,
A10.
Baur, E., E. Fischer, and F. Lenz. 1931. *Human Heredity*. New York: Macmillan.

Bayliss, H. J., District Court Judge. 1993. "Findings of Fact, Conclusions of Law and Judgment: *Evans vs. Romer,*" Transcript of Colorado Amendment, 2 Trial. Civil Action #92, CV7223.

Beckwith, J. 1983. "Gender and Math Performance: Does Biology Have Implications for Educational Policy?" *Journal of Education* (Boston University) 165:158–74.

———. 1991. "The Human Genome Initiative: Genetics' Lightning Rod." *American Journal of Law and Medicine* 17:1–14.

———. 1993. "A Historical View of Social Responsibility in Genetics." *BioScience* 43, no. 5:327–33.

———. 1997. "The Responsibilities of Scientists in the Genetics and Race Controversies." In *Plain Talk about the Human Genome Project,* ed. E. Smith and W. Sapp, pp. 83–94. Tuskegee: Tuskegee University Press.

———, and J. S. Alper. 1997. "Human Behavioral Genetics." *The Genetic Resource* 11:5–9.

Berg, P. 1991. "The Human Genome Project: Biological Nature and Social Opportunities." Talk presented at the *Stanford Centennial Symposium,* January 11.

Bernhardt, B.A. 1997. "Empirical Evidence That Genetic Counseling Is Directive: Where Do We Go from Here?" *American Journal of Human Genetics* 60:17–20.

Billings, P. R., J. Beckwith, and J. S. Alper. 1992. "The Genetic Analysis of Human Behavior: A New Era?" *Social Science and Medicine* 35:227–38.

Botstein, D. 1997. "Of Genes and Genomes." In *Plain Talk about the Human Genome Project,* ed. E. Smith and W. Sapp, pp. 201–14. Tuskegee: Tuskegee University Press.

Bouchard, T. J. Jr., D. T. Lykken, M. McGue, N. L. Segal, and A. Tellegen. 1990. "Sources of Human Psychological Differences: The Minnesota Study of Twins Reared Apart." *Science* 250:223–28.

Boyd, R. 1995. "Observations, Explanatory Power, and Simplicity: Toward a Non-Humean Account." In *The Philosophy of Science,* ed. R. Boyd, P. Gasper, and J. D. Trout, pp. 349–78. Cambridge: MIT Press.

Burian, R. M., and J. Gayon. 1999. "The French School of Genetics: From Physiological and Population Genetics to Regulatory Molecular Genetics." *Annual Review of Genetics* 33:313–49.

Butler, D. 1996. "French Scientists Rally against Racist Claim." *Nature* 383:369.

Carlier, M. 1999. "Le contexte actuel des controverses sur les différences entre races: analyse de quelques évènements récents." *Psychologie Française* 44:107–11.

Cavalli-Sforza, L. L. 1997. "Race Differences: Genetic Evidence." In *Plain Talk about the Human Genome,* ed. E. Smith and W. Sapp, pp. 51–58. Tuskegee: Tuskegee University Press.

Charles, G., and F. Harrois-Monin. 1993. "Il faut croire en l'homme." *L'Express International,* November 4, p. 31.

Chase, A. 1977. *The Legacy of Malthus: The Social Costs of Scientific Racism.* New York: Knopf.

Cohen, D. 1993. *Les gènes de l'espoir.* Paris: Robert Laffont.

Cook-Deegan, R. 1994. *The Gene Wars: Science, Politics, and the Human Genome.* New York: Norton.

Crew, F. A. E., J. B. S. Haldane, S. C. Harland, L. T. Hogben, J. S. Huxley, H. J. Muller, and J. Needham. 1939. "Men and Mice at Edinburgh." *Journal of Heredity* 30:371–73.

DelGuercio, G. 1987. "Designer Genes." *Boston Magazine,* August, 79.

Devlin, B., Resnick, D. P., Fienberg, S. E., Roeder, K., eds. 1997. *Intelligence, Genes and Success: Scientists Respond to The Bell Curve.* New York: Springer.

Feldman, M. W., S. P. Otto, S. I. Greenspan, L. J. Kamin, A. Falek, L. F. Jarvik, G. E. McClearn, F. Ahern, B. Johansson, S. Berg, N. L. Pedersen, S. A. Petrill, and R. Plomin. 1997. "Twin Studies, Heritability and Intelligence." *Science* 278:1383–87.

Feldman, M. W., and R. C. Lewontin. 1975. "The Heritability Hang-up." *Science* 190:1163–68.

Galton, F. 1884. *Hereditary Genius*. New York: Appleton.

Gaudillière, J.-P. 1998. "Les racines de l'exception Française." *La Recherche* no. 311 (August): 89–92.

Goleman, D. 1996. "Forget Money; Nothing Can Buy Happiness, Some Researchers Say." *New York Times*, July 6, C1,C9.

Gould, S. J. 1994. "Curve Ball." *New Yorker* 70 (39):139–49.

Hamer, D., and P. Copeland. 1998. *Living with Our Genes*. New York: Doubleday.

Hamer, D. H., S. Hu, V. L. Magnuson, N. Hu and A. M. L. Pattatucci. 1993. "A Linkage between DNA Markers on the X Chromosome and Male Sexual Orientation." *Science* 261:321–27.

Herbert, W. 1997. "How the Nature vs. Nurture Debate Shapes Public Policy—and Our View of Ourselves." *U.S. News and World Report*, April 21, 72–80.

Herrnstein, R. J., and C. Murray. 1994. *The Bell Curve*. New York: Free Press.

Holden, C. 1995a. "Behavior geneticists shun colleague." *Science* 270:1125.

———. 1995b. "Specter at the feast." *Science* 269:35.

Holtzman, N. A. 1989. *Proceed with Caution: Predicting Genetic Risks in the Recombinant DNA Era*. Baltimore: Johns Hopkins University Press.

Jacob, F. 1979. "Biologie et société." *Le Monde*, November 14–16, pp. 1, 16.

———. 1980. "Eugénisme aux États-Unis: germe et prix Nobel." *Le Monde*, March 5, pp. 1, 11.

Jacquard, A. 1994. *Les Hommes et Leurs Gènes*. Paris: Flammarion.

Jaroff, L. 1989. "The Gene Hunt." *Time*, March 20, p. 67.

Joseph, J. 2001. "Separated Twins and the Genetics of Personality Differences: A Critique." *American Journal of Psychology* 114:1–30.

Katz, J. 1972. *Experimentation with Human Beings*. New York: Russell Sage Foundation.

Kevles, D. 1985. *In the Name of Eugenics: Genetics and the Uses of Human Heredity*. Berkeley: University of California Press.

Kitcher, P. 1996. *Lives to Come: The Genetic Revolution and Human Possibilities*. New York: Simon and Schuster.

Kolata, G. B. 1980. "Math and Sex: Are Girls Born with Less Ability?" *Science* 210:1234–35.

Koshland, D. 1991. "The Human Genome Project: Biological Nature and Social Opportunities." Paper presented at the *Stanford Centennial Symposium*, January 11.

Kuhn, T. S. 1970. *The Structure of Scientific Revolutions*. Chicago: University of Chicago Press.

Lauria, D. P., M. J. Webb, P. McKenzie, and R. Hagerman. 1993. "The Economic Impact of the Fragile X Syndrome on the State of Colorado." In *1992 International Fragile X Conference Proceedings*, pp. 393–405.

Leo, J. 1987. "Exploring the Traits of Twins." *Time*, January 12, p. 63.

Levins, R., and R. Lewontin. 1985. *The Dialectical Biologist*. Cambridge: Harvard University Press.

Lewontin, R. C. 1976. "The Fallacy of Biological Determinism." *The Sciences* 16, no. 2: 6–10.

Longino, H. E. 1990. *Science as Social Knowledge*. Princeton: Princeton University Press.

Ludmerer, K. 1972. *Genetics and American Society*. Baltimore: Johns Hopkins University Press.

Michie, S., F. Bron, M. Bobrow, and T. M. Marteau. 1997. "Nondirectiveness in Genetic Counseling: An Empirical Study." *American Journal of Human Genetics* 60:40–47.

Montagu, A. 1963. "The UNESCO Statements on Race." In *Race, Science and Humanity*, pp. 178–83. Princeton: D. Van Nostrand Co.

Paul, D. B. 1998. *The Politics of Heredity*. Albany: State University of New York Press.

Pinholster, G. 1994. "SIDS Paper Triggers a Murder Charge." *Science* 264:199–98.

———. 1995. "Multiple 'SIDS' Case Ruled Murder." *Science* 268:494.

Rabinow, P. 1999. *French DNA*. Chicago: University of Chicago Press.

Rogers, L. 1999. "Having Disabled Babies Will Be 'Sin', Says Scientist." *Sunday Times (London)*, July 4, p. 28.

Roubertoux, P., and M. Carlier. 1996a. *Intelligence et Hérédité*. Paris: Flammarion, Dominos.

———. 1996b. "Le QI est-il héritable? Le consensus inventé par certains anglo-saxons n'existe pas." *La Recherche* 283:70–78.

Shaw, M. 1984. "To Be or Not to Be." *American Journal of Human Genetics* 36:1, 9.

Steinschneider, A. 1972. "Prolonged Apnea and the Sudden Infant Death Syndrome: Clinical and Laboratory Observation." *Pediatrics* 50:646–54.

Stoltenberg, S. F. 1997. "Coming to Terms with Heritability." *Genetica* 99:89–96.

Strohman, R. C. 1993. "Ancient Genomes, Wise Bodies, Unhealthy People: Limits of a Genetic Paradigm in Biology and Medicine." *Perspectives in Biology and Medicine* 37:112–45.

Suzuki, D., and Knudson, P. 1988. *Genethics:The Ethics of Engineering Life*. Toronto: Stoddart.

Todd, A. 1973. "Le racisme, a-t-il des fondements scientifiques?" *Le Nouvel Observateur*, September 10, pp. 36–39.

Watson, J. D. 1997. "President's Essay: Genes and Politics." *Cold Spring Harbor Laboratory Annual Report*, 1–20.

Weiss, R. 1994. "Born to Be Fat." *Washington Post Health*, December 6, pp. 10–13.

Wertz, D. C. 1997. "Is There a 'Women's Ethic' in Genetics: A 37-Nation Survey of Providers." *Journal of the American Medical Women's Association* 52:33–38.

———, and J. C. Fletcher. 1998. "Ethical and Social Issues in Prenatal Sex Selection: A Survey of Geneticists in 37 nations." *Social Science and Medicine* 46:255–73.

Wolf, U. 1995. "The Genetic Contribution to the Phenotype." *Human Genetics* 95:127–48.

CHAPTER THREE

Genetics and Behavior in the News

Dilemmas of a Rising Paradigm

Peter Conrad

In the past two decades genetics has re-entered the public discourse in terms of explanations for a variety of behaviors and human problems (Nelkin and Lindee, 1995; Condit, 1999). I see genetics as a rising paradigm that is increasingly applied to a range of human behavior. One of the main vehicles for the dissemination of genetics findings and claims to the public is the news media.

This chapter examines some issues that stem from the way genetic research on behavior is presented in the news. The data come primarily from a study of how findings related to behavioral genetics (e.g., alcoholism, homosexuality, and depression and schizophrenia) have been reported in five major newspapers and three news magazines, along with other print media, over a

An earlier version of this chapter appeared as "Media Images, Genetics, and Culture: Potential Impacts of Reporting Scientific Findings on Bioethics" in Barry Hoffmaster, ed., *Bioethics in Context* (Philadelphia: Temple University Press, 2001). This chapter was partially supported by a grant from the Ethical, Legal, and Social Implications section of the Human Genome Project of the National Institutes of Health (1R55 HGO0849–01A1). The research assistance of Dana Weinberg, Nancy Martin, Ben Davidson, and Sarah Marin is gratefully acknowledged. My thanks to Diane Beeson, Barry Hoffmaster, and members of the Genetic Screening Study Group for comments on an earlier version of this chapter.

thirty-year period (1965–95).* The print press can be seen as an exemplar of the news media; television and radio news tend to cover less science news in general and probably less about genetics as well. In addition to examining the actual news articles, I have interviewed fifteen science reporters about their work. Examples from this study are supplemented with data on press coverage of genes for breast cancer to illustrate some ways in which presentations in the news media can shape the public discourse on genetics.

Science in the News

The news media are a critical vehicle for disseminating new scientific find-ings into the culture. The popular press has increasingly reported on science and health, both as part of general reportage and in special science and health sections (Klaidman, 1991). While the news media report on only a very limited selection of the scientific findings published in professional journals (Houn et al., 1995; Conrad and Weinberg, 1996; Conrad, 1997), this coverage still ac-counts for a significant amount of information conveyed to the public through the media. Science and health have become important beats for newspapers. The *New York Times*, for example, employs more than a dozen science and health reporters and publishes health and science news every day, frequently more than one article. While there has been little specific research on how this dissemination of scientific knowledge is interpreted by readers, it is clear that the press is one of the most accessible means for transmitting new scientific and medical findings to the lay public.

Science and medical reporters tend to monitor a few of the most prestigious professional journals, which are then overwhelmingly represented in the news: *Science, Nature, New England Journal of Medicine, Journal of the American Medical Association (JAMA), National Academy of Sciences, Nature Genetics,* and the *Lancet*. While other journals are occasionally reported, these pres-tigious journals dominate the medical and science news. For example, in a study of the press coverage of the association between alcohol and breast

---

*The newspaper sample includes the *New York Times*, the *Boston Globe*, the *Washington Post*, the *Wall Street Journal*, and the *Los Angeles Times*, which represent some of the largest and most influen-tial newspapers in the United States. For homosexuality, the *San Francisco Chronicle* was added. The news magazines included *Time, Newsweek*, and *U.S. News and World Report*. Representatives of the gay press were largely drawn from the same cities as those of the mainstream press and included the *New York Native, Bay Windows*, the *Washington Blade*, the *San Francisco Sentinel*, and the *Bay Area Reporter* (see Conrad and Markens, 2001).

cancer over a thirteen-year period, 88 percent of the news stories came from studies reported in *JAMA* or the *New England Journal of Medicine* (Houn et al., 1995). Reporters believe this handful of journals usually publish the most consequential scientific research and presume the scientific findings are more likely to be of high quality because of the journals' reputation for rigorous peer review. While science reporters recognize that important research is also published elsewhere, it simply does not usually come across their radar screen. This narrow focus suggests that science reporting presents a very selective slice of biomedical research.

News science writing is not a straightforward process of "reporting" the facts of a study garnished with a few quotations from the researchers or other scientists. Science reporters, like other journalists, select, shape, and frame stories into news. Science and medical stories are difficult to present accurately and in an accessible manner. Journalists often need to convert complex and ambiguous scientific findings into nontechnical, compelling, and readable stories. This requires reporters to simplify findings and to present them in ways that are comprehensible to a lay readership. A few studies have examined how medical science has been presented in the media. Dorothy Nelkin (1987) argues that science reporting tends to be uncritical and engages largely in "selling science" to the public. Medical and science newswriting often frames stories as "a new breakthrough in medicine" or depicts the newsworthiness of a story as "scientists report for the first time." There is some evidence that only studies with positive findings become news and that there is a bias against negative studies (Koren and Klein, 1991). Negative studies and disconfirmations of previous findings are a crucial part of the development of scientific knowledge and important to obtaining accurate scientific understanding, but they are less likely to be reported in the news.

The New Genetics

Genetics is becoming an increasingly dominant explanation in medicine and science. People have long noted that some disorders ran in families, and scientists have proffered hereditary theories of various diseases, conditions, and behaviors. Eugenics was popular among scientists and lay people alike through the early part of this century (Kevles, 1985) but fell into disfavor owing to the paucity of valid scientific evidence and the horrors of Nazi genocide. With the study of DNA's structure, a new genetics has emerged in recent decades. Along with producing some remarkable discoveries, the new genetics has also engendered fresh concerns about legal and ethical issues (Kevles and Hood, 1992; Kitcher, 1996)

In recent decades, molecular biology and medical genetics have moved to the cutting edge of science. Important new discoveries involving genes for cystic fibrosis, Huntington disease, fragile X syndrome, Duchenne muscular dystrophy, and types of breast and colon cancer, among others, have been reported. Many of these received widespread notice in the news media.

The advent of the Human Genome Project in 1989, the largest biological project in history (Kevles, 1992), has further fueled genetic research. The genome project is a fifteen-year international research initiative with the aim of sequencing all 3 billion base pairs of the human genetic structure. The project is proceeding ahead of schedule, and a "rough draft" of the genome sequencing was presented in 2000. This information will be used to find the chemical or genetic basis for the two thousand or so genetic diseases that affect humans, with the ultimate hope of producing new preventions and cures. The genome map will allow genetic research to progress more rapidly; this undoubtedly means that new claims about genetic associations and linkages with diseases, conditions, and behaviors will be increasingly forthcoming over the next decade.

The mapping of the human genome has been the object of several provocative metaphors, including a search for the "holy grail" (Gilbert, 1992), investigating the "the essence of human life," and decoding "the book of life." The genome project itself has been called biology's equivalent to the World War II Manhattan Project. Others have suggested that the gene is becoming a cultural icon in American society (Nelkin and Lindee, 1995), invested with almost mystical powers. Critics contend that the "geneticization" of human problems has expanded beyond scientific knowledge (Lippman, 1992) and that a kind of "genetic fatalism"—an assumption that a genetic association is deterministic and means a trait or behavior is unchangeable—underlies much public discourse about genetics (Alper and Beckwith, 1995). What is clear is that genetic research is relevant to an increasing number of diseases, conditions, and behaviors and that the genetic "frame" is commonly employed for explaining a wider range of human problems.

Simply put, an increasing amount of genetic research is being reported in the news (Nelkin and Lindee, 1995; Conrad, 1997; Van Dijck, 1998; Condit, 1999). In 1996, for example, news articles reported research associating genetics with breast and colon cancer, diabetes, Alzheimer disease, homosexuality, "novelty-seeking" personality traits, bed-wetting, and obesity, among numerous other characteristics and conditions. Often these stories are highlighted on the front page of newspapers (most of those mentioned above were) because genetics seems to make good news. Stories about new findings are legion, so much so that it sometimes appears as if we're seeing announcements of "gene of the week" discoveries.

While ethicists and others have raised issues concerning the potential harm of genetic screening and its impact on decision making, the privacy and confidentiality of genetic information, the prospect of genetic discrimination, the dangers of coercion, and the revival of eugenics (e.g., Bartels et al., 1993), less attention has been paid to the effect of the public's understanding of genetics and its implications.

In this chapter, I will briefly examine two science reporting issues that have social and bioethical implications, what I call "finding and losing genes" and "the OGOD assumption" (one gene, one disease) (see Conrad, 1999). For each issue I will present two cases of genetic news presentations in some detail, to illustrate the specifics of reporting and different facets of each problem, followed by a discussion of some implications of these presentations for the public understanding of genetics.

Finding and Losing Genes

Articles reporting significant new genetic research are typically reported in prominent places in newspapers or magazines. Yet if subsequent research does not replicate the findings or disconfirms the first study's results, how does the news media cover the dissenting studies? The way the media reports on such subsequent studies contributes to an information flow problem in public discourse.

The Old Order Amish and a Gene for Manic Depression

In February 1987 major newspapers featured a front-page story reporting the discovery of a marker linked to a gene for manic-depressive illness. Janice Egeland and her colleagues (Kelsoe et al., 1989) had identified the genetic marker based on research involving extended families with a high incidence of the disorder among the Old Order Amish of Pennsylvania, a group with a stable and closed gene pool who keep good genealogical records. A genetic marker is a specific genetic pattern (or difference) found in individuals with a certain disorder; researchers then assume the problematic gene is in the general vicinity of the marker. While the actual gene linked to manic-depressive disorder had not been located, the research indicated it was a dominant gene (i.e., it could be inherited from either parent) and pointed to its location (on the tip of the short arm of chromosome 11). The *New York Times'* headline was "Defective Gene Tied to Form of Manic Depressive Illness." The news story announced a breakthrough finding: "Scientists have discovered the first proof that some cases of manic-depressive illness are linked to a specific gene defect" (*New York Times,* February 26, 1987, p. 1).

A month later newspapers reported on an Israeli study of three large Jewish families that linked another genetic marker (this time on the X chromosome) with the development of manic-depressive illness. The *New York Times* headline announced, "Second Genetic Defect Linked to Illness: Manic-Depressive Disorders Traced to Faulty Gene on X Chromosome" (*New York Times,* March 19, 1987, p. A20).

Estimates suggest that 2 million Americans have manic-depressive illness. It has long been observed that the disorder has a propensity to run in families, and thus it was thought to be at least partly hereditary. The news articles sometimes offered new hope to people with the disorder and their families. "Once the faulty gene is identified," Dr. Risch, one of the study's authors added, "physicians should be able to help guide high-risk people in developing a strategy for a satisfactory way of life. It might also help in devising a treatment that would minimize the risk of manic-depressive attacks, he said" (ibid.).

Two years later the Amish study was disconfirmed. In November 1989, scientists, including some from the original research team, published a paper reporting that continuing research among the Amish led them to conclude that the genetic marker probably was not significant in identifying manic-depressive illness. In one particularly important change, two subjects from the original study who didn't have the chromosome 11 pattern and had shown no signs of mental disorder subsequently developed the illness. With the small sample size of these family pedigree studies, this shift invalidated the statistical significance of the study (Kelsoe et al., 1989).

To its credit, the *New York Times* reported this disconfirmation in the medical science section with the headline "Scientists Now Doubt They Found Faulty Gene Linked to Mental Illness" (November 7, 1989, p. C20). Several of the other newspapers did not report the new disconfirming evidence at all or only mentioned it years later as part of another article. The *Times* story outlined how the new study "cast serious doubt on the conclusions of [the first] study that linked a faulty gene to manic-depressive illness." It discussed the difficulty of assigning specific causes to complex and variable illnesses. The news story ended by noting that the Israeli study linking a suspected gene on the X-chromosome to manic-depressive illness "still seems to be unchallenged." In 1993, however, a research paper reported that after more exhaustive analysis of the Israeli data the X-chromosome link could not be confirmed. The *Times* reported this in the health and medicine section with the headline "Scientists Now Say They Can't Find a Gene for Manic-Depressive Illness," while three of the four other newspapers in our sample never reported the disconfirmation. The *Times* story described how, in the wake of this disconfirmation and an additional one involving a gene on chromosome 5 thought linked to schizophrenia, scientists now believed that there was no single gene for mental disorders. Rather, it was likely that the interplay of a number of genes, in interaction with an individual's environment, might produce a disorder. Again, the article ended on an upbeat note for genetics by quoting one of the study's authors, "Nevertheless, Dr. Baron remains optimistic that scientists will tease out the genes that go afoul in mental disease, if only they are meticulous in their hunt" (January 13, 1993, p. D12).

Alcoholism and the D2 Dopamine Receptor

A similar situation occurred with alcoholism and the dopamine D2 receptor gene. In April 1990 the *Journal of the American Medical Association* (*JAMA*) published an article by Kenneth Blum, Ernest P. Noble, and associates that reported, for the first time, an allelic (specific-gene) association with alcoholism. Based on cadaver brain research with samples from alcoholics and nonalcoholics, the authors found that "the presence of the A1 allele of the dopamine D2 receptor (DRD2) gene correctly classified 77% of alcoholics, and its absence classified 72% of nonalcoholics." The authors concluded they had found a marker for a specific gene in a specific location (q22-q23 region of chromosome 11) that "confers susceptibility to at least one form of alcoholism" (Blum et al., 1990: 2055).

This study was widely reported in the news. All five major newspapers in my study sample reported the Blum-Noble findings on April 18, and all three news magazines reported it in the April 30 issue. The *New York Times* and the *Boston*

Globe printed stories on page one, and the other papers ran them in prominent locations like page three. Headlines announced "Alcoholism Is Linked to a Gene" (*Wall Street Journal*) and "Scientists Link Alcoholism to Gene Defect" (*Boston Globe*). The newspapers reported it as a major breakthrough. The *New York Times*, for example, wrote: "A gene that puts people at risk for becoming alcoholics has been identified for the first time." The newspaper stories were optimistic, stating that this discovery strengthens the growing conviction that heredity plays a key role in alcoholism and that new drugs for alcoholism treatment could eventually emerge. The news magazines all reported the study but were somewhat more temperate with their optimism. While the news media did note some reservations about the study (e.g., its sample size and the unclear role of environment), the tenor of the reporting presented the discovery of a gene linked to alcoholism as a major breakthrough for medicine.

Eight months after publishing the Blum-Noble finding, *JAMA* published a study that essentially found no significant genetic differences between alcoholics and controls (Bolos et al., 1990): the DRD2 gene for alcoholism was not confirmed. This inability to replicate the findings received some attention from the press but much less than the Blum-Noble study. While four of the five newspapers in our study carried some report of the nonreplication, none of the news magazines did. The dissenting reports were also considerably shorter than those for the original study and were located in less prominent places (e.g., p. 20, p. 59). Typical headlines were "Researchers Cannot Confirm Link to Alcoholism" (*New York Times*) and "A Disputed Study of Alcoholics Finds No Genetic Pattern" (*Boston Globe*). While there was some reporting of the disconfirming study, often the stories were written in a manner that still affirmed a genetic basis for alcoholism. Both the *Times* and the *Boston Globe*, for example, quoted Blum as saying the gene was still relevant and that other studies supported their claim. An overall reading of the news coverage of these and related studies suggests the news media continued to emphasize a genetic link for alcoholism in their reporting, despite a prominent failure to replicate. The news magazines did not report the dissenting studies at all. (See Conrad and Weinberg, 1996.)

These two cases indicate that science reporting on genetics maintains a bias toward positive reports, those suggesting genetic associations with behaviors or diseases. This is not surprising, given that others have reported that the media has a bias against negative studies (Koren and Klein, 1991). In addition, genetic discoveries may pass for good news among all the bad news like crimes and routine news like business and politics. But while the discoveries are trumpeted to the public with front-page stories, the dissenting or disconfirming studies are noted (if at all) in smaller back-page items. This kind of reporting is likely to convey the impression that this or that gene has been found, but is unlikely to correct that view once they are lost.

This of course is the logic of news: finding something new is news, but not finding it may not be. Nevertheless, science is always provisional. Disconfirmations and modifications are to be expected as part of the scientific process, even if such complexities don't always make good news. Moreover, news writing often has to simplify to the extent that many of the scientific caveats or qualifications may be lost. And, it seems, the press considers discoveries important news, while disconfirmations or failures to replicate are treated as inherently less important or uninteresting (or perhaps the media simply believe the public takes that view). This parallels crime reporting: Arrests or indictments for a crime may be front-page news, but dismissal of charges or an acquittal get far less attention and my be reported in back pages, if at all. Putative discoveries are news; their negation rarely is.

The OGOD Assumption

News media use catch phrases to signify complex phenomena, from *White-water* to *Generation X* to the *tobacco wars*. This is especially evident in headlines, but it permeates reporting as well. Genetic influence is complex, multifaceted, and indirect, yet it is often presented in the news as if a single gene is responsible for a behavior or condition, be it a gay gene, a breast cancer gene, or a fat gene (Conrad, 1999). We might call this the OGOD model—for "one gene, one disease." The assumption here, of course, is that a single gene determines the disease or trait.

BRCA1 as the Breast Cancer Gene

Breast cancer is the most common cancer for women. It is usually estimated that one in eight women (12%) will contract it, and that forty-six thousand women in the United States die from it each year. In late 1990 Mary-Claire King of the University of California, Berkeley, announced that her lab had identified a marker for some forms of breast cancer somewhere on the lower end of chromosome 17. This discovery was based on research with families that had multiple cases of breast (and ovarian) cancer (Hull et al., 1990). The genetic susceptibility for women in families prone to breast cancer is estimated to be strikingly high—perhaps ten to twenty times higher than for women without the susceptibility.

With this genetic signpost, a number of labs worldwide raced to identify the actual gene, now dubbed BRCA1. In the fall of 1994 Mark Skolnick and his colleagues at the University of Utah reported in *Science* that they had isolated BRCA1 (Miki et al., 1994). In a very unusual course of events, an announcement of the discovery was released three weeks before the publication date of the scientific journal article, in large part due to an *NBC News* report and persistent rumors of the impending discovery. On September 15, all major newspapers carried the story, most of them on the front page. Headlines announced: "Gene for Inherited Form of Breast Cancer Is Located" (*Washington Post*); "Scientists Identify a Mutant Gene Tied to Hereditary Breast Cancer" (*New York Times*); and "Scientists Say They've Found Gene That Causes Breast Cancer" (*Wall Street Journal*). The news stories were quite detailed, describing the BRCA1 gene as a tumor-suppressing gene and circumscribing indications that this gene was implicated in only about half of all hereditary incidence and perhaps in only 5 percent of the total incidence of breast cancer. All women have the BRCA1 gene, but only a small percentage seem to have the mutated version that makes them more susceptible to breast cancer. For the women with the BRCA1 mutation, researchers claimed there was an 80 percent likelihood of getting breast cancer by age 70 and a 50 percent chance of developing it by age 50. Natalie Angier of the *New York Times* pointed out that roughly six hundred thousand women carry the genetic defect.

This was unquestionably a major discovery, depicted by some scientists and reporters as a window to understanding all breast cancer. Early reports following the BRCA1 discovery implicated the gene only with inherited forms of breast cancer in highly susceptible families, that is, a defective BRCA1 gene was deemed to cause only a small proportion of all breast cancer. Yet if one examines the press coverage of this and subsequent findings, BRCA1 is frequently referred to as "the breast cancer gene." Taking headlines as an indicator, we see many designations of it as such, some beginning even before its actual discovery; for example: "The Breast Cancer Gene: A Women's Dilemma" (*Time*, Janyary 17, 1994, p.1); "Vexing Pursuit of Breast Cancer Gene" (*New York Times*,

July 12, 1994, p. C1); "Breast Cancer Gene's Impact Limited" (*Washington Post*, September 20, 1994, p. 7); and "Return of the Breast Cancer Gene" (*Newsweek*, November 13, 1995, p. 72).

It is important to note that while BRCA1 and the subsequently discovered BRCA2 (on chromosome 13) are genes linked to breast cancer, they account for only a small percentage of all cases. The BRCA1 defect is present in roughly 5 percent of breast cancer cases, hardly sufficient to be deemed "the breast cancer gene." Research subsequent to the original BRCA1 report has suggested that a BRCA1 mutation may be more prevalent among Ashkenazi Jews (as high as 1 in 100 compared to perhaps 1 in 800 among the general population) (Struewing et al., 1995), and BRCA1 mutations have been found in some non-inherited tumors. Yet even with these additional studies it is probably most appropriate to call the mutated BRCA1 a gene that indicates a specific, very high-risk breast cancer among families with a history of breast and ovarian cancer. It is important to keep in mind that an overwhelming proportion of breast cancer, at least at this point, appears to be noninherited. This is not to say that future scientific findings could not implicate BRCA1 or other mutations in a wider range of breast cancer causation, but current evidence does not warrant designating it the breast cancer gene.

Why should this apparent journalistic shorthand matter? In the most general sense, calling BRCA1 the breast cancer gene (quotes are never used here) suggests that inherited genes are the main cause of breast cancer, which is not the case. While the environment as a factor in breast cancer is discussed in both the scientific and news media articles, focus on the breast cancer gene turns our attention away from environmental sources to germ-line DNA.

Focusing on breast cancer genes raises a number of issues. First, calling a disease agent the breast cancer gene may lead women, understandably anxious about the disease, to request tests for the gene from their physicians. It is not clear what, if any, relevance BRCA1 mutations at this time has for women without family histories of breast cancer. Thus far the gene's explanatory power is limited to high-risk families. Yet many other women will want to know whether they are free of the gene defect. Would a negative test lull women into a false sense of security about their risk for breast cancer, perhaps leading them to neglect breast self-exams or appropriate mammograms? Second, testing for BRCA1 is an imperfect predictor. Some women in high-risk families who test positive for the gene defect may choose to undergo "prophylactic bilateral mastectomies," a radical operation removing both breasts, which, while reducing risk, still does not guarantee protection from breast cancer. Likewise, those who test negatively, while justifiably relieved, still carry at least an average risk for breast cancer, a one in eight lifetime prevalence. Third, even for high-risk families, locating the gene does not necessarily allow prediction of the course of the disease or lead directly to treatment. The gene for Huntington's disease, which was discovered several years ago, has had little clinical impact on that disorder so far.

In the near term, given the potential genetic testing market, we are beginning to see that commercial products allowing for the easy testing for BRCA genes will become readily available (see Kolata, 1996). While virtually all the news articles noted that the discovery of the gene would have no immediate impact on treatment or even on prevention and detection, some were more optimistic about the implications. One reporter, for example, suggested that the discovery "sets the stage for a blood test, probably in a year or two, that would identify women who would benefit from intensive monitoring and preventive treatments" (Saltus, 1994, p. 1). Another science writer was much more cautious, however. "Even when a test goes on the market, only a fraction of the women who believe they are members of families high for breast or ovarian cancer should consider it" (Brownlee and Watson, 1994, p. 78). This writer suggests that only women with two or more first-degree relatives (mother, daughter, sister) with breast or ovarian cancer, or those with multiple family members stricken with breast cancer before age 40, should be tested when such a test becomes available.

More than a year after the discovery, Francis Collins, director of the Center for Human Genome Research and himself a genetic researcher studying breast cancer, suggested that for a variety of scientific, ethical, and social reasons, BRCA1 testing should only be done in the context of a research setting (Collins, 1996). If the *breast cancer gene* becomes part of the common parlance, then many more people beyond those in high-risk families may want to be tested. Even putting aside the potential cost of unnecessary testing, what impact will a negative BRCA test have on women in a society in which breast cancer risk is still so high?

It may someday turn out that BRCA1, BRCA2, and other genes yet to be discovered are parts of a collection of gene mutations that cause breast cancer. It is also possible that scientists will discover that genes and the environment interact in subtle ways to produce breast cancer or that some breast cancers are fundamentally environmental. As important as the discovery of the BRCA1 gene is, journalists and scientists should avoid simplistic designations that misinform and potentially misguide people about the risk of breast cancer.

"Gay Genes"

Scientists and physicians have offered theories about a hereditary predisposition toward, or a congenital nature of, homosexuality for more than a century (Greenberg, 1988). In July 1993 Dean Hamer, a neurogeneticist at the National Institutes of Health, published an article in *Science* reporting the discovery of a genetic marker associated with homosexuality. Hamer and his colleagues traced the family pedigrees of seventy-six homosexual men and found that 13.5 percent of brothers, 7.3 percent of maternal uncles, and 7.7 percent of maternal cousins were homosexual. They then conducted a DNA linkage analysis on forty pairs of gay brothers and found that thirty-three pairs shared genetic markers on the Xq28 region of the X chromosome. Hamer and his colleagues concluded that "at least one subtype of male sexual orientation is genetically influenced" and inherited through the maternal line (Hamer et al., 1993, p. 321).

Our research examined how five studies linking biology and homosexuality, published between 1990 and 1993, were reported in the mainstream and gay press (see Conrad and Markens, 2001). Most of these studies received substantial media attention, although the discussion here will be limited to Hamer's research because it is the only study to claim to have located a specific genetic marker.

Hamer's research was widely reported. It was on the front page of five of the six newspapers we studied (we added the *San Francisco Chronicle* to our sample for reporting on homosexuality; the *Wall Street Journal* ran it on page B1). Three of the papers ran two stories on the study; typically, one reporting the findings and a second focusing on reactions or potential implications. All three news magazines covered the story, including *Newsweek*, which featured a nine-page cover story.

The lead in the *Washington Post* (July 16, 1993, p. 1) story was typical: "Scientists at the National Institutes of Health have discovered evidence that some gay men have inherited one or more genes that predisposed them to being homosexual." This was usually followed by a more detailed description of the study and its findings. But for the first time, several articles began to use the term *gay gene* to describe the findings (even though Hamer explicitly noted that it is unlikely a single gene is responsible for homosexuality). For example, in three of the headlines, the term *gay gene* was used: "Research Points to Gay Gene" (*Wall Street Journal*); "New Evidence of 'Gay Gene' in Some Men" (*San Francisco Chronicle*); and "Coming to Grips with Finding the Gay Gene" (*San Francisco Chronicle*). In 1993 the *San Francisco Chronicle* was the only paper to use the term in both the headline and the article.

The gay press, at least as represented by the six gay newspapers we examined, also reported Hamer's study. They gave this study more coverage than they had the previous studies but relatively less attention than the mainstream press had given it. Only one editorial used the term *gay gene*, although other headlines implicitly referred to gay genes: "It's in the Genes" or "Gays with Designer Genes."

But within two years the term *gay gene* had become more common. Hamer and a journalist coauthored a book about the research leading to the discovery of the Xq28 association with homosexuality, the subtitle of which was "The Search for the Gay Gene and the Biology of Behavior," and the term *gay gene* was used frequently in the book (Hamer and Copeland, 1995). When Hamer published a second study in 1995 (Hu, et al., 1995), refining and replicating his research with a different sample, the news media again reported it. By then the term *gay gene* was common currency; headlines included "Search for a Gay Gene" (*Time,* June 12, 1995, p. 60); "New Evidence of a 'Gay Gene'" (*Time,* November 13, 1995); "Is There a 'Gay Gene'?" (*U.S. News and World Report,* November 13, 1995); "In Search of the Gay Gene" (*Advocate,* December 26, 1995, cover); and "Study Provides New Evidence of 'Gay Gene'" (*Washington Post,* October 31, 1995, p. 1). Even a news item in *Science* had the headline "NIH's 'Gay Gene' Study Questioned" (June 30, 1995, p. 1841). The writers also used the term *gay gene* much more frequently in the articles. David Miller (1995) notes it is regularly used by the press in the United Kingdom as well.

There are some stylistic issues here worth noting. On the one hand, it simply may be a journalistic shortcut to use the term *gay gene* instead of saying *marker for a gene for homosexuality*—the former certainly has a more catchy sound to it. At the same time, the use of the term *gay gene* may indicate an increasing acceptance of the existence of genetic causes of homosexuality. Recall that both of Hamer's studies located only a section of the X chromosome (Xq28) that has a marker associated with homosexuality. At best, the researchers have discovered the approximate location where a "gay gene" might reside. It also makes a difference whether the term *gay gene* is set off in quotes. Placing it in quotation marks flags the point that it is merely a term that is in use (like saying "so-called gay gene"). Without quotes, use of the term suggests that there is such an entity—even though no such gene has yet been isolated.

It is also important to note that some writers designate it *a* gay gene, while others call it *the* gay gene. While neither is scientifically accurate, the latter is more problematic. Hamer's studies are based on researching a very specialized sample of homosexual men: gay men who have brothers who are also gay, both of whom are willing to go public about it. Neither Hamer nor any other researcher claims that this or any other gene is likely to be *the* cause of homosexuality, yet calling it *the* gay gene suggests that it is the cause. Not all gay men have the marker on the Xq28 region (most probably don't), so clearly there are other causes, be they environmental, psychological, or genetic (caused by other genes). And there is no evidence that whatever gene resides on Xq28 is deterministic; is it still "the gay gene" if there are individuals who have it and are not homosexual? At the very least, it is misleading to call this marker the gay gene. The more the news media uses such terms, the wider the dissemination of the image of homosexuality as a genetically driven phenomenon, with all this implies.

One other point should be mentioned here. Scientists are not neutral figures in relation to the media. Some scientists have become very media savvy and know how to promote their research and ideas in the news. Dean Hamer is both a scientist and an entrepreneur for the idea that homosexuality has a genetic basis. He has appeared on radio, on television, and in documentaries advocating this idea and has written two books promoting a genetic view of human behavior (Hamer and Copeland, 1995, 1998). While Hamer's popular writing may be an extreme example of a scientist attempting to promote a viewpoint, scientists frequently use the media to infuse their ideas or views into the public sphere. The optimism about genetics in the news is not always a creation of the media; it is also a reflection of the scientists. (To cite another example, Ernest Noble has been a steadfast supporter of the genetic approach to alcoholism, even in the wake of critical and disconfirming research.)

There is a difference of opinion in the gay community about whether finding genetic links to homosexuality is good, bad, or irrelevant for gays. Some suggest that linking homosexuality to genes shows that homosexual orientation is "natural" and implies that gays shouldn't been blamed, stigmatized, or discriminated against for an orientation that arises from their genetic makeup. Individuals who take this view argue that if the public understood a gay orientation to be an innate characteristic, like skin color, then our society would realize that gays deserved legal protection against discrimination. The t-shirt that proclaims "Gay by Nature, Proud by Choice" represents this viewpoint. In contrast, there are people in the gay community who are less sanguine about the finding. They are concerned that finding a gene for homosexuality would lead to a remedicalization of homosexuality. Possible "treatments" for the "defect," such as testing fetuses and aborting those with the implicated genes, or possibly even "eugenic" interventions (e.g., as depicted in the play *Twilight of the Golds*) might follow. Others have suggested that it is not sensible to base rights on biology, and thus finding genes for homosexuality is irrelevant to justice (Nardi, 1992).

While Hamer replicated his own study with a different sample, George Ebers and his associates (Rice et al., 1999) were unable to replicate Hamer's findings and concluded that the Xq28 marker is not proven to be linked to male homosexuality. While it is not in our realm to adjudicate the science, current claims about "the gay gene" are best seen as contentious. At this moment, "the gay gene" is more a social construction than a biological reality. Nevertheless, its designation in the public sphere may be having an impact on how we think about homosexual orientation and how we treat people who are gay.

In the next section I outline some broader ramifications of the presentation of genetic findings in the news.

Implications

Embedded in the ways genetics is reported in the news are an array of implications for the public understanding of genetics. This chapter has only begun to articulate these, but it seems clear that the way problems are constructed in the culture and the common knowledge around them affect people's perceptions and what they do about those problems. We can identify a number of specific issues.

1. *Genetic optimism and raising public expectations.* Genetic associations with human behavior are regularly reported prominently in the press (often on page one). The tone of this reporting reflects a genetic optimism, which comprises beliefs that genes are causally related to human behavior, that scientists will discover these relationships, and that these discoveries will lead to treatments or the reduction of suffering (see also Conrad, 2000). Reporters

covering studies on genetic molecular biological associations try to be up-beat and leave the reader with the idea that the discovery of gene linkages is "good news." This stance is manifested in the ways the stories are written, and, specifically, in cases of disconfirmation or nonreplication, the way the last word emphasizes that better science or more research will eventually find the genes.

Genetic optimism reinforces the "magic bullet" conception of medicine—that, if we just identify the right gene for an ailment, science will come up with a specific biomedical treatment for it. Demands for genetic tests may increase, although their medical purpose remains questionable. As the discoveries of genetic linkages to Alzheimer or Huntington disease have shown, treatments don't necessarily follow from gene identification. This type of genetic opti-mism, even when tempered by discussions about social implications (e.g., stigma or the potential loss of insurance) or by the knowledge that genetic tests or treatments are not yet available, pervades the news reporting of genetics. Despite these caveats, the tone of the reporting is likely to raise the public's expectation of what will come from genetic discoveries.

2. *Disconfirmations and cultural residues.* Scientific findings are provisional and always subject to modification; failure to replicate results can lead to new understanding. The two examples of disconfirmation or nonreplication pre-sented (and to these one could add the discovery and disconfirmation of a gene for schizophrenia on chromosome 5 and several others) raise several issues around science reporting. Discoveries of genetic associations for common human problems are deemed important enough to become front-page news and are presented in a positive light. Yet if subsequent research disconfirms the original study the press allocates far less space and attention to the contradict-ing findings, often completely ignoring them. Thus genetic discoveries receive wide play and are infused into the culture, but if they are disconfirmed fewer people know about it. This creates a progenetic bias in the news and ulti-mately becomes a vehicle for misinformation. The public is left with mis-taken ideas about the relationship of genes to problems, and patients or fami-lies may become frustrated when the medical profession cannot deliver on the media's promise.

The press's neglect of disconfirmations can produce errant cultural resi-dues, obsolete ideas that remain part of public knowledge. The news media are the major avenue by which information about genetics enters the culture. Without proper reporting of disconfirmations, outdated or false ideas can become fossilized in the culture. For example, in the late 1960s the news media widely reported the putative relationship between the XYY chromosome and criminal behavior (Green, 1985). This connection was disconfirmed in the 1970s. Yet when asked if they knew about XYY, some of my undergraduate students, who had not even been born at the time of this controversy, replied, "Isn't that the criminal gene?" Without clear and proper reporting of disconfirmations, genetic information (correct or incorrect) will linger and misinform those who encounter it. This may play a part in decision making for medical services as well as shaping how society (e.g., employers or insurance companies) respond to the particular disorders. Moreover, the fact that "successes" become news and "failures" do not reinforces the idea that genetics can explain more of the world.

3. *The OGOD model and the overgeneticization of human problems.* When news reporters use terminological short cuts such as *gay gene, breast cancer gene, obesity gene,* or *thrill-seeking gene,* it oversimplifies complex issues. These simplified terms are especially common in headlines, but they appear frequently in the news stories as well. They overgeneticize the issues they describe: genes are depicted as if they were the most significant factor causing a phenomenon, when they may be only a piece. Such terms convey the notion that single genes can cause diseases, which may be appropriate for cystic fibrosis or Huntington disease (see also Chapter 1 in this volume; Conrad, 1999), but this single-gene model does not suit most behaviors or even diseases like cancer. Calling a discovery "the breast cancer gene" suggests it is at least involved with most breast cancer, when it actually is linked to only 5 percent of the incidence. In other cases, such as homosexuality or alcoholism, no "gene" was ever isolated; rather, researchers only identified genetic markers that suggest genes involved are probably located nearby. Strictly speaking, there is no "gay gene" at this time.

In short, by terming a finding "the" gene, news media give the impression that genetics is the primary cause of the phenomenon, which may not be the case. It privileges genetics in public discourse and reinforces ideas of "genetic essentialism" (Nelkin and Lindee, 1995), the idea that human beings are fundamentally products of their DNA. In its extreme, this can become a type of "genetic fatalism," whereby genetic associations to behaviors or conditions are pessimistically deemed to be deterministic and unchangeable (Alper and Beckwith, 1993), an unintended and unarticulated result of geneticization.

4. *Geneticization and the shift to individual responsibility.* When genes are

implicated in behavior, conditions, or diseases, we often see a shift in responsibility. Behaviors or traits can be attributed to the individual's DNA, with certain consequences. On the one hand, many in the gay community believe that if genetics are associated with sexual orientation, then they will not be "blamed" for their difference and laws will be passed to protect them from discrimination (see Chapter 9). Assuming this is a valid argument—and there are those who would question it—what might this same notion mean for individuals and families suffering from alcoholism? On the other hand, when we deem breast cancer a "genetic disease," we shift responsibility for cause and prevention. If genetics is seen as the first cause, then we minimize attention to environmental factors that are associated with breast cancer and invest fewer resources in identifying environmental contributions to the disease. If the idea of breast cancer as genetic disease gains common currency, it may affect whether women conduct self breast exams and seek out mammograms. And, as mentioned earlier, even in the cases where a BRCA1 mutation is identified, it is not clear what steps women with the gene can take to prevent the onset of the disease. Is it not premature and problematic to present breast cancer as if it were predominantly a genetic disease?

This shift in responsibility from society to the individual aligns with our current political climate, which increasingly blames individuals rather than social conditions for human problems. Thus genetics could become part of an ideological shift away from environmental and social analyses of problems, fostering the decline of public responsibility for human misfortune and misery. To the extent that news reporting privileges genetics in its coverage, the media contribute to this shift in the public eye.

Conclusion

The media's coverage of genetics—whatever excellence is achieved in terms of information, technical accuracy, and clarity of presentation—manifests journalistic conventions that ultimately misrepresent the role of genetics in human behavior. Not to imply that they necessarily treat genetics differently than they treat other scientific and medical topics—while that may very well be the case, I have no comparative evidence to substantiate such a claim. Rather, I do contend that because the media function the way they do, and because genetic information has particular potential impact, the implications of genetics news raise significant social concerns. News conventions, such as those leading writers to ignore disconfirmations and depict discoveries of "the" gene, compromise the accuracy of science reporting. Perhaps inadvertently, the media reinforce simplistic notions of how genes affect behavior or contribute to diseases. These may affect public attitudes and engender new cultural myths about the role of genetics in explaining and addressing human problems.

In recent years we have observed at least one promising change in the reporting of genetics. Reporters, perhaps chastened by the prospect of disconfirmations and failures to replicate, now frequently mention that though a finding may be interesting and provocative, it still must be replicated by other studies. By the time Hamer's first study was published (1993), all the articles pointed out that these findings needed to be confirmed, and at least four specifically noted that scientific reports of genes for schizophrenia, manic-depression, and alcoholism were later discredited (*Los Angeles Times, Boston Globe, New York Times, Washington Post*). This small change at least informs the public about the provisional nature of scientific findings and the need to be alert to replications and disconfirmations. But it will also be important for the media to report on further research, as important claims that have been widely reported are modified.

All of these examples raise issues about how genetics has been "packaged" in the media and how it affects what people think about particular problems. Media presentations of genetics are the raw materials by which individuals and communities create their own understandings of the role of genes in disease and behavior. While communities select and interpret from various presentations of cultural information, news depictions are a key source for shaping public understanding. To the degree that this source utilizes conventions that misrepresent genetic reality, community perceptions will reflect a partial and inevitably biased perspective of the role of genes in life's problems.

REFERENCES

Alper, J. S., and J. Beckwith. 1993. "Genetic Fatalism and Social Policy: The Implications of Behavior Genetics Research." *Yale Journal of Biology and Medicine* 66:511–24.
Bartels, D. M., S. L. Bonnie, and A. L. Caplan, eds. 1993. *Genetic Counseling.* New York: Aldine DeGruyter.
Blum, K., E. P. Noble, P. J. Sheridan, A. Montgomery, T. Ritchie, P. Jagadeeswaran,

H. Nogami, A. H. Briggs, and J. B. Cohen. 1990. "Allelic Association of Human Dopamine D2 Receptor Gene and Alcoholism." *JAMA* 263:2055–60.

Bolos, A. M., M. Dean, S. Lucas-Derse, M. Ramsbury, G. L. Brown, and D. Goldman. 1990. "Population and Pedigree Studies Reveal Lack of Association between the Dopamine D2 Receptor Gene and Alcoholism." *JAMA* 264: 3156–60.

Brownlee, S., and Watson, T. 1994. "Hunting a Killer Gene." *U.S. News and World Report,* September 24, pp. 76–78.

Collins, F. S. 1996. "RCA1—Lots of Mutations, Lots of Dilemmas." *New England Journal of Medicine* 334:186–89.

Condit, C. 1999. *The Meanings of the Gene: Public Debates about Human Heredity.* Madison: University of Wisconsin Press.

Conrad, P. 1997. "Public Eyes and Private Genes: Historical Frames, News Constructions and Social Problems." *Social Problems* 44:139–54.

———. 1999. "A Mirage of Genes." *Sociology of Health and Illness* 21:228–41.

———. 2000. "Genetic Optimism: Framing Genes and Mental Illness in the News." *Culture, Medicine, and Psychiatry* 25:225–47.

———, and S. Markens. 2001. "Constructing the 'Gay Gene' in the News: Optimism and Skepticism in the American and British Press." *Health* 5:373–400.

———, and D. Weinberg. 1996. "Has the Gene for Alcoholism Been Discovered Three Times since 1980? A News Media Analysis." *Perspectives in Social Problems* 8:3–24.

Gilbert, W. 1992. "A Vision of the Grail." In *The Code of Codes,* ed. D. Kevles and L. Hood, pp. 83–97. Cambridge: Harvard University Press.

Green, J. 1985. "Media Sensationalization and Science: The Case of the Criminal Chromosome." In *Expository Science: Forms and Functions of Popularization,* ed. T. Shinn and R. Whitley, pp. 139–61. Boston: D. Reidel.

Greenberg, D. 1988. *The Construction of Homosexuality.* Chicago: University of Chicago Press.

Hamer, D., S. Hu, V. L. Magnuson, N. Hu, and A. M. L. Pattatucci. 1993. "A Linkage between DNA Markers on the X Chromosome and Male Sexual Orientation." *Science* 261:321–27.

Hamer, D., and P. Copeland. 1994. *The Science of Sexual Desire: The Search for the Gay Gene and the Biology of Behavior.* New York: Simon and Schuster.

Hamer, D., and P. Copeland. 1998. *Living with Our Genes.* New York: Doubleday.

Houn, F., M. A. Bober, E. E. Huerta, S. D. Hursting, S. Lemon, and D. L. Weed. 1995. "The Association between Alcohol and Breast Cancer: Popular Press Coverage of Research." *American Journal of Public Health* 85:1082–86.

Hu, S., A. M. L. Pattatucci, C. Peterson, L. Li, W. Fulker, S. S. Cheney, L. Kruglyak, and D. H. Hamer. 1995. "Linkage between Sexual Orientation and Chromosome Xq28 in Males but Not in Females." *Nature Genetics* 11:248–56.

Hull, J. M., M. K. Lee, B. Newman, J. E. Morrow, et al. 1990. "Linkage of Early-Onset Familial Breast Cancer to Chromosome 17q21." *Science* 250:1684–89.

Kelsoe, J. R., E. I. Ginns, J. A. Egeland, et al. 1989. "Re-evaluation of the Linkage Relationship between Chromosome 11p loci and the Gene for Bipolar Affective Disorder in the Old Order Amish." *Nature* 342:238–42.

Kevles, D. J. 1985. *In the Name of Eugenics: Genetics and the Uses of Human Heredity.* Berkeley: University of California Press.

———. 1992. "Out of Eugenics: The Historical Politics of the Human Genome." In *The*

Code of Codes, ed. D. J. Kevles and L. Hood, pp. 3–36. Cambridge: Harvard University Press.

———, and L. Hood, eds. 1992. *The Code of Codes*. Cambridge: Harvard University Press.

Kitcher, P. 1996. *The Lives to Come: The Genetic Revolution and Human Possibilities.* New York: Simon and Schuster.

Klaidman, S. 1991. *Health in the Headlines*. New York: Oxford.

Kolata, G. 1996. "Breaking Ranks, Lab Offers Test to Assess Risk of Breast Cancer." *New York Times,* April 1, 1996, A1.

Koren, G., and N. Klein. 1990. "Bias against Negative Studies in Newspaper Reports of Medical Research." *JAMA* 266:1824–26.

Lippman, A. 1992. "Led (Astray) by Genetic Maps: The Cartography of the Human Genome and Health Care." *Social Science and Medicine* 35:1469–76.

Miki, Y., J. Swanson, D. Shattuck-Eidens, P.A. Futreal, et al. 1994. "A Strong Candidate for Breast and Overian Cancer Susceptibility Gene BRCA1." *Science* 266:66–71.

Miller, D. 1995. "Introducing the 'Gay Gene': Media and Scientific Representations." *Public Understanding of Science* 4:269–84.

Nardi, P. 1992. "Gays Should Lean on Justice, Not Science." *Los Angeles Times,* August 6, B7.

Nelkin, D. 1987. *Selling Science: How the Press Covers Science and Technology.* New York: W. H. Freeman.

———, and M. S. Lindee. 1995. *The DNA Mystique: The Gene as a Cultural Icon.* New York: W. H. Freeman.

Rice, G., C. Anderson, N. Risch, and G. Ebers. 2000. "Male Homosexuality: Absence of Linkage to Microsatellite Markers at Xq28." *Science* 284:265–67.

Saltus, R. 1994. "Mutated Gene Tied to Early Breast Cancer." *Boston Globe,* September 15, p. 1.

Struewing, J. P., D. Ableiovich, J. Peretz, N. Avishai, et al. 1995. "The Carrier Frequency of the BRCA1 185delAG Mutation Is Approximately 1 Percent in Ashkenazi Jewish Individuals." *Nature Genetics* 11:198–200.

Van Dijck, J. 1998. *Imagenation: Popular Images of Genetics.* New York: New York University Press.

CHAPTER FOUR

Advocacy Groups and the New Genetics

Alan Stockdale and Sharon F. Terry

Genetic research commands great attention from the general public and advocacy groups, perhaps unjustifiably. Many advocacy groups strive to play a role in advancing gene discovery, with the hope that such knowledge will bring expanded research programs, genetic testing, and improved treatment options. However, for people living with a genetic disease, genetic knowledge and research is often of limited immediate value and may even be problematic. There are medical, social, and psychological issues associated with the use of genetic testing technologies. And gene therapy research, initially portrayed as being on the verge of offering breakthrough treatments, has so far been a source of more disappointment than therapy. Advocacy groups therefore must decide how to effectively balance research, with its potential for long-term benefits, with the immediate social and medical issues inherent in living with a genetic condition. This chapter explores these issues by focusing on advocacy organizations associated with two genetic diseases, cystic fibrosis (CF) and pseudoxanthoma elasticum (PXE), the former from the perspective of a social scientist and the latter from the perspective of a parent who founded an advocacy organization.

We begin with a few general comments. First, we have decided to use the term *advocacy groups,* though terms such as *consumer groups, support groups,* and *patient organizations* are also in use. It is not our wish to debate the correctness of these terms. As Hilda Bastian, who prefers the term *consumer,* notes, each term is "weighed down by a lot of ideological baggage" (1998, p. 3). The use of different terms reflects changing attitudes and realities about the roles of individuals living with genetic conditions, their families, and their friends in relation to the condition or disability, researchers, clinicians, other professionals, genetic technologies and services, and society. Since the 1960s, a number of societal changes have been a catalyst for increasing activist consumer involvement in health care and the proliferation of advocacy groups. These changes include: the disability rights movement, based on a social understanding of disease and disability that sees solutions not in treatment or cure but in antidiscrimination and societal inclusion of people regardless of impairment (Chapter 6); increased concern with the ethical, social, and legal implications of research and clinical trials; consumerism; self-help movements; and the influence on research and policy achieved by AIDS and breast cancer groups. The character of more recent advocacy groups is thus very different from that of medical charities of the 1950s and 1960s.

Not everyone with a genetic condition becomes involved with an advocacy organization. Several studies have noted that it is often white and middle-class individuals who become involved in advocacy and support (Epstein, 1995; Rapp, 1999). Some may avoid advocacy groups because they do not want a medical condition to define their identity, or they might be uncomfortable with the orientation of advocacy groups, or they might fear discrimination. At the other extreme are individuals who become actively involved in advocacy activities, redefining their lives around their condition and even founding new organizations where they perceive a need.

A shared genetic condition does not imply shared attitudes and perspectives. People living with the same genetic condition may have significant disagreements about the relative importance and characteristics of the challenges they face and how to address them. Some may wish to invest in research for improved treatment or a "cure," which may not result in benefits for many years. This may be particularly true for those who have more to gain in such a scenario because of factors such as age and health status. Others may be more inclined to focus on education, support, and services that are of immediate benefit. Still others may focus on rights and justice issues.

Advocacy organizations may try to address a broad range of different member needs, or they may emphasize a more narrowly defined agenda. They may not necessarily be representative of even most people with the condition. The range of potential services and functions includes fundraising, public education and awareness, informational support, emotional support, the organization and improvement of clinical services, research advocacy, support and conduct of research through funding and collaboration, and rights advocacy. Striking a balance between research and services, including the new services necessitated by genetic medicine itself, poses a challenge to advocacy organizations, particularly in this era of rapidly expanding genetic research programs and widely held expectations that genetic research will eventually "revolutionize" medicine.

Cystic Fibrosis

With the support of a powerful advocacy group, cystic fibrosis (CF) has played a trail-blazing role in molecular research over the last couple of decades. The gene associated with CF was one of the first major discoveries resulting from breakthrough molecular techniques developed in the 1980s, and an enormous amount of effort has since been devoted to using this discovery to help develop new diagnostic and therapeutic applications. Now, nearly a dozen years after the discovery of the gene, CF may instead serve as an example of the consequences of focusing extensive resources almost exclusively on basic research. One of the most striking results is how little impact the discovery has had so far on the prevention, diagnosis, and clinical management of CF. In the meantime, other issues, such as ready access to affordable medications and care, receive less attention than they might warrant. Moreover, genetic testing and gene therapy research have generated new educational and support needs. These receive little recognition and are poorly mediated because of a narrow focus on "curing" CF.

CF is a single-gene disease most commonly found among Caucasians. Approximately 1 in every 2,500 children is born with CF. It is a recessive disease, so to develop it a child must inherit a copy of the deleterious gene from each parent. The disease results from a malfunction of a cell membrane protein, the most obvious manifestations of which are abnormal functioning of the sweat glands in the skin, inhibition of enzyme secretion necessary for digestion, and chronic bacterial infections in the respiratory system. Accumulated damage to the lungs resulting from chronic infection eventually causes lung failure and premature death in the majority of people with CF.

A threefold treatment strategy of airway-clearing techniques, antibiotics to control bacterial infection, and digestive enzymes to maintain nutrition has remained largely unchanged since the 1950s. While focused on symptoms, this strategy has been enormously successful over the last forty years, extending the median survival age of a person with CF from a few years to the early 30s. In the 1980s, the development of powerful new molecular tools opened up the possibility of tracking down the responsible gene and understanding the underlying disease processes. When researchers eventually identified the cystic fibrosis transmembrane conductance regulator (CFTR) gene in 1989, it was followed by an enormous expansion of research and development activity in the 1990s.

The Cystic Fibrosis Foundation, formed by physicians and parents in 1955 (Morrison and Morrison, 1993), has played a prominent role in the development of CF treatment and research. In the 1950s, most physicians had little or no awareness of the disease and treatment options were very limited. There was a pressing need to educate both medical professionals and the public and to promote both clinical and basic research. To address these needs, a network of CF centers was set up at hospitals across the United States, where children with CF could obtain care from knowledgeable physicians and physicians could readily conduct research. There are now more than one hundred foundation-accredited centers delivering care to some twenty thousand patients across the United States. Establishment of a national network of chapters that promoted awareness of the disease and fundraised provided further support for research and education.

During the 1980s, the foundation became an increasingly research-oriented organization. The foundation, along with other national associations such as the Canadian Cystic Fibrosis Foundation and the United Kingdom's Cystic Fibrosis Trust, played an important role in the search for the gene. By centralizing financial control, the foundation was able to focus its energies on research and actively draw in the best researchers by concentrating funds in a few key research centers and extending the period of grant support. As its fundraising activities became more professional, the foundation was also able to effectively capitalize on the discovery of the CFTR gene. Walk-a-thons, dinner dances, and golf tournaments supported by celebrities and large corporate sponsors successfully expanded funding to support further research activities. Between 1989 and 1999 the foundation's annual income grew from approximately $50 million to $150 million, making it as important a fund-provider to CF research as the National Institutes of Health (NIH) during the 1990s. In fact, the foundation collaborated with NIH to fund NIH's designated gene therapy research centers and important research NIH would otherwise have not been able to support. In recent years, the foundation has also invested huge amounts of capital into research and development relationships with biotechnology companies.

The foundation plays an important role as a broker of the relationships essential to the research enterprise. It links researchers at medical schools and biotechnology companies and facilitates relationships between these groups and the NIH, the Food and Drug Administration (FDA), and legislators. A key component of this strategy has been two annual conferences: the North American Cystic Fibrosis Conference, a large annual event attended by medical professionals and researchers, and the Williamsburg Conference, a small annual meeting of invited researchers and key officers at the FDA and the NIH. The foundation also plays an important lobbying role, making frequent representation to and appearances before congressional committees. In this capacity, it serves to protect NIH funding, orphan drug legislation, patenting, control over pharmaceutical pricing, and other legislative matters of importance to researchers.

The foundation has been enormously successful at devising an extremely aggressive and ambitious research program to exploit the CFTR gene discovery, but its focus on therapeutic research has not been without consequences. Twelve years after the discovery of the gene, there have, as yet, been few tangible clinical benefits for people living with CF. In the meantime, the foundation has not been very effective at mediating the genetic testing technologies and gene therapy research that followed the gene discovery, although both these developments have considerable consequences for people living with CF. Moreover, one of the costs of focusing on the search for improved therapies has been that other issues of immediate importance for people with CF, such as access to existing drugs and quality treatment and the needs of the rapidly growing adult population with CF, have received less attention (Duster and Beeson, 1997, pp. 45–52; Stockdale, 1999, pp. 588–89). Some people with CF even consider the foundation's position on patenting, drug pricing, and healthcare reform to be at odds with their interests.

The need to understand and make decisions regarding the use of genetic testing technologies confronts adults with CF, and parents of children with CF, unlike nearly any other group in American society. Since the mid-1980s, and especially following the discovery of the CFTR gene in 1989, individuals with CF and their families have witnessed the development and broad application of genetic testing technologies. But medical professionals and ethicists involved have largely focused their attention on the use of genetic screening services to identify CF carriers in the general population. Initially, it was thought that general population screening for carriers would begin rapidly after the discovery of the gene; but this did not happen, since the genetics of CF proved much more complicated than expected, and it quickly became apparent that there were significant barriers to providing informed and responsible testing to large numbers of people.

Soon after the discovery of the gene, a number of professional groups issued statements that opposed general carrier screening in the United States because of the potential risks associated with misunderstanding and the psychological impact of test results (Caskey et al., 1990; National Institutes of Health, Workshop on Population Screening, 1990; American Society of Human Genetics, 1992). All these statements recommended that genetic testing be restricted to individuals who have a close relationship to someone who had already been diagnosed with CF. This position was maintained until 1997, when an NIH panel recommended offering genetic testing to any couples considering pregnancy (National Institutes of Health, 1997).

The recommendations to restrict testing to family members of affected individuals are at odds with studies that have examined the impact of genetic testing on those families. Two important research groups, one examining "high-risk" families (Duster and Beeson, 1997) and the other, siblings of people with CF (Fanos and Johnson, 1995a, 1995b), have shown that within families that have members diagnosed with CF, prenatal genetic testing to detect affected fetuses and genetic testing to identify carriers can have serious implications for family dynamics and personal identity. These recommendations, particularly the one resulting from the 1997 meeting, whose participants had access to the results of these studies, appear to have been driven by a biomedical perspective and agenda, not the perspectives and interests of those living with CF. This is an issue on which the foundation has failed to take a position, although it was represented at the NIH meeting in 1997.

There are numerous issues associated with the use of genetic testing for families with CF. Carrier testing of family members may be problematic when different mutations are *perceived* by family members to be associated with different degrees of severity and when testing reveals that different sides of the family contributed different mutations (Duster and Beeson, 1997, p. 35). Healthy siblings of people with CF often develop mistaken beliefs about their carrier status as a result of guilt, depression, and anxiety. Beliefs about carrier status and transmission may play an important role in helping siblings cope. (Fanos and Johnson, 1995a, 1995b). The availability of preimplantation genetic testing and prenatal diagnosis may also involve parents in difficult decisions that cannot be separated from feelings about an existing child or children with CF. Based on a study of 180 families living with CF in California, Duster and Beeson found that the "successful functioning of high-risk families rests on their acknowledgment of the value of the lives and contributions of their members with genetic disease," hence the "closer people are to someone with a genetic disease, the more problematic and usually *unacceptable* genetic testing is as a strategy for dealing with the issue" (1997, p. 83; emphasis in the original). For this reason, they argue, a common medical rationale for offering testing to these families—that it will assist in reproductive decision making—is invalid.

Some people living with CF are also uneasy about genetic testing for the general population for reproductive decision making and critical of their exclusion from policy making on this issue. Barbara Palys, the chair of the International Association of Cystic Fibrosis Adults, had these comments on the NIH Consensus Conference: "There was precious little discussion about quality of life and, in fact, no individual with CF was invited to address this issue at the meeting. . . . My concern is that genetic applications like genetic testing are advancing faster than society's ability to understand, assess and provide safety-nets for those stigmatized with a genetic disease or predisposition to a genetic disease. Screening for CF is a glaring example. With barely a whimper, a small gathering decided that it was viable to screen for CF. While mention was made of the fact that 35% of the USA's CF population are adults living functional lives (with this number expected to grow increasingly), there was no debate or even awareness of the precedent being established" (Palys, 1997, p. 24). Like people affected by other genetic disabilities (see the discussion of statements by Little People of America and the National Down Syndrome Congress, Chapter 6 in this volume), some adults with CF are concerned that couples will make decisions based on insufficient knowledge and that the medical focus will shift from treatment to prevention.

Another testing application that has attracted little attention but may be significant is the genotyping of individuals already diagnosed with CF. As part of the collection of epidemiological data on CF patients for research purposes by the foundation and other groups, there have been efforts to genotype everyone with the disease. This testing has been perceived as innocuous, given that the person undergoing testing is already aware that he or she has CF; however, given what we know from the studies cited above, there is reason to suspect that this type of testing may also have psychological repercussions for some. Individuals may *perceive* genotype information as either reinforcing or contradicting beliefs about the severity of their disease and the likely effectiveness of potential treatments. For example, the identification of one or two copies of the most common mutation associated with CF may have psychological consequences for someone who has developed a coping strategy built around a "mild case" identity, despite other genetic and nongenetic factors that generally affect the disease course in unpredictable ways.

A key issue given the studies of families cited above is the general lack of genetic education and counseling. There are very few quality educational materials on CF genetics specifically developed for people with CF and their families. Genetic knowledge by itself is insufficient. Effective education depends on addressing the psychological and social issues within these families, as ignorance and misunderstanding of genetic information may be an active response that helps some families and individuals cope with their situation (Richards, 1996; Turney, 1996). Moreover, access to professional counseling is generally limited. Foundation-accredited CF centers are not required to have genetic counselors on the CF care team, and so few do. Most counseling on genetic issues is provided by CF physicians, generally pediatric pulmonologists or other care-team professionals who are generally not trained in either genetics or counseling. Skills and knowledge aside, the financial pressures under which many CF centers operate may limit the availability of staff to provide these types of services.

The foundation has little involvement in genetic diagnostics, aside from the collection of genetic information on people diagnosed with CF. Although it has sent representatives to many of the key policy meetings, such as the NIH CF Genetic Testing Consensus Development Conference, it has not been an active participant in these matters. The foundation's official position is that its mission is the promotion of research into the development of better therapies for the treatment of CF; therefore involvement in genetic testing issues, as with other issues, would be a distraction. Others have suggested that the foundation has avoided testing issues because of the potential political cost of any association with the highly contentious issue of abortion (Cook-Deegan, 1994, pp. 243–44).

After the discovery of the gene, the foundation focused its efforts on improved therapies, particularly gene therapy. (Note that this research focus was broadened substantially in the late 1990s as it became clear that the development of an effective gene therapy for CF was much more difficult than initially anticipated.) At the time of the discovery, gene therapy clinical trials were just beginning, and with the confident backing of the foundation CF rapidly became one of the principal research targets, with the first CF gene therapy clinical trials beginning in early 1993.

Gene therapy research potentially impacts a host of important decisions. The possibility of effective gene therapy may reinforce negative feelings regarding the use of genetic testing in reproductive decision making (Duster and Beeson, 1997). Gene therapy may also have an impact on care, possibly affecting decisions about lung transplantation or teenage compliance with existing therapy. Accurate information also has an important direct bearing on decisions about participation in gene therapy clinical trials (Churchill et al., 1998). However, the nature of CF gene therapy's effects and the research process are complex, unfamiliar, and have been difficult for some people with CF and their families to fully comprehend (Stockdale, 1999).

The difficulty in understanding gene therapy—what it does, what its risks and limitations might be, and its likelihood of success—has been compounded by research hype and often exaggerated media coverage, both negative and positive. From the early 1990s to mid-1990s, researchers, biotechnology companies, the Cystic Fibrosis Foundation, and the media often gave the impression that CF might be "cured" in a few years. As a result, many families living with CF developed very high expectations in the years immediately after the discovery of the gene (Duster and Beeson, 1997, pp. 52–53). By 1995, more skeptical media coverage was appearing; in some cases, coverage moved to the other extreme and declared gene therapy a failure. A more reasoned response was contained in an NIH report released in December 1995, which was very critical of the "overselling" of gene therapy research and its potentially damaging impact on research programs and families. The authors expressed concern about "the possibility that patients, their families, and health providers may make unwise decisions regarding treatment alternatives, holding out for cures that they mistakenly believe are 'just around the corner.' For instance, patients with cystic fibrosis may be less vigilant about pulmonary management or a couple at risk for producing a child with a life threatening genetic disorder may base reproductive decisions on unrealistic expectations of gene therapy" (Orkin and Motulsky, 1995).

The images used to promote investment in gene therapy research have further exacerbated the impact of the hype surrounding gene therapy research. Promotion often plays optimistic promises of research breakthroughs against negative portrayals of the present experience living with CF. For example, in the early 1990s one of the slogans used by the foundation in its fundraising literature was "We're fighting a child killer. And winning." Although not uncommon among medical charities, this is a controversial strategy, as its representations of people living with a condition may be a partial truth at best, may be upsetting and detrimental to coping, and may be perceived as patronizing (Stockdale, 1999, pp. 589–99). The image of the passive child victim awaiting a scientific breakthrough, often in contrast with dynamic images and heroic accounts of researchers, rarely reflects reality. More than one-third of the population with CF are adults, many of whom, by their own accounts, are living rich and rewarding lives despite the demands of living with CF.

Education to help patients and families realistically evaluate the hype surrounding gene therapy has also been lacking. The foundation's interest in funding and promoting gene therapy research is, if anything, antithetical to the genuine education of patients and families. Such educational efforts have been lacking despite the recommendation of a panel appointed by the NIH director in 1995 that efforts be undertaken to better inform the public about gene therapy research (Orkin and Motulsky, 1995). Recently, in response to the much-publicized death of a patient with a different genetic disease while participating in gene therapy research, another NIH advisory group has recommended that NIH "should target education efforts at specialty clinical centers where gene transfer studies are likely to be conducted or subjects recruited, such as CF centers or hemophilia clinics" (Advisory Committee to the Director, 2000).

One important aspect of the education issue is that there has been relatively little contact between people living with CF and those supporting and undertaking the research enterprise (Stockdale, 1999), although both researchers and people living with CF would clearly benefit by better understanding the issues and concerns of the other (Terry and Boyd, 2001). Conferences, one of the main ways these groups could interact with each other, have been largely closed for this purpose in the United States. The few parents of affected children or adults with CF who attend the North American Cystic Fibrosis Conference do so on their own initiative rather than as invited participants. In 1996, the foundation denied consumers the right to registration because of concerns that lay attendance might inhibit open discussion among medical and research professionals (Stockdale, 1999). This situation is in stark contrast to conferences held by other CF associations in Canada and Europe, where people with CF and their advocacy groups generally play a more significant role.

Meanwhile, other organizations have been formed to fill gaps in services needed by people with CF and their families, and these groups undertake grassroots educational efforts to better inform people about genetics and gene therapy. Some, such as Cystic Fibrosis Research Incorporated (CFRI) in northern California, are former chapters of the foundation that broke away to gain local control over financial resources and services. Adults have also formed a number of organizations such as the International Association of Cystic Fibrosis Adults (IACFA), the United States Adult Cystic Fibrosis Association, and CF Network. All these organizations publish newsletters that address education issues as well as a broad spectrum of other issues of concern to adults with CF. In particular, IACFA, founded in Europe but with many American members, has undertaken to work with physicians and researchers to educate the readers of its newsletter about CF genetics, testing technologies, and gene therapy research (e.g., Parad, 1995; Williamson, 1995). CFRI, sometimes in conjunction with IACFA, also runs the only conference in the United States for people with CF and their families. This has been one of the few public forums for critical discussions about genetics and gene therapy that has included researchers, physicians, and people living with CF. It is unfortunate that many of these smaller organizations, who might broaden the spectrum of perspectives on CF, have had limited national visibility and therefore lack influence with policy makers.

Cystic fibrosis is a disease for which the agenda has been set and dominated by one advocacy group that has narrowly focused on genetic research to "cure" it. Among people with CF there is widespread support for research that might result in improved treatments, but other concerns and needs are also prominent. Many of these needs, as well as those who would give voice to them, have been marginalized in the pursuit of a genetic research agenda. Moreover, the educational and support needs necessitated by new and emerging genetic technologies have been inadequately addressed.

Pseudoxanthoma Elasticum

Lay advocacy groups that formed in the 1990s benefit from the experience of older groups but are also highly susceptible to the exaggerated promise of genetic research. This era of a pervasive "genetic" perspective of biomedical research and groundbreaking consumer involvement in genetics holds both promise and peril. With the ability to easily connect affected individuals through the use of electronic technology and the sexiness of often-publicized genetic "solutions" to genetic conditions, neophyte groups must be very cautious as they structure their mission and activities to meet the needs of those affected by the condition. PXE International, a lay advocacy organization for those with pseudoxanthoma elasticum (PXE), came into being in the crux of this tension.

Pseudoxanthoma elasticum (PXE) is a rare, autosomal recessive genetic disorder that causes mineralization of elastic tissue, primarily in the skin, retina, and arteries. Skin can become folded and wrinkled, and individuals may experience cardiovascular complications. The most severe complication of the condition is loss of central vision because of retinal hemorrhage, secondary to mineralization of the membrane behind the retina. The phenotype is extremely varied.

The founders of PXE International, Sharon and Patrick Terry, entered the world of genetics, research, and lay advocacy groups when their two children were diagnosed with PXE, a few days before Christmas 1994. The diagnosing dermatologist, Lionel Bercovitch, M.D., spent Christmas Eve explaining the consequences of the disorder to them: central vision loss; loose and hanging skin on the neck, underarms, behind the knees; and perhaps several other problems pertaining to the cardiovascular and gastrointestinal systems.

The Terrys received the news of the children's diagnosis with tremendous anguish and responded to it by seeking support and information, heading to local medical school libraries to research PXE. Neither had a background in biology, and they also needed to buy medical dictionaries and primary textbooks on basic biology and genetics. Nevertheless, what struck the Terrys most forcibly was that little research was being conducted on the disorder and there was no clear understanding of how the disorder progressed. They wondered if a cure could be around the corner in this newly dawning age of genetics. At the same time, they also began to see that research on rare disorders was a highly unorganized activity and was apparently disconnected from the real needs of those affected. They were surprised to find a lack of coordination and consensus in the research community, not understanding at first that there was no mechanism for such organization. At the same time, the hype around genetic research made it difficult to sort out what was possible from what was mere fantasy. For example, a few months after the children were diagnosed a researcher told the Terrys that he had an article in press describing the PXE gene and to watch a particular journal for publication. Each month the Terrys went to medical libraries and searched for the article. It later became clear that the researcher had not discovered the gene and had no publication in press. Experiences like this caused the Terrys to wonder if the promise of genetics was mostly hype.

It also became clear that there were no adequate support services for individuals affected with the various signs and symptoms of PXE. Most had never had contact with another person with the condition. The Terrys founded PXE International in 1995 with a three-pronged focus: support for affected individuals, clinicians, and research. In the first few weeks of the foundation's existence, the board of directors, composed primarily of adults affected by vision loss, emphasized the importance of a dynamic balance between services for affected individuals and support for research, ensuring that the lived experience of affected individuals informed the founding of PXE International.

One of the first things the foundation did was establish an e-mail list to listen to the needs of the individuals living with PXE. In addition, it held small regional meetings around the country and in Europe to help formulate the mission and goals of PXE International. The services provided grew to include three e-mail lists to meet the varying needs of individuals interested in the condition. PXE Announcements is an announcement-only service (offering no discussion) for those interested in news blurbs only. PXE Information is a service for those interested in detailed discussions about living with PXE and its ramifications. PXE Chat is for those who wish to talk about everything and anything, supporting each other in more than the ways relating to how PXE touches their lives.

As a result of listening to affected individuals, PXE International was faced with the challenge of balancing the needs of adults who already had vision loss with those of other adults who had not yet lost vision. Adults losing vision in their mid-thirties and forties seek help dealing with the loss of employment and abilities to read and drive a car; those that have not yet lost vision seek treatments that will slow down or halt the progression of PXE. Additionally, the parents of the very few children who manifest symptoms at an early age (children represent only 40 of 2,500 registered affected individuals) seek a cure.

The Terrys contacted the Genetic Alliance (then known as the Alliance for Genetic Support Groups) to ask how they might be able to accelerate both support for individuals with PXE and meaningful research on the disease. Staff at the Genetic Alliance connected them with a number of resources, including other lay advocacy groups and the Ethical, Legal, and Social Implications Research Program of the National Human Genome Research Institute at NIH. The Terrys' interaction with the Genetic Alliance was the main catalyst in their vision of a lay advocacy group. Staff at the Genetic Alliance involved with groups such as Neurofibromatosis, Inc., and Little People of America helped impress upon the Terrys the importance of services as a central hub for a lay advocacy group, as well as the importance of those services being determined by those living with the condition. Coming into existence in this new genetics age, PXE International responded judiciously to the lure of seeing genetic research as *the* solution. It chose not seek a genetic cure but instead look for ways to give its members options, simultaneously working to connect affected individuals to existing resources and to establish treatments.

PXE International embraced the following critical concepts in the formulation of its mission and goals:

— a central and commanding respect for the lived experience of affected individuals
— recognition of the urgent need for improved clinical services, health insurance issues, and so on, and action to alleviate some of these issues
— attention to disability rights issues (e.g., discrimination against people with PXE in employment) and access to treatments, giving rise to activism designed to alleviate these problems
— an interdisciplinary approach, encouraging the interaction of many specialties, including service providers, clinicians, and researchers, in

the quest to meet the broad needs of the community and protect research participants
— a broad base of affiliations with researchers, allowing for the creation
  of consortia to pool resources rather than confine them to one lab or
  another
— a grounding in the philosophy that basic research on any disorder will
  lead to discoveries for others, an approach that encourages working
  diligently with the Genetic Alliance and other coalitions
— facilitating clinician referral and peer consultation.

PXE International developed a series of electronic and printed publications
for both lay persons and medical professionals. These discuss various aspects
of PXE and give suggestions for monitoring, treating, and adapting to its
effects. In addition, PXE International publishes a quarterly newsletter that
provides information about low-vision clinics, programs, adaptive software,
and the like. Periodic regional, national, and international conferences feature speakers and exhibitors from foundations and companies involved in
low-vision services. Other workshops deal with psychosocial aspects of health
and illness and integrating life changes. PXE International has made a conscious decision to draw upon the resources of the service community rather
than try to provide vision and psychosocial services in its place. In addition, these conferences offer innovative information about current PXE and
related research.

While much of the day-to-day work of PXE International involves services
for and with those affected by the condition, resources are also dedicated to
research, including genetic research. This aspect of PXE International's mission rests on the premise that involvement of affected individuals will alleviate
some of the usual challenges of human research and at the same time assure
consumer-centered and focused research. PXE International involves individuals in understanding the need for data collection, in receiving updates and
information as it is discovered, and in contributing their own insights into the
research process. For example, women with PXE wanted to know why their
mammograms continually showed microcalcification. The involvement of
these women led to research on PXE and mammograms, resulting in recommendations specific to their care.

As a lay volunteer–lay advocacy organization, PXE International has established a registry of twenty-five hundred affected individuals, served by more

than fifty offices worldwide. In addition, it has collected more than one thousand pedigrees, created the PXE International Blood and Tissue Bank, housing fifteen hundred DNA samples and one hundred tissue samples, collected detailed epidemiological data from six hundred affected individuals, initiated several research projects, and described these and other projects to research participants in a direct and expedient manner. This lay foundation acts as a firewall between the sample donors and the researchers, ensuring confidentiality to minimize the risk of discrimination to research participants and at the same time facilitating ethical research by providing a safe pathway to recontacting donors for more information or samples. PXE International funds research in seven countries and has branches of the blood and tissue bank in South Africa and Italy.

Human samples are available to any research group that has a solid research project, Institutional Review Board approval, and the willingness to share resulting discoveries with PXE International. Researchers using the bank sign an agreement that recognizes PXE International's role as a full collaborator in the discovery process. PXE International and researchers collaborate on the research, discussing methods, analyzing results, and engaging together in discovery. Sharon Terry, executive director of PXE International, is coauthor of two gene discovery papers (Bergen et al., 2000; Le Saux et al., 2000) and helped facilitate submission of both papers to *Nature Genetics,* where they were published back-to-back in June 2000. She has also filed a patent application with the other discoverers of the PXE gene.

Ms. Terry has assigned her rights to the patent to PXE International. The organization has made it very clear that their goals with regard to patenting and licensing are to facilitate useful, timely treatments and to make all tests and treatments accessible and affordable. Unlike some lay advocacy groups, it does not oppose patenting. On a BBC broadcast (Terry, 2000), Sharon Terry was asked why the gene should be patented at all. She sees the need arising out of the current intellectual property practice and the need to hold the patent in order to encourage research that may produce more immediate results and protect access to the products and services that will arise from the gene discovery. Again, as custodian of the gene for the brief period the patent is held, PXE International has had the foresight to plan ways to keep the research and its results focused on the needs of the affected individuals. It is notable that some other groups that have supported genetic research have ended up in conflict with researchers over intellectual property rights, although PXE International was not aware of these cases when it conceived its approach to property rights. The most striking case has been the legal battles between the Canavan Foundation and Miami Children's Hospital over genetic testing royalties that the Canavan Foundation sees as restrictive.

PXE International believes that in some instances it is necessary to offer a restrictive license in order to provide incentives for the development of treatments. In the BBC interview Ms. Terry said, "In an ideal world, it would be best to have it all in the public domain, available to everyone equally. But in a market economy, we can ensure greater access, more focused research, and affordable testing and treatments by giving PXE International the power to make decisions regarding licensing and royalties" (Terry, 2000).

PXE International is able to broker a strong and viable collaboration between researchers, serving as a vehicle for coordination and communication. A lay advocacy group that is attentive to the needs of its members, educated with regard to the science, and able to remain somewhat objective can greatly facilitate the science surrounding a disease, providing and ethical framework that can be beneficial for all involved. When asked if every group should materially participate in research and hold the patent to their gene, the Terrys respond that they do not think that is necessary. Many possibilities for benefit-sharing arise through productive relationships between lay advocacy groups and researchers. Research, funding, and participant issues often delineate cultures that share some commonality but diverge in significant ways. Nevertheless, gains can be made that protect the interests of all the players and allow each culture, through compromise, to reap the "profits" it needs. This might include embargoing information to allow researchers to publish, allowing restrictive licensing to provide incentive for drug development, and sharing benefits of testing and treatments by lowering costs for participants and their family members.

Genetic testing for PXE is not yet available. PXE International is working to establish a central lab for testing, requiring that it be coupled with genetic counseling and appropriate services. Individuals may face some of the same issues that people with CF face. Because PXE has wide phenotypic variability, there will be an attempt to correlate phenotype with genotype. This could result in individuals trying to predict the course of the disease and what ramifications it will have for their lives. Education, counseling, and support will be critical. The strongest desire for genetic testing comes not from affected individuals but from their relatives, who want to know if they are carriers, or have PXE, or both. PXE International is educating its members about these issues through its newsletter, in anticipation of the genetic test's availability. The organization will try to balance its expenditures on genetic testing and continued involvement in making sure that various clinical aspects of PXE are studied.

Conclusion

We have provided two examples of the role of advocacy groups in the new genetics, illustrative of some of the issues that arise for these groups in the context of genetic research. An important caveat is that these two cases are not representative of genetic advocacy groups in general. Rather, what we have tried to lay out are the important roles these groups sometimes play in genetic research, the support of individuals and families living with genetic conditions, and some of the tensions that result from these different roles.

Advocacy groups often play a pivotal role in advancing research and treatment for genetic conditions, which may otherwise languish in research and clinical backwaters because of their relative rarity. CF is unusual in that it has been a major focus of gene therapy research. On the whole there has been little gene therapy research on rare genetic diseases; most such research focuses on the development of treatment for more common diseases such as AIDS and cancer, for which there are potentially large, profitable markets. One of the reasons that CF has attracted so much research attention is that the Cystic Fibrosis Foundation has worked forcefully to build the relationships and gather the funding necessary to support and sustain a large, ambitious research program. Similarly, in the case of PXE, PXE International offers a particularly important example in the way an advocacy organization has been able to both rapidly facilitate research and position itself at the center of that research so as to maintain control over the products and benefits for affected families. Many small advocacy groups have not been able to organize as effectively.

Genetic research can be a double-edged sword for people living with genetic conditions; it raises issues advocacy groups may have difficulty addressing. In the case of CF, some of the issues associated with the use of genetic testing technologies in families living with CF have been underaddressed because they are perceived as distracting from therapeutic research. PXE International's position is that they must offer genetic testing along with comprehensive information about its limitations, particularly its inability to predict the morbidity or progression of the disorder.

Genetic testing applications open up a number of possibilities that might be seen as beneficial to some individuals and families but may be disturbing and threatening to others. For example, in cases where the condition is severe and results in very premature death, attitudes toward the use of testing technologies for reproductive choice may be more positive than in the case of CF, described above. On the other hand, some advocacy groups take the position that prenatal genetic testing reinforces a medical model of disability, when the issue from their perspective is discrimination and stigmatization (Parens and Asch, 1999). A widespread concern of people with genetic disabilities is that parents and medical professionals often have a limited understanding of life with a disability or preconceived notions that bear little relation to the experience of people living with a disability; therefore they are in no position to either provide adequate counseling or make a reasoned decision about pregnancy termination. For example, Little People of America, a group that represents people with dwarfism, see that their members might benefit from the genetic testing technologies to prevent "fatal, traumatic birth outcomes" but worry about the general public using the technology to terminate nonfatal births of dwarf children (Ricker, 1995).

Therapeutic research also raises a number of issues. Greatly improved therapies are the Holy Grail for some genetic advocacy groups, such as those described here, but it is unlikely that genetic research will result in many new therapies in the near future. Even once a gene has been identified, there are often enormous complexities and technological hurdles that inevitably result in a long lag between gene discovery and effective new therapeutics—assuming new therapies are eventually developed at all. In the meantime, people with genetic conditions have to live in an overheated environment of rapid research advances and biotechnology investment that has a well-established history of overpromising. It is quite possible, maybe even likely, that research programs like that of the Cystic Fibrosis Foundation will eventually result in much improved therapies that will dramatically aid the treatment of people with many genetic conditions. However, this is far from what we see in the present, since, as in the case of CF, people now have to live with both their disease and frequent overblown predictions of dramatic therapeutic advances and cures.

The word *cure* is misleading and much overused in the context of genetic research. While the benefits of research advances and the hope they provide should not be understated, grossly inflating the expectations of people living with genetic conditions is not productive and may cause harm. PXE International feels very strongly that hype is detrimental to both services and research. Instead, they have chosen to focus on directing individuals affected by the disorder to appropriate services and support.

Genetic research programs are particularly problematic when they reduce the needs of people with a genetic disease to the search for a cure. There is an enormous contradiction in gene therapy research, which, if successful, would result in treatments that cost tens of thousands of dollars a year, when many individuals with genetic conditions currently have difficulty gaining access to quality care and affording existing drug treatments. It is quite likely that many of the people living with genetic conditions now have very little to gain from future therapies because of their age or health status. These people may have a much greater interest in access to affordable quality health care, affective measures against discrimination, and other immediate concerns. Other areas of research that are currently underemphasized may also be significant. In the case of CF, for example, adults who have accumulated significant lung damage may have little to gain from gene therapy research but might benefit significantly from research to improve lung-transplant procedures and postoperative care. Likewise, for individuals who have lost central vision as a result of PXE, gene therapy or even mitigating treatments will not restore vision.

Many of the issues we have touched on in this paper are issues of education—for people living with genetic conditions, service providers, researchers, and the general public—and informed public discussion. Both education and discussion have been lagging far behind genetic science and technology. As the representatives of people on the front line of the new genetic services, genetic advocacy groups should play an important role in addressing education issues and enabling informed public debate. Their input could provide for a broader and more grounded perspective on the impact of the "genetic revolution." Greater support of the services and programs provided by umbrella organizations such as the Genetic Alliance could greatly expand the ability of advocacy groups to deliver high-quality services to address these issues. Another important step would be greater involvement of lay advocates in key policy groups. Recently, there have been attempts to involve consumers and advocates to a greater degree, in the wake of a report issued by the Institute of Medicine that criticized the lack of genuine public participation in setting NIH policy (In-

stitute of Medicine, 1998). However, in too many cases there are token consumer advocates and no real attempt to solicit a broad spectrum of consumer
perspectives in a way that actually brings about meaningful change.

REFERENCES

Advisory Committee to the Director, Working Group on NIH Oversight of Clinical
Gene Transfer Research. 2000. "Enhancing the Protection of Human Subjects in
Gene Transfer Research at the National Institutes of Health." National Institutes of
Health, July 12. http://www.nih.gov/about/director/07122000.htm.
American Society of Human Genetics. 1992. "Statement of the American Society of
Human Genetics on Cystic Fibrosis Carrier Screening." *American Journal of Human
Genetics* 51 (6):1443–44.
Bastian, H. 1998. "Speaking Up for Ourselves: The Evolution of Consumer Advocacy in
Health Care". *International Journal of Technol Assess Health Care* 14, no. 1 (winter):3–
23.
Bergen, A. A., A. S. Plomp, E. J. Schuurman, S. Terry, M. Breuning, H. Dauwerse,
J. Swart, M. Kool, S. van Soest, F. Baas, J. B. ten Brink, and P. T. de Jong. 2000.
"Mutations in ABCC6 Cause Pseudoxanthoma Elasticum." *Nature Genetics* 25, no. 2
(June):228–31.
Caskey, T., M. M. Kaback, and A. L. Beaudet. 1990. "American Society of Human
Genetics Statement on Cystic Fibrosis Screening." *American Journal of Human Ge-
netics* 46:393.
Churchill, L., M. L. Collins, N. M. P. King, S. G. Pemberton, and K. A. Wailoo. 1998.
"Genetic Research as Therapy: Implications of 'Gene Therapy' for Informed Con-
sent." *Journal of Law, Medicine and Ethics* 26 (1):38–47.
Cook-Deegan, R. 1994. *Gene Wars: Science, Politics, and the Human Genome.* New York:
W. W. Norton.
Duster, T., and D. Beeson. 1997. "Pathways and Barriers to Genetic Testing: Molecular
Genetics in the 'High-Risk Family.' " Report published by the Institute for the Study
of Social Change, University of California–Berkeley.
Epstein, S. 1995. "The Construction of Lay Expertise: AIDS Activism and the Forging of
Credibility in the Reform of Clinical Trials." *Science, Technology, and Human Values*
20:408–37.
Fanos, J., and J. Johnson. 1995a. "Barriers to Carrier Testing for Adult Cystic Fibrosis
Sibs: The Importance of Not Knowing." *American Journal of Medical Genetics* 59
(1):85–91.
———. 1995b. "Perception of Carrier Status by Cystic Fibrosis Siblings." *American Jour-
nal of Human Genetics* 57 (2):431–38.
Institute of Medicine, Committee on the NIH Research Priority-Setting Process. 1998.
*Scientific Opportunities and Public Needs: Improving Priority Setting and Public Input
at the National Institutes of Health.* Washington, D.C.: National Academy Press.
Le Saux, O., Z. Urban, C. Tschuch, K. Csiszar, B. Bacchelli, D. Quaglino, I. Pasquali-

Ronchetti, F. M. Pope, A. Richards, S. Terry, L. Bercovitch, A. de Paepe, and C. D. Boyd. 2000. "Mutations in a Gene Encoding an ABC Transporter Cause Pseudoxanthoma Elasticum." *Nature Genetics* 25, no. 2 (June):223–27.

Morrison, C., and R. Morrison. 1993. "National and International Cystic Fibrosis Associations." In *Cystic Fibrosis: Current Topics*, vol. 1, ed. Dodge, J. A., D. J. H. Brock, and J. H. Widdicombe. Chichester: John Wiley.

National Institutes of Health, CF Genetic Testing Consensus Development Panel. 1997. *Consensus Development Statement: Genetic Testing for Cystic Fibrosis*. National Institutes of Health, April 14–16.

National Institutes of Health, Workshop on Population Screening for the CF Gene. 1990. "Statement from the National Institutes of Health Workshop on Population Screening for the Cystic Fibrosis Gene." *New England Journal of Medicine* 323:70–71.

Orkin, S., and A. Motulsky. 1995. *Report and Recommendations of the Panel to Assess the NIH Investment in Research on Gene Therapy*. National Institutes of Health, December 7. http://www.nih.gov/news/panelrep.html.

Palys, B. 1997. "Genetic Screening for Cystic Fibrosis: Establishing a New Precedent?" *IACFA Newsletter* 49.

Parad, R. 1995. "Applications of Genetic Information Regarding the Gene Responsible for Cystic Fibrosis," *IACFA Newsletter* 40, 41.

Parens, E., and A. Asch. 1999. "The Disability Rights Critique of Prenatal Testing: Reflections and Recommendations." *Hastings Center Report*, Special Supplement 29 (5):S1–22.

Rapp, R. 1999. *Testing Women, Testing the Fetus: The Social Impact of Amniocentesis in America*. New York: Routledge.

Richards, M. 1996. "Lay and Professional Knowledge of Genetics." *Public Understanding of Science* 5:217–30.

Ricker, R. 1995. "Do We Really Want This? Little People of America Inc. Comes to Terms with Genetic Testing." http://www2.shore.net/~dkennedy//dwarfism_genetics.html.

Stockdale, A. 1999. "Waiting for the Cure: Mapping the Social Relations of Gene Therapy Research." *Sociology of Health and Illness* 21:579–96.

Terry, S. F. 2000. BBC Interview. BBC World Service, Science and Technology, October 27th.

———, and C. Boyd. 2001. "Researching the Biology of PXE: Partnering in the Process." *American Journal of Medical Genetics (Semin. Med. Genet.)* 106 (3): 177–84.

Turney, J. 1996. "Public Understanding of Science." *Lancet* 347:1087–90.

Williamson, R. 1995. "Gene Therapy for Cystic Fibrosis: New Advances?" *IACFA Newsletter* 41.

CHAPTER FIVE

Invisible Women

Gender, Genetics, and Reproduction

Susan Markens

> Increased knowledge, without increased responsibility on the part of the society, translates to increased knowledge with the inevitable burden of responsibility on mothers. We are asking mothers to be the gatekeepers of life. We are individualizing social problems of disease and disability, medicalizing life itself, and doing it through the bellies of pregnant women.
>
> B. K. ROTHMAN, 1994

Introduction: Where Have All the Women Gone?

The mapping of the human genome and the potential for an increasing number of tests for genetically influenced traits poses ethical questions to society at large, as well as to specific communities. Yet, the impact of genetics is assumed to be gender-neutral (see Lippman, 1994; Mahowald, 1994, 2000), as women are often strangely neglected and invisible in the debates about the potential uses and abuses of new genetic knowledge and technologies. However, women, particularly pregnant women, are in fact the largest consumers of genetic services owing to their encounters with prenatal testing. For this reason, women's experiences must be acknowledged and understood when examining the consequences of our ever-increasing knowledge of genetics and its applications.

As a growing body of feminist research has shown (e.g., Rothman, 1986;

This chapter was supported by the National Center for Human Gene Research (1R01 HG001384–01) and a Mellon Postdoctoral Fellowship at Brandeis University. I would like to thank Carole Browner and the volume editors for thoughtful feedback on earlier drafts.

Press and Browner, 1993, 1997; Cowan, 1994; Kolker and Burke, 1994; Rothenberg and Thomson, 1994; Browner and Press, 1995, 1997; Gregg, 1995; Browner and Preloran, 1999; Markens, Browner, and Press, 1999; Rapp, 1999; Mahowald, 2000), child-bearing women are becoming "moral pioneers" (Rapp, 1999) as the increasing routinization of prenatal screening places them on the front lines of genetic decision making. While the most common type of genetic screening is newborn screening, prenatal screening is currently the most common form of adult genetic testing (Cowan, 1992; Nelkin, 1992; Spitzer, 2000), and abortion is the only "remedy" for most genetic or chromosomal abnormalities that are, or could be, detected during pregnancy. As a result, pregnant women are increasingly becoming crucial arbiters on issues of quality of life, health, disability, and "normality" as they shape future generations. Increased genetic knowledge and the routinization of prenatal testing affects the choices women must make during pregnancy. These decisions affect their "control" and accountability over a pregnancy's outcome. Feminist researchers have revealed the complexity and paradoxes of "choice" that pregnant women experience in the face of prenatal genetic diagnosis.

Despite this rich and developing feminist scholarship, a gendered analysis of the impact of new genetic knowledge is generally lacking. Gender is often ignored and women are made invisible in discussions about the impact of new genetic knowledge. This is reflected, for example, in a thirty-three-page report developed in 1999 by the Secretary's Advisory Committee on Genetic Testing of the National Institutes of Health that only devotes two paragraphs to the topic of prenatal testing (National Institutes of Health, 1999–2000). Similarly, at a conference celebrating ten years of research for the Ethical, Legal, and Social Implications Research Program of the Human Genome Project, only twelve of more than ninety papers presented addressed the issue of prenatal testing (National Institutes of Health and the Department of Energy, 2001). Even when reproduction and prenatal testing are discussed, women's bodies, views, interests, and experiences are often obscured by a discourse that revolves around "couples" (e.g., Bosk, 1992; Caskey, 1992) or, even more alarmingly, what are described as "pregnant couples" (e.g., Kevles and Hood, 1992, p. 321).

To combat this neglect of women, I review some of the recent feminist scholarship devoted to these issues. I also discuss my collaborative research based on the voices of pregnant women who were offered prenatal screening.

This research was carried out in the context of California's state-administered program for prenatal diagnosis. Since 1986, the state of California has mandated that all pregnant women who enroll in prenatal care before the twentieth week of gestation be offered maternal serum alpha-fetoprotein (AFP) screening. AFP blood screening is usually offered to pregnant women between their sixteenth and twentieth weeks of gestation, to test for several types of fetal anomalies. The test was initially developed to screen for neural tube defects (NTDs), which are serious abnormalities of the brain and spine, and currently it is commonly used to screen for Down syndrome as well. As a screening test, AFP indicates only that something may be wrong with the fetus. Women with positive test results are referred for genetic consultation and further testing at a state-approved prenatal diagnosis center. At the consultation, women are offered ultrasound and, in some cases, amniocentesis for the purpose of a more definitive genetic diagnosis. Amniocentesis involves passing a needle through the woman's abdomen into the uterine wall, to withdraw several teaspoons of amniotic fluid for laboratory analysis.

The illustrative quotes I use in this chapter are derived from interviews with 147 women of Mexican origin who came to a genetic consultation session and were offered amniocentesis after an abnormal AFP result (see Browner and Preloran, 1999, for further discussion of methods and data). Although these women are not representative of all women who confront prenatal diagnosis, the issues I discuss capture how women experience the availability of prenatal genetic technologies and knowledge. On the one hand, women often want and appreciate the knowledge available to them via prenatal genetic testing. On the other hand, complex and contradictory issues of "choice," knowledge, and control arise as a result of this prenatal genetic testing. I suggest that women's experiences with genetics, vis-à-vis opportunities for prenatal genetic testing, are, as the title of this books suggests, "double-edged." As R. Gregg (1995, p. 2) writes, "the technologies enhance the range of choices for women and the possibility of greater social control of those choices." The focus on prenatal testing and women's experiences shows that gender must be central to understandings of the impact of new genetic knowledge. A gender-neutral analysis of prenatal and genetic decision making obscures the lived and gendered biological, physical, emotional, and social realities that pregnant (or yet-to-be pregnant) women experience in the face of ever-increasing advances in biomedical and genetic technologies.

Bringing the Women Back In

Jonathan Tolin's 1993 play (later turned into a movie), *The Twilight of the Golds*, tells the story of married couple Suzanne and Rob. To their delight, as well as that of her parents, Suzanne becomes pregnant with their first child. Coincidentally, Rob works at a biotechnology company that is doing cutting-edge genetic research for the Human Genome Project. When Rob's boss finds out that Suzanne is pregnant, he urges Rob to encourage her to have an amniocentesis and test some of the company's latest diagnostic techniques. Suzanne agrees, and the couple is informed that they are having a healthy baby boy with a genetic marker for homosexuality, indicating a high likelihood the child will grow up to be gay. (As indicated in two chapters in this book, however, the notion of a "gay gene" is problematic.) This information sets in motion a cascade of crises and conflicts within the Gold family. While not certain how she feels, Suzanne is concerned about bringing a child into the world who faces possible hurdles and discrimination. Her uncertainty creates chaos within her own family: Her brother David, who is gay, is both hurt and upset that his sister would even consider terminating her pregnancy. Her parents reveal their continued ambivalence and disappointment about their own son's homosexuality. Outraged, David cuts off contact with his family. In a climactic scene, Suzanne repeatedly yells at her husband, "You're making it my problem!" as he abdicates all responsibility for the decision. Finally, Rob admits that he does not want a gay son. Suzanne first agrees to an abortion, then changes her mind. The event brings her closer to her parents and brother, but Suzanne and Rob separate before the birth of their child. Rob does have contact with his son, but Suzanne ends up a single mother, not knowing, despite the test, what the future holds.

The Twilight of the Golds brings out many key issues concerning women, genetics, and reproduction. First, we see that the woman is at the moral center of the story. She is the one who must agree to be tested. She, ultimately, is the one who has to decide what to do with the test results. And in this story she is the one who bears primary caregiving responsibility for the child who is born. In sum, this fictional story clearly reflects the fact that men and women are differentially impacted by new genetic knowledge and prenatal tests. Analyses of genetics cannot be gender neutral.

For instance, in her research on amniocentesis in New York City, anthropologist Rayna Rapp observed that many men did not accompany their pregnant
partner to the genetic consultation. Rapp also had great difficulty obtaining
interviews with the husbands of women who were offered amniocentesis. She
speculates that men's reluctance to participate in her research is attributable to
their view that pregnancy and reproductive decision making are a "woman's
topic." In fact, from the interviews she did conduct, she found that men of
different class and ethnic backgrounds often viewed pregnancy as primarily
women's domain and thus saw the use of amniocentesis as *her* decision to
make (1999, pp. 148–49, emphasis mine).

Similarly, in our research sample, only half of the women attended a genetic
consultation with the father of their child after testing positive on the AFP
screening test (Browner and Preloran, 1999; Markens, Browner, and Preloran,
n.d. b). This finding is significant, since the vast majority of women in our
study made their decision of whether or not to undergo an amniocentesis at or
right after the counseling session. Furthermore, even though most of the men
who attended the genetic consultation claimed they wanted to share in the
responsibility for this important decision, most ceded the decision to the
woman. On the one hand, these findings are encouraging, since they indicate
that many women seem to maintain significant autonomy over reproductive
decision making. On the other hand, like Suzanne in *The Twilight of the Golds*,
the *burden* of decision making usually falls on the woman as well.

This burden is illustrated by women's responses about the decision-making
process in our amniocentesis study. For instance, as one participant, Laura,[*]
explained when asked if her husband agreed with her decision: "He really . . .
didn't have a . . . he didn't really tell me yes or no, he said it was really up to me
'cause . . . I mean, he didn't really help me in the deciding." Likewise, Lily told
us why she was the one who made the decision: "He didn't say anything. It was
[up] to me. He said, 'Whatever you want to do, it's up to you.' " Thus, for the
most part, women seem to bear the responsibility for decision making about
whether to undergo prenatal genetic testing, and so they also experience more
anxiety over it.

Many women are aware that they are more anxious about such decision
making even if their husbands are involved with prenatal care. For instance,

---

[*]All names used are pseudonyms.

when asked whose opinion mattered the most, Nancy replied: "Well, I think mine and my husband's, both of ours. But because men always take these things more lightly, that is . . . he is sure that everything is fine, he doesn't worry. . . . He says everything is fine, everything is fine. I am always the one who is more worried." Similarly, Julia offered this description about her genetic consultation and subsequent decision-making process:

> Oh yes . . . when they told me about the amniocentesis . . . yes, I said, well in that moment I didn't know what to say and then the girls [medical personnel] said to me, "would you like us to find your husband to see what he thinks?" I said, "well, yes" . . . and I was crying at the time. At first they looked for him and he was not around. . . . Oh! Then I said to them, "You know what? I'm going to think about it." Shortly thereafter he [my husband] came in . . . and he was angry because it was getting late for him to go to work. Then he said, "Well, whatever you want" but at that time I felt . . . I don't know . . . like I was out in space . . . and I said that I would prefer to think about it.

In addition to experiencing more anxiety than their husbands about whether to undergo prenatal screening, women who accept are also more burdened in the event of a positive diagnosis. Expectant mothers are much more anxious than expectant fathers after receiving a positive AFP result (Keenan et al., 1991; Kolker and Burke, 1994). Furthermore, while aborting a fetus or raising a child with a chromosomal abnormality obviously affects both men and women, this impact is generally stronger on women (Kolker and Burke, 1994). Although men also mourn the loss of a wanted child when a pregnancy is aborted, it is only women who physically experience that pregnancy (Rothman, 1989). This differential impact is illustrated by Rayna Rapp's description of her own experience of a second-trimester abortion after a diagnosis of Down syndrome: "Because it happened in my body, a woman's body, I recovered much more slowly than Mike did. By whatever mysterious process, he was able to damp back the pain, and throw himself back into work after several weeks. For me, it took months. As long as I had the 14 pounds of pregnancy weight to lose, as long as my aching breasts, filled with milk, couldn't squeeze into bras, as long as my tummy muscles protruded, I was confronted with the physical reality of being post-pregnant, without a child. . . . I was still in deep mourning while he seemed distant and cured" (Rapp, 1984, p. 323). Similar gender differences in the response to an abortion after a positive diagnosis have been found in subsequent research. In particular, studies find that women grieve more, and for a longer duration, than men (Kolker and Burke, 1994; Rothman, 1994; Rapp, 1999).

These examples clearly demonstrate that, although men are affected by reproductive genetics, women must be central in discussions about the impact of genetics on society more generally. From the anxiety and burden of decision making to aborting a fetus with a genetic abnormality, it is evident that a gender-neutral analysis of the impact of genetics, particularly prenatal screening, distorts and hides how women are particularly affected by the increasing proliferation of genetic technologies.

Women's Bodies, Women's Choices?

How do women themselves think about and respond to the availability and experience of prenatal genetic testing? Women may experience genetic technologies as both an expansion of "choice" and an increase in social, and, in particular, medical control over their prenatal care and pregnancy experience. However, while women often choose to undergo prenatal testing, their choice may be based on incomplete knowledge, familial and societal pressure, or both. These aspects of prenatal testing make women's experiences with genetic technologies and knowledge "double-edged."

"Women Make Their Own Choices": Women as Active Consumers of Genetic Technologies

Many women appreciate and desire the information provided by prenatal genetic technologies. In her history of the development of prenatal diagnosis, Ruth Schwartz Cowan (1994) shows that women were important actors in the development of amniocentesis. Women were eager participants in experimental trials for amniocentesis between the 1950s and 1970s; and women sued doctors over wrongful births in the 1970s when they were *not* offered prenatal screening, which helped institutionalize amniocentesis as a part of prenatal care. Likewise, women's desire for a test that can be done earlier in pregnancy than amniocentesis facilitated the development and use of chorionic villi sampling (CVS). CVS is performed between the ninth and twelfth weeks of pregnancy. The procedure involves inserting a catheter through the woman's vagina and cervix in order to obtain outer tissue from the embryonic sac that can be analyzed in a laboratory. The history of women's involvement in and demand for prenatal genetic testing indicates that these techniques have not been simply imposed and forced onto women.

In addition, women tend to feel favorably toward and accept prenatal screening when it is offered to them. Researchers analyzing the 1996 U.S. General Social Survey found that 65 percent of women responded that they would want a prenatal test (Singer, Corning, and Antonucci, 1999, p. 437). Women's overall positive assessment of such tests plays out when they are actually confronted with the decision of prenatal genetic testing. Today more than half of all pregnant American women undergo some form of fetal screening (Meaney, Riggle, and Cunningham, 1993). In California, where the state mandates the availability of AFP screening, there was a 70 percent acceptance rate statewide in 1997 for this diagnostic technique (Cunningham, 1998), while acceptance rates as high as 82 percent have been found in specific HMOs (Browner and Press, 1995; Press and Browner, 1997). Likewise, by the late 1990s there was a 71 percent acceptance rate for amniocentesis in California from women who initially screened positive on AFP (Cunningham, 1998).

Stories from women themselves also attest to their desire to have such tests done. A colleague, hearing about my research, told me that when she was pregnant at the age of 33 she demanded to have an amniocentesis even though the procedure is generally only recommended for women 35 and over. Similarly, I have heard many accounts by and about pregnant women who insisted on an ultrasound even when it was not deemed medically necessary. These anecdotes suggest that women aren't "forced" to take prenatal tests, and in fact many of them seek out and demand such tests. Research on women's responses to opportunities for prenatal diagnosis also indicates that prenatal genetic testing is very much desired by many women. For instance, in her study, R. Gregg (1995) found at least one woman who, because of her advanced age, would not have gotten pregnant if diagnostic technology had not been available. On the other hand, Kolker and Burke (1994) found that women under 34 were among the ones most adamant about using prenatal diagnosis in order to avoid giving birth to an affected child.

These favorable attitudes toward prenatal tests, along with a seemingly high rate of acceptance when offered, suggest that women often appreciate the availability of genetic technologies. At the same time, the fact that some women do reject these tests shows that these technologies are not imposed on women. Women can and do make decisions on whether or not to make use of them, evaluating each genetic test to see whether it provides the information they want or need. They also recognize that such testing may not be medically necessary and therefore may not be worth the perceived risks (Markens, Browner, and Press, 1999). It is important to recognize that whether a particular woman accepts or refuses prenatal tests depends on her individual perception of the risks and benefits (Gregg, 1995, p. 95)

Additionally, while I argue for the necessity of a gendered analysis of genetic testing, it is also important to recognize that women of various racial-ethnic groups and classes may experience and respond to the offer of prenatal genetic testing differently. For instance, the 1996 General Social Survey found that 52 percent of whites said that "genetic testing will do more good than harm," whereas only 39 percent of nonwhites agreed with this statement (Singer, Corning, and Antonucci, 1999, p. 437). With regard to the actual decision to undergo testing, a smaller percentage of minority and lower-class women chose to be tested (Kolker and Burke, 1994; Rapp, 1999; Voogd and Hunt, 2000). For example, in California white women are more likely than Latina and black women to have an amniocentesis after testing positive on AFP screening (Cunningham, 1998). Returning once again to *The Twilight of the Golds*, it is not surprising that Suzanne readily agrees to be tested; she fits the statistical profile of those mostly likely to accept—white and middle class.

At the same time, ethnic and class differences in utilization rates do not necessarily mean that minority and working-class women are unhappy with the availability of, and their experiences with, prenatal testing. Rayna Rapp (1999) found that, among the women she interviewed, those with middle-class backgrounds were often more dissatisfied with the information available through amniocentesis than were working-class women. This was because they were disappointed with how little the test could tell them, thereby challenging their sense of "entitlement to control" (110). Additionally, white middle-class women's experience of prenatal screening must be analyzed in the context of both their greater access to medical resources and their greater susceptibility to being controlled by medical institutions (Kolker and Burke, 1994; Rapp, 1999). At the same time, less-privileged women's experience of prenatal screening must be analyzed in the context of their simultaneous neglect and exploitation by medical institutions more generally (Rosser, 1994; Voogd and Hunt, 2000), as well as the recent history of eugenics and population control targeted at their communities (Davis, 1981; Duster, 1990; Gordon, [1977] 1990; Nsiah-Jefferson, 1994; Roberts, 1997).

While ethnic and class differences with regard to attitudes toward and experiences with genetic technologies must be examined and acknowledged, we should also be careful not to focus solely on cultural explanations (Markens, Browner, and Preloran, 2001b). The institutional and organizational structure of health care must also be recognized as affecting women's differential experiences with prenatal testing. Several researchers have pointed out that unequal access, shaped by larger social inequalities of race and class, are often more significant in explaining differences between women's rates of prenatal testing than any putative cultural differences (Kolker and Burke, 1994; Nsiah-Jefferson, 1994; Rapp, 1999; Voogd and Hunt, 2000). It is clear that we must avoid essentializing gender and generalizing from white, middle-class women (Spelman, 1990; Collins, 1990); nevertheless, we must also recognize that gender does matter for all women and, in this particular case, for our understandings of the impact of genetics.

Despite their differences, women's opinions, as well as their actions, suggest generally favorable attitudes toward prenatal genetic testing. Therefore, it is important to explore *why* women usually want and agree to it. An examination of women's rationales for prenatal diagnosis, not surprisingly, reveals a range of explanations—from belief in the benefits of modern medicine to wanting control over their pregnancies—that motivate women's use of genetic technologies.

First, for many women prenatal testing is viewed as part of the process of ensuring and obtaining good prenatal care (Browner and Press, 1995). For instance, many women in our study thought not only that amniocentesis was a positive option for them but also that all pregnant women had the obligation to undergo prenatal analyses at the beginning of the pregnancy. As Danielle succinctly explained, "I think that everybody . . . every woman should go under some type of prenatal analysis." Carmen expressed a common view that prenatal testing represents an opportunity afforded to those living in a "modern" nation: "I think that . . . well many people can't do it because of their financial resources, but here in America they do it so we can have it. They give us the opportunity to do it. . . . We should take it."

Other women's explanations reveal the varied ways in which pregnant women view the information provided by prenatal genetic testing as positive opportunities for themselves and other women. For instance, some women want prenatal diagnosis because it may provide information that would determine whether or not they abort a particular pregnancy. Carla appreciated the information she could gain when there was still time to decide to terminate a pregnancy: "Well, to me I think it's a good thing because the baby could come out deformed and I wouldn't find out until I gave birth, and right now with amniocentesis they'll find out right away and there's still time for me to get an abortion done. So I'd rather have them do it to me now than wait later for the consequences I have to face."

Similarly, Marissa felt positive about information that could prevent the birth of a child who would physically suffer: "To make sure that the baby is okay and . . . like the baby, the nurse told me . . . the baby might live only a year if it had heart problems. I wouldn't bring the baby into the world to suffer. You know, she told me that there was the possibility of that happening and I wanted to know if it was going to come out with something wrong." Such sentiments reveal that many women view the availability and accessibility of prenatal genetic testing as an issue of reproductive freedom that provides them more choice and control over their pregnancies.

It is important to note, however, when talking about "control" and "choice," that many women undergo prenatal screening with no intention of aborting an affected fetus (Kolker and Burke, 1994; Press and Browner, 1997; Markens, Browner, and Preloran, 2001a; Rapp, 1999). For instance, although 74 percent of the women in our study viewed amniocentesis as a way to help themselves, 40 percent specified that it would help provide "reassurance," while 48 percent thought it was "better to know" and 56 percent wanted the information "to be prepared." Thus many women view prenatal diagnosis as providing valuable information that they feel would enable them to be prepared prior to the birth of an affected child. Helena explained why she considered prenatal analysis necessary:

My opinion on that is actually, it depends on the personality. I'm the kind of person that I like to know, be prepared for whatever, so, in my case I think it's important to find out, just because . . . if anything to be prepared to what's to come . . . so you know what's to come, you know, if you're the kind of parent that could handle a major problem, I think you should know in advance to know what to do with it. . . . It's nice to know so you don't have any surprises. You know, because I think it'd be very . . . disappointing if you go through the whole pregnancy . . . and then find out, you know, there's a problem, you know, it won't be felt the same.

Likewise, Martha was more explicit in differentiating her desire to know from her lack of willingness to abort: "No, no [she would not abort]. . . . but I did it because I'd know. I'd prepare myself to have this child in that way." In addition to wanting to be prepared, many women also want reassurance. Gloria, a devout Catholic who was unwilling to abort, told us she had an amniocentesis to be prepared but also admitted the real reason she underwent the procedure: "In the bottom of my heart, I wanted to do it because I hoped for a good result and take the worries from my head." In the end, regardless of the reasons given, many women seem to want and appreciate the knowledge prenatal genetic tests can provide them.

Perhaps ironically, while many women undergo prenatal diagnosis to be reassured (Press and Browner, 1997), prenatal tests often create the same type of anxiety that they alleviate (Beeson and Golbus, 1979; Kolker and Burke, 1994; Browner and Press, 1995, 1997; Gregg, 1995; Browner and Preloran, 1999; Rapp, 1999). Indeed, early research on amniocentesis found that women's anxiety was raised before the procedure (Beeson and Golbus, 1979). More recently, Kolker and Burke found that amniocentesis may increase rather than alleviate anxiety. They argue that "the experience of amniocentesis has the unintended consequence of dramatizing what would otherwise be diffuse, low-level anxieties" (1994, p. 76), an observation also made by several other researchers (Rothman, 1986; Gregg, 1995; Rapp, 1999). Responses by women in our amniocentesis study confirm the anxiety that accompanies women's experience of prenatal diagnosis. For instance, of the women we interviewed, 55 percent were somewhat to very worried while waiting for amniocentesis results, 57 percent were somewhat to very worried when amniocentesis was offered, and 77 percent were somewhat to very worried when they received abnormal AFP results. Connie's explanation of why she accepted an amniocentesis after testing positive on AFP is illustrative: "To tell you the truth, I think it was the fear. I think that the people there put a fear or a terror into you. I was so afraid, I thought better end this, better to know. . . . So I wanted to know because not knowing is terrifying."

Thus, while many women do seem to appreciate the availability of prenatal tests and the genetic information they can provide, access to such knowledge may not have the desired or expected consequences. From this perspective, we might view diagnostic tests as filling a need that is of their own making.

"But Not as They Please": The Social Context of Women's "Choices"

Although women seem to appreciate genetic technologies, it is also important to recognize the social context and pressures that affect women's decisions about and experiences with prenatal diagnosis. On the surface women knowledgeably and individually "choose" whether or not to make use of prenatal genetic technologies; yet it is naive to believe that such decisions are made in a social or cultural vacuum. First, there is concern about the limited and socially influenced knowledge available to women when they make decisions about prenatal diagnosis. Second, as prenatal testing becomes, and is perceived to be, a normal part of prenatal care, it raises concern about the technological imperative embedded in these techniques. In particular, the routinization of prenatal screening is viewed as part of the medicalization of pregnancy, whereby women's experiences with and decisions about their pregnancy and prenatal care are influenced and controlled by medical personnel and institutions. These issues raise questions of how free and informed women's choices and experiences actually are when confronted by prenatal genetic testing.

While prenatal genetic tests offer women previously unobtainable information, critics wonder about the extent of knowledge women have about the tests and the meaning of the test results. Such imperfect knowledge is relevant to the issue of "informed choice" (Sargent and Hunt, 2000). These concerns are not unwarranted. In our amniocentesis study we found that 51 percent agreed with statement "Prenatal testing makes your pregnancy at less risk"; 11 percent said there was the same "risk" from a high and low AFP result, and 55 percent didn't know when asked which was more of a risk; 19 percent did not know or were unsure about which disabilities amniocentesis detects; 18 percent did not know or were unsure whether amniocentesis detects spina bifida; 37 percent believed or were unsure of whether there was a cure for the conditions amniocentesis detects; and 15 percent did not know that one of the options after a positive amniocentesis result is abortion. Clearly, this last finding has an impact on "informed choice." Unfortunately, such findings are not surprising, since in our study of AFP screening we found that nurses rarely mention abortion when discussing the test (Browner and Press, 1995; Press and Browner, 1997; Markens, Browner, and Press, 1999) and the official state booklet on AFP given to all women eligible for screening does not mention abortion at all (State of California, 1998).

Women's limited knowledge about genetics and the nature of a disability can also affect their informed choice. First, as disability rights scholars and others argue, women often "choose" to be tested and to terminate pregnancies without complete knowledge of the actual effect of a particular genetic abnormality and the resources available to families (Saxton, 1984; Kaplan, 1994; Press et al., 1998; Rapp, 1999; also see chapter 6 in this volume). Second, women's knowledge is limited to the extent that the genetic information is itself limited or inaccurate. For example, most genetic tests are probabilistic, not predictive. Even when the expression of a specific trait is certain, as in the case of Down syndrome, a genetic determination of an anomaly cannot predict its severity.

Finally, the medicalization of pregnancy increases the likelihood that the authority of doctors and technology will affect decision making. As noted earlier, women appreciate new medical technologies, but the rationales for using prenatal diagnosis must be examined critically. For instance, research has found that women's decisions about whether to accept or refuse amniocentesis after a positive AFP test is affected by their desire to be "compliant patients" (Sargent and Hunt, 2000). As a result, "many women experience prenatal testing not as an option but as a requirement" (Kolker and Burke, 1994, p. 5). Remarkably, in some cases doctors scheduled women for amniocentesis *prior* to any prenatal visit and consultation (Gregg, 1995).

These findings challenge the idea that women do not experience coercion in the process of making decisions regarding genetic testing. This coercion may not even be perceived. In our research on AFP screening in California, we found that close to 85 percent of those accepting the test said they did not think much before deciding (Browner and Press, 1995; Press and Browner, 1997; Markens, Browner, and Press, 1999). Of significance, their reasons for acceptance were similar to those of women in our amniocentesis study. For example, Betty explained that she thought prenatal analysis was necessary "because it is part of prenatal care." Such sentiments reveal that, even though testing is optional, the power of medical authority shapes women's experiences with and choices about prenatal diagnosis.

The desire to be a compliant patient is exemplified by Barbara. She explained how her faith in doctors influenced her acceptance: "I wanted to do what doctors recommend I do . . . if not, what is the purpose of going to the doctor?" Likewise, Julia revealed a faith in the authority of doctors when she clearly stated, "It's better to do what the doctor says." Later, when probed about her views on this issue, she expressed belief in the authoritative knowledge of physicians because of their training, as well as confidence in the ability of medical technology to provide wanted and reliable information:

Q: You said before that we have to do what the doctor says. Is that always?
Julia: In this, I think so.
Q: Why?

Julia: They have all these things now, like the ultrasound, where they can see with much more clarity what is inside.

Q: And with the amnio?

Julia: They know with that, they are doctors for a reason, they have studied, this is why they can tell us if the baby is fine or not.

Acquiescence to medical authority is also illustrated in the following excerpt from an interview with Tina, who expressed not just trust in her medical providers but her desire to please them with her decisions.

Q: So you trust in tests and medicine?

Tina: Sure, this is why I come to the clinic, I believe they offer the best for me and the baby, and I don't think they would be pleased if I didn't trust them.

Of possible significance then in understanding *why* most women accept prenatal genetic analysis is our finding that, although 89 percent of the women in our study said they did not feel pressure from the genetic counselor, 39 percent did think that the genetic counselor wanted them to accept testing. Connie's explanation of these dynamics is quite revealing: "They say one can say yes or no, but I believe that they want you to do it. Because, look, it's that they say, 'I want you to do this,' but . . . first I said, 'No, I don't want to do it.' But she said, 'There is very little risk, very little pain, it's like having an injection.' . . . I don't know how to explain it, but I believe they say, it's you who decides, but I don't know, it seems to me that if I had refused the test they would have said, 'Oh, this woman is ignorant, she knows nothing.'"

These findings suggest that women's general acceptance of prenatal testing should be understood with respect to their desires to take what they and others view as a medically and maternally responsible course of action. In particular, to ignore how deeply entrenched beliefs about maternal responsibility for children informs and shapes choices about prenatal genetic testing obscures why pregnant women do and do not have prenatal screening and what they think about the tests, as well as others' reactions to their decisions. As Gregg (1995, p. 127) writes, "The tendency to 'blame Mom' is nothing new, but the advent of procreative technologies has meant an extension of maternal responsibility and an attendant expansion of potential maternal guilt and social censure." In other words, women may be held accountable if they give birth to children with genetic abnormalities if they were "at risk" (because of maternal age, family history, etc.) and did not opt for prenatal genetic screening. As a result, women may feel compelled to undergo genetic testing that is considered "a normal part of prenatal care" in order to present themselves as good mothers who are maternally accountable (Charo and Rothenberg, 1994; Markens, Browner, and Press, 1999).

So, along with being offered more "choices" thanks to new genetic knowledge and technologies, women may also be held responsible for giving birth to babies with genetic anomalies. This responsibility is often internalized. Fifty percent of the women in our amniocentesis study said that they felt responsible for the outcome of their pregnancy, although most factors that affect pregnancy outcome are beyond their individual control. Therefore, although many women do seem to want prenatal genetic testing, the "choices" they make regarding the use of such technologies must be analyzed with a recognition of the gendered context in which individual women's decisions are made. This context ranges from an increasing emphasis on maternal responsibility and the medicalization of the pregnant female body to the gender dynamics, roles, and power within heterosexual couples.

Conclusion: Brave New Women

It has been fifteen years since sociologist Barbara Katz Rothman wrote one of the first social science accounts of the impact of prenatal screening on women. In her book, *The Tentative Pregnancy,* she documented how the increasing use of prenatal genetic testing was transforming women's experience of pregnancy. Since its publication, reproductive and genetic technologies have continued to develop, but the basic reproductive and biological capacities of men and women have not changed—and probably never will. As a result, we can continue to expect that women and their bodies will be uniquely affected by increased knowledge of and developments in genetics.

The purpose of this chapter was to show that women are particularly affected by genetic knowledge and testing precisely because of their unique role in biological reproduction. In addition, "being developed in a world that is gendered, the genetic and other reproductive technologies cannot escape gendered use, use that reflects prevalent ideas about women" (Lippman, 1994, pp. 9–10). Therefore, gender as an analytic category must be fully integrated into accounts of the applications, experiences, and implications of genetic information and technologies.

What would a gendered analysis of genetics entail? Any discussion of the impact of new genetic knowledge must include, if not make central, the specific use of prenatal testing, given its common use. However, focusing on the prenatal testing process itself is not enough. A gendered analysis must also take into account that only women become pregnant, and thus only women are subjected to prenatal testing. We must also recognize the gender dynamics that occur within individual couples that influence women's decisions about prenatal diagnosis (Markens, Browner, and Preloran, 2001b). For instance, since social science research continues to find a persistent gender gap in domestic responsibilities, with women still responsible for and performing the majority of the "second shift" of domestic work (DeVault, 1991; Hochschild, 1989; Perkins and DeMeis, 1996; Press and Townsley, 1998), we must explore how resulting gendered balances of power within families affect women's choices about prenatal diagnosis. Similarly, we need to look at how gender inequalities and biases within medical institutions, as well as within doctor-patient interactions, can shape women's experiences and decisions. Finally, we must examine how cultural attitudes toward women, particularly dominant discourses on motherhood, influence the use of prenatal diagnosis.

Fetal genetic screening presents pregnant women with two sets of "choices." First, a woman can decide whether to gain genetic information about her fetus. Second, if a woman receives a positive prenatal diagnosis for a genetic abnormality, she must decide whether or not to terminate the pregnancy. The freedom to act on these "choices" is qualified, since they are affected by the various familial, community, economic, political, and of course gendered contexts in which individual women are situated. Prenatal genetic testing places pregnant women in yet another arena in which they must struggle to present themselves as "good mothers" in a culture that continues to place a strong emphasis on maternal responsibility. Additionally, the increasing research into genetics and the application of genetic technologies shifts the health focus toward the fetus and away from the mother (Petchesky, 1987; Daniels, 1993; Duden, 1993; Kolker and Burke, 1994; Lippman, 1994; Markens, Browner, and Press, 1997; Casper, 1998).

There are no simple, easy answers to whether prenatal testing and genetic technologies are "good" or "bad." However, it is clear that with the increasing routinization of prenatal screening, and because of women's unique role in reproduction, gender-neutral analyses of genetics are inadequate. Instead, women must be visible and central in examining the impact of genetics on themselves and on society.

REFERENCES

Beeson, D., and M. Golbus. 1979. "Anxiety Engendered by Amniocentesis." *Birth Defects* 15:191–97.
Bosk, C. 1992. *All God's Mistakes: Genetic Counseling at a Pediatric Hospital.* Chicago: University of Chicago Press.
Browner, C. H., and H. M. Preloran. 1999. "Male Partners' Role in Latinas' Amniocentesis Decisions." *Journal of Genetic Counseling* 8:85–107.
Browner, C. H., and N. Press. 1995. "The Normalization of Prenatal Diagnostic Testing." Pp. 307–22 in *The Politics of Reproduction: The Global Politics of Reproduction,* ed. F. Ginsburg and R. Rapp. Berkeley: University of California Press.
———. 1997. "The Production of Authoritative Knowledge in American Prenatal Care." Pp. 113–31 in *Childbirth and Authoritative Knowledge: Cross-Cultural Perspective,* ed. R. E. Davis-Floyd and C. F. Sargent. Berkeley: University of California Press.
Caskey, C. T. 1992. "DNA-Based Medicine: Prevention and Therapy." Pp. 112–35 in *The Code of Codes: Scientific and Social Issues in the Human Genome Project,* ed. D. J. Kevles and L. Hood. Cambridge: Harvard University Press.
Casper, M. 1998. *The Making of the Unborn Patient: A Social Anatomy of Fetal Surgery.* New Brunswick, N.J.: Rutgers University Press.
Charo, A., and K. Rothenberg. 1994. " 'The Good Mother': The Limits of Reproductive Accountability and Genetic Choice." Pp. 105–30 in *Women and Prenatal Testing: Facing the Challenges of Genetic Technologies,* ed. K. H. Rothenberg and E. J. Thomson. Columbus: Ohio State University Press.
Collins, P. H. 1990. *Black Feminist Thought: Knowledge, Consciousness and the Politics of Empowerment.* Boston: Unwin Hyman.
Cowan, R. 1992. "Genetic Technology and Reproductive Choice: An Ethics for Autonomy." Pp. 244–65 in *The Code of Codes: Scientific and Social Issues in the Human Genome Project,* ed. D. J. Kevles and L. Hood. Cambridge: Harvard University Press.
———. 1994. "Women's Roles in the History of Amniocentesis and Chronic Villi Sampling." Pp. 35–48 in *Women and Prenatal Testing: Facing the Challenges of Genetic Technologies,* ed. K. H. Rothenberg and E. J. Thomson. Columbus: Ohio State University Press.
Cunningham, G. C. 1998. *An Evaluation of California's Public-Private Maternal Serum Screening Program.* Ninth International Conference on Prenatal Diagnosis and Therapy. Los Angeles.
Daniels, C. 1993. *At Women's Expense: State Power and the Politics of Fetal Rights.* Cambridge: Harvard University Press.
Davis, A. 1981. *Women, Race, and Class.* New York: Random House.

DeVault, M. 1991. *Feeding the Family: The Social Organization of Caring as Gendered Work.* Chicago: University of Chicago Press.

Duden, B. 1993. *Disembodying Women: Perspectives on the Unborn.* Cambridge: Harvard University Press.

Duster, T. 1990. *Backdoor to Eugenics.* New York: Routledge.

Gordon, L. [1977] 1990. *Woman's Bodies/Woman's Rights: Birth Control in America.* New York: Penguin Books.

Gregg, R. 1995. *Pregnancy in a High-Tech Age: Paradoxes of Choice.* New York: New York University Press.

Hochschild, A. R. 1989. *The Second Shift.* New York: Avon Books.

Kaplan, D. 1994. "Prenatal Screening and Diagnosis: The Impact on Persons with Disabilities." Pp. 49–61 in *Women and Prenatal Testing: Facing the Challenges of Genetic Technologies,* ed. K. H. Rothenberg and E. J. Thomson. Columbus: Ohio State University Press.

Keenan, K. L., D. Basso, J. Goldkrand, and W. Butler. 1991. "Low Level of Maternal Serum Alpha-Fetoprotein: Its Associated Anxiety and the Effects of Genetic Counseling." *American Journal of Obstetrics and Gynecology* 164:54–56.

Kevles, D. J., and L. Hood. 1992. "Reflections." Pp. 300–328 in *The Code of Codes: Scientific and Social Issues in the Human Genome Project,* ed. D. J. Kevles and L. Hood. Cambridge: Harvard University Press.

Kolker, M., and A. Burke. 1994. *Prenatal Testing: A Sociological Perspective.* Westport, Conn.: Bergin & Garvey.

Lippman, A. 1994. "The Genetic Construction of Prenatal Testing: Choice, Consent, or Conformity for Women?" Pp. 9–34 in *Women and Prenatal Testing: Facing the Challenges of Genetic Technologies,* ed. K. H. Rothenberg and E. J. Thomson. Columbus: Ohio State University Press.

Mahowald, M. B. 1994. "Reproductive Genetics and Gender Justice." Pp. 67–87 in *Women and Prenatal Testing: Facing the Challenges of Genetic Technologies,* ed. K. H. Rothenberg and E. J. Thomson. Columbus: Ohio State University Press.

———. 2000. *Genes, Women, Equality.* New York: Oxford University Press.

Markens, S., C. H. Browner, and H. M. Preloran. 2001a. " 'I'm Not A Doctor But I Know How I Feel': The Intersection of Embodied and Authoritative Knowledge in Amniocentesis Decisions." Paper presented at the American Sociological Association Annual Meeting, Anaheim, Calif., August 11–14.

———. 2001b. " 'I'm Not the One They're Sticking the Needle Into': Latino Couples, Fetal Diagnosis and the Discourse of Reproductive Rights." Paper Presented at the Ethical, Legal, and Social Issues of the Human Genome Project Conference, Washington, D.C., January 16–18.

Markens, S., C. H. Browner, and N. Press. 1997. "Feeding the Fetus: On Interrogating the Notion of Maternal-Fetal Conflict." *Feminist Studies* 23:351–72.

———. 1999. "Because of the Risks: How U.S. Pregnant Women Account for Refusing Prenatal Screening." *Social Science and Medicine* 49:359–69.

Meaney, F. J., S. M. Riggle, and G. C. Cunningham. 1993. "Providers and Consumers of Prenatal Genetic Testing Services: What Do the National Data Tell Us?" *Fetal Diagnosis and Therapy* 8:18–27.

National Institutes of Health. 1999–2000. Secretary's Advisory Committee on Genetic Testing. *A Public Consultation on Oversight of Genetic Tests.*

———, and the Department of Energy. 2001. *A Decade of ELSI Research: Abstracts.* National Institutes of Health, Bethesda, Md., January 16–18.

Nelkin. D. 1992. "The Social Power of Genetic Information." Pp. 177–90 in *The Code of Codes: Scientific and Social Issues in the Human Genome Project,* ed. D. J. Kevles and L. Hood. Cambridge: Harvard University Press.

Nsiah-Jefferson, L. 1994. "Reproductive Genetic Services for Low-Income Women and Women of Color: Access and Sociocultural Issues." Pp. 234–59 in *Women and Prenatal Testing: Facing the Challenges of Genetic Technologies,* ed. K. H. Rothenberg and E. J. Thomson. Columbus: Ohio State University Press.

Perkins, H. W., and D. DeMeis. 1996. "Gender and Family Effects on the 'Second-Shift' Domestic Activity of College-Educated Young Adults." *Gender and Society* 10 (1):78–93.

Petchesky, R. 1984. *Abortion and Woman's Choice: The State, Sexuality and Reproductive Freedom.* Boston: Northeastern University Press.

———. 1987. "Foetal Images: The Power of Visual Culture in the Politics of Reproduction." Pp. 57–80 in *Reproductive Technologies: Gender, Motherhood and Medicine,* ed. M. Stanworth. Minneapolis: University of Minnesota Press.

Press, J., and E. Townsley. 1998. "Wives' and Husbands' Housework Reporting: Gender, Class and Social Desirability." *Gender and Society* 12 (2):188–218.

Press, N., and C. H. Browner. 1993. "'Collective Fictions': Similarities in Reasons for Accepting MSAFP Screening among Women of Diverse Ethnic and Social Class Backgrounds." *Fetal Diagnosis and Therapy* 8:97–106.

———. 1997. "Why Women Say Yes to Prenatal Screening." *Social Science and Medicine* 45:979–89.

Press, N., C. H. Browner, D. Tran, D. Morton, and B. Le Master. 1998. "Provisional Normalcy and 'Perfect Babies': Pregnant Women's Attitudes toward Disability in the Context of Prenatal Testing." Pp. 46–65 in *Reproducing Reproduction: Kinship, Power and Technological Innovation,* ed. S. Franklin and H. Ragone. Philadelphia: University of Pennsylvania Press.

Rapp, R. 1984. "XYLO: A True Story." Pp. 313–28 in *Test-Tube Women: What Future Motherhood?,* ed. R. Arditti, R. D. Klein, and S. Minden. Boston: Pandora Press.

———. 1999. *Testing Women, Testing the Fetus: The Social Impact of Amniocentesis in America.* New York: Routledge.

Roberts, D. 1997. *Killing the Black Body: Race, Reproduction, and the Meaning of Liberty.* New York: Pantheon Books.

Rosser, S. 1994. *Women's Health: Missing from U.S. Medicine.* Bloomington: Indiana University Press.

Rothenberg, K. H., and E. J. Thomson, editors. 1994. *Women and Prenatal Testing: Facing the Challenges of Genetic Technologies.* Columbus: Ohio State University Press.

Rothman, B. K. 1986. *The Tentative Pregnancy: Prenatal Diagnosis and the Future of Motherhood.* New York: Viking Penguin.

———. 1989. *Recreating Motherhood: Ideology and Technology in a Patriarchal Society.* New York: W. W. Norton & Co.

———. 1994. "The Tentative Pregnancy: Then and Now." Pp. 260–70 in *Women and Prenatal Testing: Facing the Challenges of Genetic Technologies,* ed. K. H. Rothenberg and E. J. Thomson. Columbus: Ohio State University Press.

Sargent, J., and L. Hunt. 2000. "Client Perspectives on Amniocentesis Decision Making: The Experiences of 29 Low Income Latinas." Paper presented at the Society for Applied Anthropology Meeting, San Francisco, Calif., March 22.

Saxton, M. 1984. "Born and Unborn: The Implications of Reproductive Technologies for People with Disabilities." Pp. 298–312 in *Test-Tube Women: What Future for Motherhood?*, ed. R. Arditti, R. D. Klein, and S. Minden. London: Pandora Press.

Singer, E., A. D. Corning, and T. Antonucci. 1999. "Attitudes toward Genetic Testing and Fetal Diagnosis, 1990–1996." *Journal of Health and Social Behavior* 40:429–45.

Spelman, E. 1990. *Inessential Woman: Problems of Exclusion in Feminist Thought.* Boston: Beacon.

Spitzer, Kathryn. 2000. Director of Genetic Counseling Program, Brandeis University. Personal communication.

State of California, Department of Health Services, Genetic Disease Branch. 1998. *The California Expanded AFP Screening Program Update.*

Voogd, K. B., and L. M. Hunt. 2000. "What Would You Tell Your Sister to Do?: Offering Prenatal Genetic Screening to Low-Income Latina Women." Paper presented at the Society for Applied Anthropology Meeting, San Francisco, Calif. March 22.

CHAPTER SIX

Prenatal Diagnosis and Selective Abortion

A Challenge to Practice and Policy

Adrienne Asch

Although sex selection might ameliorate the situation of some individuals, it lowers the status of women in general and only perpetuates the situation that gave rise to it. . . . If we believe that sexual equality is necessary for a just society, then we should oppose sex selection.

D. C. WERTZ AND J. C. FLETCHER, 1992

The very motivation for seeking an "origin" of homosexuality reveals homophobia. Moreover, such research may lead to prenatal tests that claim to predict for homosexuality. For homosexual people who live in countries with no legal protections these dangers are particularly serious.

U. SCHUKLENK ET AL., 1997

The tenor of the preceding statements may spark relatively little comment in the world of health policy, the medical profession, or many contemporary readers, because many recognize the dangers of using the technology of prenatal testing in order to use selective abortion based on the characteristic of fetal sex. Similarly, members of the medical and psychiatric professions, and those in public health, have aided in the civil rights struggle of gays and lesbians by insisting that homosexuality is not a disease. Consequently, many readers would concur with those who question the motives behind searching for the causes of homosexuality, motives that might lead scientists to develop a pre-

An earlier version of this chapter appeared in *American Journal of Public Health* 89, no. 11 (November 1999):1649–57, © 1999 by the American Public Health Association.

natal test for that characteristic, as discussed in more detail by William Byne, Udo Schuklenk, Mitchell Lasco, and Jack Drescher, in Chapter 9 in this volume, and C. Phoebe Lostroh and Amanda Udis-Kessler, in Chapter 10 in this volume. Many in our society, however, have no such misgivings about prenatal testing for characteristics regarded as genetic or chromosomal diseases, abnormalities, or disabilities:

> Human mating that proceeds without the use of genetic data about the risks of transmitting diseases will produce greater mortality and medical costs than if carriers of potentially deleterious genes are alerted to their carrier status and *encouraged* to mate with non-carriers or to use other reproductive strategies. (U.S. Congress, Office of Technology Assessment, 1988, p. 84 [emphasis added])

> Attitudes toward congenital disability per se have not changed markedly. Both premodern as well as contemporary societies have regarded disability as undesirable and to be avoided. Not only have parents recognized the birth of a disabled child as a potentially divisive, destructive force in the family unit, but the larger society has seen disability as unfortunate. . . . Our society still does not countenance the elimination of diseased/disabled people; but it does urge the termination of diseased/disabled fetuses. The urging is not explicit, but implicit. (Retsinas, 1991, pp. 89, 90)

Writing in the *American Journal of Human Genetics* about screening programs for cystic fibrosis, A. L. Beaudet acknowledged the tension between the goals of enhancing reproductive choice and preventing the births of children who would have disabilities: "Although some would argue that the success of the program should be judged solely by the effectiveness of the educational programs (i.e., whether screenees understood the information), it is clear that prevention of [cystic fibrosis] is also, at some level, a measure of a screening program, since few would advocate expanding the substantial resources involved if very few families wish to avoid the disease" (1990, p. 603).

Prenatal tests designed to detect the condition of the fetus include ultrasound, maternal serum alpha-fetoprotein screening, chorionic villus sampling, and amniocentesis. Some tests, such as ultrasound screenings, are routinely performed regardless of the mother's age and provide information that she may use to guide her care throughout pregnancy; others, such as chorionic villus sampling or amniocentesis, do not influence the woman's care during pregnancy but provide information intended to help her decide whether to continue the pregnancy if fetal impairment is detected. Amniocentesis, the test that detects the greatest variety of fetal impairments, is typically offered to women who will be 35 years old or older at the time they are due to deliver, but recently commentators have urged that the age threshold be removed and that the test be available to women regardless of age (Kuppermann et al., 1999). Such testing is increasingly considered a standard component of prenatal care for women whose insurance covers these procedures, including women using publicly financed clinics in some jurisdictions (Rapp, 1999).

Although widely accepted by those in the field of bioethics, clinicians, public health professionals, and the general public (as discussed in more detail by Susan Markens, Chapter 5 in this volume), these tests have nonetheless occasioned some concern among students of women's reproductive experiences; they find that women do not uniformly welcome the expectation that they will undergo prenatal testing or the prospect of making decisions depending on the test results (Rothenberg and Thomson, 1994). Less often discussed by clinicians is the view, expressed by a growing number of individuals and groups, that the technology is itself based on erroneous assumptions about the adverse impact of disability on life. Argument from this perspective focuses on what is communicated about societal and familial acceptance of diversity in general and disability in particular (Fine and Asch, 1982; Saxton, 1984; Finger, 1987; Asch, 1989; Hubbard, 1990; Lippman, 1991; Miringoff, 1991; Field, 1993; Kaplan, 1994; Shakespeare, 1995, 1998; Asch and Geller, 1996; Dunne and Warren, 1998; Disabled Peoples International Europe, 2000). Like other women-centered critiques of prenatal testing, this chapter assumes a pro-choice perspective but suggests that unreflective uses of testing could diminish, rather than expand, women's choices. Like critiques stemming from concerns about the continued acceptance of human differences within the society and the family, this critique challenges the view of disability that lies behind social endorsement of such testing and the conviction that women will, or should, end their pregnancies if they discover that the fetus has a disabling trait.

If public health practitioners frown on efforts to select for gender and would oppose future efforts to select for sexual orientation, but they promote people's efforts to avoid having children who would have disabilities, it is because those in medicine and public health view disability as extremely different from—and worse than—these other forms of human variation. At first blush, this view may strike one as self-evident. To challenge it might even appear to be questioning our professional mission. Characteristics such as chronic illnesses and disabilities (discussed together throughout this chapter) do not resemble traits such as sex, sexual orientation, or race, because the latter are not in themselves perceived as inimical to a rewarding life. Disability is thought to be just that—incompatible with life satisfaction. In fact, it is worth noting that some who oppose selective abortion for fetal sex (Wertz and Fletcher, 1992) or for sexual orientation (Stein, 1998), differentiate between these traits as *socially disabling,* as contrasted with medically disabling traits, for which they endorse prenatal testing and selective abortion. When public health officials consider matters of sex, sexual orientation, or race, they examine how factors in social and economic life pose obstacles to health and to health care and champion actions to improve the well-being of those disadvantaged by the discrimination that attends minority status. By contrast, those in public health fight to eradicate disease and disability or to treat, ameliorate, or cure these when they occur. For medical and public health professionals, disease and disability is the problem to solve, and so it appears natural to use prenatal testing and abortion as one more means of minimizing the incidence of disability.

In the remainder of this chapter I argue, first, that most of the problems associated with having a disability stem from discriminatory social arrangements that are changeable, just as much of what has, in the past, made the lives of women or homosexuals difficult has been the set of social arrangements they have faced (and which they have begun to dismantle). After discussing ways in which the characteristic of disability resembles and differs from other characteristics, I discuss why I believe the technology of prenatal testing followed by selective abortion is unique among means of preventing or ameliorating disability and why it offends many people who are untroubled by other disease-prevention and health-promotion activities. I conclude by recommending ways health practitioners and policy makers could offer this technology so that it promotes genuine reproductive choice and helps families and society to flourish.

Contrasting Medical and Social Paradigms of Disability

The definitions of terms such as *health, normality,* and *disability* are not clear, objective, and universal across time and place. Individual physical characteristics are evaluated with reference to a standard of normality, health, and what some commentators term "species-typical functioning" (Daniels, 1985;

Boorse, 1987). These writers point out that within a society at a particular time, there is a shared perception of what is typical physical functioning and role-performance for a girl or boy, woman or man. Boorse's definition of an undesirable departure from species-typicality focuses on the functioning of the person rather than the cause of the problem: "[A] condition of a part or process in an organism is pathological when the ability of the part or process to perform one or more of its species-typical biological functions falls below some central range of the statistical distribution for that ability" (1987, p. 370). Daniels writes, "Impairments of normal species functioning reduce the range of opportunity open to the individual in which he may construct his plan of life or conception of the good" (1985, p. 27).

Chronic illness, traumatic injury, and congenital disability may indeed occasion departures from "species-typical functioning," and these conditions do constitute differences from both a statistical average and a desired norm of well-being. Certainly society prizes some characteristics, such as intelligence, athleticism, and musical or artistic skill, and rewards people with more than the statistical norm of these attributes; I will return to this point later. Norms on many health-related attributes also change over time; as the life span for people in the United States and Canada increases, conditions that often lead to death before 40 years of age (e.g., cystic fibrosis) may become even more dreaded than they are today. The expectation that males will be taller than females and that adults will stand more than five feet in height leads to a perception that departures from these norms are not only unusual but undesirable and unhealthy. Not surprisingly, professionals who have committed themselves to preventing illness and injury, or to ameliorating and curing people of their illnesses and injuries, are especially attuned to the problems and hardships that affect the lives of their patients. Such professionals, aware of the physical pain or weakness and the psychological and social disruption caused by acute illness or sudden injury, devote their lives to easing the problems that these events impose.

What many scholars, policy makers, and activists in the area of disability contend is that medically oriented understandings of the impact of disability on life contain two erroneous assumptions with serious adverse consequences: first, that the life of a person with a chronic illness or disability is forever disrupted, as one's life might be temporarily disrupted as a result of a back spasm, an episode of pneumonia, or a broken leg; second, that if a disabled person experiences isolation, powerlessness, unemployment, poverty, or low social status, these are inevitable consequences of biological limitation. Body, psyche, and social life do change immediately following an occurrence of disease, accident, or injury, and professionals in medicine, public health, and bioethics all correctly appreciate the psychological and physical vulnerability of patients and their loved ones during immediate medical crises. These professions fail people with disabilities, however, by concluding that because there may never be full physical recovery there is never a regrouping of physical, cognitive, and psychological resources with which to participate in a rewarding life. Chronic illness and disability are not equivalent to acute illness or sudden injury, in which an active disease process or unexpected change in physical function disrupts life's routines. Most people with conditions such as spina bifida, achondroplasia, Down syndrome, and many other mobility and sensory impairments perceive themselves as healthy, not sick, and describe their conditions as givens of their lives—the equipment with which they meet the world. The same is true for people with chronic conditions such as cystic fibrosis, diabetes, sickle cell disease, hemophilia, and muscular dystrophy. These conditions include intermittent flareups requiring medical care and adjustments in daily living, but they do not render the person as unhealthy as most of the public—and members of the health profession—imagine.

People with disabilities are thinking about a traffic jam, a disagreement with a friend, which movie to attend, or which team will win the World Series—not just about their diagnosis. Having a disability can of course intrude into a person's consciousness if events bring it to the fore: if two lift-equipped buses in a row fail to stop for a man using a wheelchair, if the theater ticket agent insults a patron with Down syndrome by refusing to take money for her ticket, if a hearing-impaired person misses a train connection because he did not know that a track change had been announced.

The second way in which those in medicine, bioethics, and public health typically err is by viewing all problems that occur to people with disabilities as attributable to the condition itself rather than to external factors. When ethicists, public health professionals, and policy makers discuss the importance of health care, urge accident prevention, or promote healthy lifestyles, they do so because they perceive a certain level of health not only as intrinsically desirable but as a prerequisite for an acceptable life. One commentator describes such a consensual view of types of life in terms of a "normal opportunity range": "The normal opportunity range for a given society is the array of life plans reasonable persons in it are likely to construct for themselves." Health care includes that which is intended to "maintain, restore, or provide functional equivalents where possible, to normal species functioning" (Daniels, 1985, pp. 33, 32).

According to the paradigm of medicine, the gaps in education, employment, and income that persist between adults with disabilities and those without disabilities are inevitable because the impairment precludes study or limits work. The alternative paradigm, which views people with disabilities in social, minority-group terms, examines how societal arrangements—rules, laws, means of communication, characteristics of buildings and transit systems, the typical eight-hour workday—exclude some people from participating in school, work, civic, or social life. This newer paradigm is reflected in the Individuals with Disabilities Education Act and the Americans with Disabilities Act, and it is behind the drive to ensure that employed disabled people will keep their access to health care through Medicaid or Medicare. This paradigm, which is still more accepted by people outside medicine, public health, and bioethics than by those within these fields, questions whether there is an inevitable, unmodifiable gap between people with disabilities and people without disabilities. Learning that in 1999, nine years after the passage of laws to end employment discrimination, millions of people with disabilities are still out of the workforce, despite their readiness to work (National Organization on Disability, 1999), the social paradigm asks what remaining institutional factors bar people from the goal of productive work. These issues then raise ethical and policy questions in regard to the connection that does or should exist between health and the range of opportunities open to people in the population.

Commitments to alleviate the difficulties arising from chronic illness and disability and efforts to promote healthy lifestyles throughout the population need not lead to a devaluation of the members of society who do not meet our typical understanding of health. Nevertheless, people with disabilities have indeed been subject to systematic segregation and second-class treatment in all areas of life. It is possible to appreciate the norm of having two arms without being repelled by a woman with one arm, yet social science, autobiography, legislation, and case law reveal that people with both visible and "invisible" disabilities lose opportunities to study, work, live where and with whom they choose, attend religious services, and even vote (Goffman, 1963; Schneider and Conrad, 1983; Brightman, 1984; Gartner and Joe, 1987; Bickenbach, 1993; Hockenberry, 1996; Russel, 1998).

The Americans with Disabilities Act, signed into law in 1990, is a ringing indictment of the nation's history with regard to people with disabilities:

Congress finds that . . . (3) discrimination against individuals with disabilities persists in such critical areas as employment . . . education, recreation . . . health services . . . and access to public services; . . . (7) individuals with disabilities are a discrete and insular minority who have been faced with restrictions and limitations, subjected to a history of purposeful unequal treatment, and relegated to a position of political powerlessness . . . , based on characteristics that are beyond the control of such individuals and resulting from stereotypic assumptions not truly indicative of the individual ability of such individuals to participate in, and contribute to, society. (Americans with Disabilities Act; 1990)

Eight years after the passage of the Americans with Disabilities Act, disabled people reported some improvements in access to public facilities and stated that things are getting better in some areas of life, but major gaps between the disabled and the nondisabled still exist in income, employment, and social participation. For example, to dramatically underscore the prevalence of social stigma and discrimination, "fewer than half (45%) of adults with disabilities say that people generally treat them as an equal after they learn they have a disability" (National Organization on Disability, 1999).

It is estimated that 54 million people in the United States have disabilities, the most well-known of which are impairments of mobility, hearing, vision, and learning; arthritis; cystic fibrosis; diabetes; heart conditions; and back problems (National Organization on Disability, 1999). Thus, in discussing discrimination, stigma, and unequal treatment for people with disabilities, we are considering a population that is larger than the known gay and lesbian population or the African American population. These numbers take on new significance when we assess the rationale behind prenatal diagnosis and selective abortion as a desirable strategy to deal with disability.

Prenatal Diagnosis for Disability Prevention

If some forms of disability prevention are legitimate medical and public health activities, and if people with disabilities use the health system to improve and maintain their own health, there is an acknowledgment that the characteristic of disability may not be desirable. Although many within the disability rights movement challenge prenatal diagnosis as a means of disability prevention, no one objects to public health efforts to clean up the environment, encourage seat-belt use, reduce tobacco and alcohol consumption, and provide prenatal care to all pregnant women. All these activities deal with the health of existing human beings (or fetuses expected to come to term) and seek to ensure their well-being. What differentiates prenatal testing followed by abortion from other forms of disability prevention and medical treatment is that this strategy is intended not to prevent the disability or illness of a born or future human being but to prevent the birth of a human being who will have one of these undesired characteristics. In reminding proponents of the Human Genome Project that gene therapy will not soon be able to cure disability, James Watson declared, "We place most of our hopes for genetics on the use of antenatal diagnostic procedures, which increasingly will let us know whether a fetus is carrying a mutant gene that will seriously proscribe its eventual development into a functional human being. By terminating such pregnancies, the threat of horrific disease genes contributing to blight many family's prospects for future success can be erased" (Watson, 1996, p. 19).

But Watson errs in assuming that tragedy is inevitable for the child or for the family. When physicians, public health experts, and bioethicists promote prenatal diagnosis to prevent future disability, they let disability become the only relevant characteristic and suggest that it is so problematic that people eagerly awaiting a new baby should terminate the pregnancy and "try again" for a healthy child. Professionals fail to recognize that along with whatever impairment may be diagnosed come all the characteristics of any other future child. The health professions suggest that once a prospective parent knows of the likely disability of a future child there is nothing else to know or imagine about who the child might become: in short, disability subverts parental dreams.

My concern here is not with the decision made by the pregnant woman or by the woman and her partner. I focus on the view of life with disability that is communicated by society's efforts to develop prenatal testing and urge it on every pregnant woman. If public health officials espouse goals of social justice and equality for people with disabilities, as they have worked to improve the status of women, gays and lesbians, and members of racial and ethnic minorities, they should reconsider whether they wish to continue endorsing the technology of prenatal diagnosis. If there is an unshakable commitment to the technology in the name of reproductive choice, those in public health should work with practitioners to change the way that information about impairments detected in the fetus is delivered.

Rationales for Prenatal Testing

The medical professions justify prenatal diagnosis and selective abortion on the grounds of the *costs* of childhood disability—the costs to the child, to the family, and to the society. Some Human Genome Project proponents from the fields of science and bioethics argue that in a world of limited resources we can reduce disability-related expenditures if all diagnoses of fetal impairment are followed by abortion (Shaw, 1984).

On both empirical and moral grounds, endorsing prenatal diagnosis for societal reasons is dangerous. Only a small fraction of total disability can now be detected prenatally, and, even if future technology enables the detection of predisposition to diabetes, forms of depression, Alzheimer disease, heart disease, arthritis, or back problems—all more prevalent in the population than many of the currently detectable conditions—we will never manage to detect and prevent most disability. Rates of disability increase markedly with age, and the gains in life span guarantee that most people will deal with disability in themselves or someone close to them. Laws and services to support people with disabilities will still be necessary, unless society chooses a campaign of eliminating disabled people in addition to preventing the births of those who would be disabled. Thus, there is small savings in money or in human resources to be achieved by even the vigorous determination to test every pregnant woman and abort every fetus found to exhibit disabling traits.

My moral opposition to prenatal testing and selective abortion flows from the conviction that life with disability is worthwhile and the belief that a just society must appreciate and nurture the lives of all people, whatever the endowments they receive in the natural lottery. I hold these beliefs because—as I show throughout this chapter—there is abundant evidence that people with disabilities can thrive even in this less-than-welcoming society. Moreover, people with disabilities do not merely take from others, they contribute as well—to families, to friends, to the economy. They contribute neither in spite of nor because of their disabilities but because along with their disabilities come other characteristics of personality, talent, and humanity that render people with disabilities full members of the human and moral community.

Implications for People with Disabilities

Implications of prenatal testing for children and adults with disabilities, and for their families, warrant more consideration. Several prominent bioethicists claim that to knowingly bring into the world a child who will live with an impairment (whether it be a "withered arm," cystic fibrosis, deafness, or Down syndrome) is unfair to the child because it deprives the child of the "right to an open future" by limiting some options (Feinberg, 1980). Ronald Green's words represent a significant strand of professional thinking: "In the absence of adequate justifying reasons, a child is morally wronged when he/she is knowingly, deliberately, or negligently brought into being with a health status likely to result in significantly greater disability or suffering, or significantly reduced life options relative to the other children with whom he/she will grow up" (1996, p. 10). Green is not alone in his view that it is irresponsible to bring a child into the world with a disability (Purdy, 1995; Davis, 1997).

The biology of disability can affect people's lives, and not every feature of life with a disability is socially determined or mediated. People with cystic fibrosis cannot now expect to live to age 70. People with type 1 diabetes can expect to have to use insulin and think carefully and continuously about diet, rest, and exercise, far more than typical sedentary people who are casual about the nutritional content of their food. People who use a wheelchair for mobility might not climb mountains; people with the intellectual disabilities of Down syndrome or fragile X syndrome are not likely to read this chapter and engage in debate about its merits and shortcomings. Yet, such limitations do not preclude a whole class of experiences, only certain instances in which these experiences might occur. People who move through the world in wheelchairs may not be able to climb mountains, but they can and do participate in other athletic activities that are challenging and exhilarating and call for stamina, alertness, and teamwork. Similarly, people who have Down syndrome or fragile X syndrome are able to have other intellectual experiences as they weigh important questions and make distinctions and decisions. They exercise capacities for reflection and judgment even if not in the rarified world of abstract verbal argument.

The child who will have a disability may have fewer options for the so-called open future that philosophers and parents dream of for children. Yet I suspect that disability precludes far fewer life possibilities than members of the bioethics community claim. The fact that many people with disabilities find their lives satisfying has been documented. For example, more than half of people with spinal cord injury (paraplegia) reported feeling more positively about themselves since becoming disabled (Ray and West, 1984, p. 83). Similarly, Canadian teenagers who had been extremely low-birthweight infants, when compared with nondisabled teens, were found to resemble them in terms of their own subjective ratings of quality of life. "Adolescents who were [extremely low-birthweight] infants suffer from a greater burden of morbidity, and rate their health-related quality of life as significantly lower than control teenagers. Nevertheless, the vast majority of the [extremely low-birthweight] respondents view their health-related quality of life as quite satisfactory and are difficult to distinguish from controls" (Saigal et al., 1996, p. 453).

Professionals faced with such information often dismiss it and insist that happy disabled people are the exceptions (Tyson and Broyles, 1996). Here again, James Watson expresses a common view when he asks, "Is it more likely for such children to fall behind in society or will they through such afflictions develop the strengths of character and fortitude that lead . . . to the head of their packs? Here I'm afraid that the word handicap cannot escape its true definition—being placed at a disadvantage. From this perspective seeing the bright side of being handicapped is like praising the virtues of extreme poverty. To be sure, there are many individuals who rise out of its inherently degrading states. But we perhaps most realistically should see it as the major origin of asocial behavior" (Watson, 1996, p. 19).

I now return to the points made earlier regarding how many of the supposed limits and problems associated with disability are socially, rather than biologically, imposed. The 1998 survey of disabled people in the United States conducted by Louis Harris Associates found gaps in education, employment, income, and social participation between people with disabilities and people without disabilities, and it noted that fewer disabled than nondisabled people were "extremely satisfied" with their lives. However, the reasons for dissatisfaction did not stem from anything inherent in the impairments; they stemmed from disparities in attainments and activities that are not inevitable in a society that takes into account the needs of one sixth of its members. Only 29 percent of people with disabilities work full- or part-time, yet, of disabled working-age people surveyed who were unemployed, more than 70 percent would prefer to work and most did not perceive their disability as precluding them from productive employment. Unemployment, and the resulting inadequate income, coupled with problems obtaining health insurance or having that insurance pay for actual disability-related expenses, accounts for the problems most commonly described by disabled people as diminishing life satisfaction (National Organization on Disability, 1999).

For children whose disabling conditions do not cause early degeneration, intractable pain, and early death, life offers a host of interactions with the physical and social world—a world in which people can be involved to their and others' satisfaction. Autobiographical writings and family narratives testify eloquently to the rich lives and the even richer futures that are possible for people with disabilities today (Brightman, 1984; Turnbull and Turnbull, 1985; Ferguson, Gartner, and Lipsky, 2000).

I do not deny that disability can entail physical pain, psychic anguish, and social isolation—even if much of the psychological and social pain can be attributed to human cruelty rather than to biological givens. In order to imagine bringing a child with a disability into the world when abortion is possible, prospective parents must be able to imagine saying to a child, "I wanted you enough and believed enough in who you could be that I felt you could have a life you would appreciate, even with the difficulties your disability causes." If parents and siblings, family members and friends can genuinely love and enjoy the child for who he or she is and not lament what he or she is not; if child care centers, schools, and youth groups routinely include disabled children; if television programs, children's books, and toys take children with disabilities into account by including them naturally in programs and products, the child may not have to live with the anguish and isolation that have marred life for generations of disabled children.

Implications for Family Life

Many who concede that people with disabilities could have lives they themselves would enjoy nonetheless argue that the cost to families of raising them justifies abortion. Women are seen to carry the greatest load for the least return in caring for such a child. Proponents of using technology to avoid the births of children with disabilities insist that raising a disabled child epitomizes what women have fought to change about their lives as mothers: unending labor, the sacrifice of their work and other adult interests, loss of time and attention for the other children in the family as parents juggle resources to give this disabled child the best available support, and uncertain recompense in terms of the mother's relationship with the child (Wertz and Fletcher, 1993).

Writing in 1995 on justifications for prenatal testing, J. Botkin proposed that only conditions that impose "burdens" on parents equivalent to those of an unwanted child warrant society-supported testing.

> The parent's harms are different in many respects from the child's, but include emotional pain and suffering, loss of a child, loss of opportunities, loss of freedom, isolation, loneliness, fear, guilt, stigmatization, and financial expenses. . . .

Some conditions that are often considered severe may not be associated with any experience of harm for the child. Down syndrome is a prime example. Parents in this circumstance are not harmed by the suffering of a child . . . but rather by their time, efforts, and expenses to support the special needs of an individual with Down syndrome. . . . It might also be added that parents are harmed by their unfulfilled expectations with the birth of an impaired child. In general terms, the claim is that parents suffer a sufficient harm to justify prenatal testing or screening when the severity of a child's condition raises problems for the parents of a similar magnitude to the birth of an unwanted child. . . . Parents of a child with unwanted disability have their interests impinged upon by the efforts, time, emotional burdens, and expenses added by the disability that they would not have otherwise experienced with the birth of a healthy child. (Botkin, 1995, pp. 36–37)

I believe the characterizations found in the writings of D. C. Wertz and J. C. Fletcher (1993) and J. Botkin (1995) are at the heart of professionals' support for prenatal testing and deserve careful scrutiny. Neither Wertz and Fletcher nor Botkin offer citations to literature to support their claims of family burden, changed lifestyle, disappointed expectations, or additional expenses, perhaps because they believe these claims are indisputable. Evaluating them, however, requires recognizing an assumption implied in them: that there is no benefit to offset the "burden," in the way that parents can expect rewards of many kinds in their relationship with children who do not have disabilities. This assumption, which permeates much of the medical, social science, and bioethics literature on disability in relation to family life and disability in general, rests on a mistaken notion. As rehabilitation psychologist Beatrice Wright has long maintained (1983, 1988), people imagine that incapacity in one arena spreads to incapacity in all—the child with cystic fibrosis is always sick and can never play; the child who cannot walk cannot join classmates in word games, parties, or sleepovers; someone who is blind is also unable to hear or speak. Someone who needs assistance with one activity is perceived to need assistance in all areas and to contribute nothing to the social, emotional, or instrumental aspects of family life.

Assuming for a moment that there are "extra burdens" associated with certain aspects of raising children with disabilities, consider the "extra burdens" associated with raising other children: those with extraordinary (above statistical norm) aptitude for athletics, art, music, or mathematics. In a book on gifted children, Ellen Winner writes, "All the family's energy becomes focused on this child. . . . Families focus in two ways on the gifted child's development: either one or both parents spend a great deal of time stimulating and teaching the child themselves, or parents make sacrifices so that the child gets high-level training from the best available teachers. In both cases, family life is totally arranged around the child's needs. Parents channel their interests into their child's talent area and become enormously invested in their child's progress" (Winner, 1996, p. 187).

Parents, professionals working with the family, and the larger society all value the gift of the violin prodigy, the talent of the future Olympic figure skater, the aptitude of a child who excels in science and who might one day discover the cure for cancer. They perceive that all the extra work and rearrangement associated with raising such children will provide what people seek in parenthood: the opportunity to give ourselves to a new being who starts out with the best we can give, who will enrich us, gladden others, contribute to the world, and make us proud.

If professionals and parents believed that children with disabilities could indeed provide their parents with many of the same satisfactions as any other child in terms of stimulation, love, companionship, pride, and pleasure in influencing the growth and development of another, they might reexamine their belief that in psychological, material, and social terms, the burdens of raising disabled children outweigh the benefits. A vast array of literature, both parental narrative and social science quantitative and qualitative research, powerfully testifies to the rewards, typical and atypical, of raising children with many of the conditions for which prenatal testing is considered de rigeur and abortion is expected—Down syndrome, hemophilia, and cystic fibrosis, to name only a few (Massie and Massie, 1975; Walker, Ford, and Donald, 1987; Van Riper, Ryff, and Pridham, 1992; Turnbull et al., 1993; Berube, 1996; Taanila, Kokkonen, and Jarvelin, 1996; Beck, 1999; Ferguson, Gartner, and Lipsky, 2000). Yet professionals in bioethics, public health, and genetics remain woefully—scandalously—oblivious, ignorant, or dismissive of any information that challenges the conviction that disability dooms families.

Two years before the gene mutation responsible for much cystic fibrosis was identified, Lynn Walker and her colleagues published their findings about the effects of cystic fibrosis on family life. They found that mothers of children with cystic fibrosis did not differ from mothers of children without the condition on measures of

Child dependency and management difficulty, limits on family opportunity, family disharmony, and financial stress. The difference between the two groups of mothers almost reached statistical significance on a fifth subscale, Personal Burden, which measured the mother's feeling of burden in her caretaking role. . . . The similarities between mothers of children with cystic fibrosis and those with healthy children were more apparent than the differences. Mothers of children with cystic fibrosis did not report significantly higher levels of stress than did the control group mothers of healthy children. Contrary to suggestions that mothers of children with cystic fibrosis feel guilty and inadequate as parents, the mothers in this study reported levels of parenting competence equal to those reported by the mothers of healthy children. (Walker, Ford, and Donald, 1987, pp. 242–43)

The literature on how disability affects family life is, to be sure, replete with discussions of stress; anger at unsupportive members of the helping professions; distress caused by hostility from extended family, neighbors, and strangers; and frustration that many disability-related expenses are not covered by health insurance (Massie and Massie, 1975; Lipsky, 1985; Walker, Ford, and Donald, 1987; Van Riper, Ryff, and Pridham, 1992; Turnbull et al., 1993; Berube, 1996; Taanila, Kokkonen, and Jarvelin, 1996; Beck, 1999). These and other writers increasingly try to distinguish why—under what conditions—some families of disabled children founder and others thrive. Contrary to the beliefs still much accepted in medicine, bioethics, and public health, recent literature does not suggest that, on balance, families raising children who have disabilities experience more stress and disruption than any other family (Ferguson, Gartner, and Lipsky, 2000).

Implications for Professional Practice

Reporting in 1997 on a five-year study of how families affected by cystic fibrosis and sickle cell anemia viewed genetic testing technologies, Troy Duster and Diane Beeson learned, to their surprise, that the closer the relationship between the family member and the affected individual, the more uncomfortable the family member was with the technology.

[The] closer people are to someone with genetic disease the more problematic and usually unacceptable genetic testing is as a strategy for dealing with the issues. . . . The experience of emotional closeness to someone with a genetic

disease reduces, rather than increases, the acceptability of selective abortion. A
close relationship with an affected person appears to make it more difficult to
evaluate the meaning or worth of that person's existence solely in terms of their
genetic disease. Family members consistently affirm the value of the person's life
in spite of the disorders, and see value for their family in their experiences with
(and of) this member, and in meeting the challenges the disease poses. (Duster
and Beeson, 1997, p. 43)

This finding is consistent with other reports that parents of children with
disabilities generally reject the idea of prenatal testing and abortion of subsequent fetuses, even if those fetuses are found to carry the same disabling trait
(Evers-Kiebooms, Denayer, and Van den Berghe, 1990; Wertz, 1992; Beeson
and Duster, Chapter 7 in this volume).

Professionals charged with developing technologies, offering tests, and interpreting results should reassess their current assumptions and practice in
light of the literature on disability and family life and data about how such
families perceive selective abortion. Of the many implications of such data, the
first is that familiarity with disability as one characteristic of a loved child
changes the meaning of disability for parents contemplating a subsequent
birth. The disability, instead of being the child's sole, or most salient, characteristic, becomes only one of the child's characteristics, along with appearance,
aptitudes, temperament, interests, and quirks. The typical woman or couple
discussing prenatal testing and possible pregnancy termination knows very
little about the conditions for which testing is available, much less what these
conditions might mean for the daily life of the child and the family. People
who do not already have a child with a disability and who are contemplating
prenatal testing must learn considerably more than the names of some typical
impairments and the odds of their child's having one.

To provide ethical and responsible clinical care for anyone concerned about
reproduction, professionals themselves must know far more than they now do
about life with disability; they must convey more information, and different
information, than they now typically provide. After being shown a film about
the lives of families raising children with Down syndrome, nurses and genetic
counselors—but not parents—described the film as unrealistic and too positive
a portrayal of family life (Cooley et al., 1990). Whether the clinician is a
genetics professional or (as is increasingly the case) an obstetrician promoting
prenatal diagnosis as routine care for pregnant women, the tone, timing, and
content of the counseling process cry out for drastic overhaul.

Many discussions of genetic counseling suggest that counselors, even graduates of master's-level genetic counseling programs, are ill equipped by their own training and norms of practice to provide any insights into disability in today's society. Most graduate programs in genetic counseling do not include courses in the social implications of life with disability for children and families, nor do they include contact between counselor trainees and disabled children and adults outside clinical settings. They also do not expose counselors to the laws, disability rights organizations, and peer support groups that constitute what is described as the disability rights and independent living movement. Often, if providers seek a "consumer" perspective on genetic issues, they consult organizations that focus on genetic research and cure, and they generally have taken a medical, rather than social, approach to improving life for people with genetic conditions (for more on advocacy groups' differing approaches to disability, see the discussions of the Cystic Fybrosis Foundation and PXE International in Stockdale and Terry, Chapter 4 in this volume). Reviews of medical school curricula suggest that medical students do not receive formal instruction on life with disability, instruction that would remind them that the people with disabilities they see in their offices have lives outside those offices.

Until their own education is revamped, obstetricians, midwives, nurses, and genetics professionals cannot properly counsel prospective parents. With broader exposure themselves, they would be far more likely to engage in discussions with their patients that would avoid problems such as those noted by Abby Lippman and Benjamin Wilfond in a survey of genetic counselors. These researchers found that counselors provided far more positive information about Down syndrome and cystic fibrosis to parents already raising children diagnosed with those conditions than they did to prospective parents deciding whether to continue pregnancies in which the fetus had been found to have the condition.

> At the least, we must recognize that every description of a genetic disorder is a story that contains a message. The story is the vehicle through which complex and voluminous information is reduced for the purposes of communication between health-care provider and health-care seeker. The message is shaped as the storyteller selects what to include and what to exclude to reduce the amount of information. . . . Should we strive to tell the same story to families considering carrier testing and prenatal diagnosis and to families who receive a postnatal

diagnosis? . . . Is telling the same story required if we are to provide sufficiently balanced information to allow potential parents to make fully informed family-planning decisions? (Lippman and Wilfond, 1992, pp. 936–37)

Lippman and Wilfond question the disparity in information provided; I call for change to ensure that everyone obtaining testing or seeking information about genetic or prenatally diagnosable disability receives sufficient information about predictable difficulties, supports, and life events associated with a disabling condition to enable them to consider how a child's disability would fit into their own hopes for parenthood. Such information for all prospective parents should include, at a minimum, a detailed description of the physical, sensory, cognitive, or psychological impairments associated with specific disabilities, and what those impairments imply for day-to-day functioning; a discussion of the laws governing education, entitlements to family support services, access to buildings and transportation, and financial assistance to disabled children and their families; and literature by family members of disabled children and by disabled people themselves.

If prenatal testing indicates a disabling condition in the fetus, the following disability-specific information should be given to the prospective parents: information about services to benefit children with the diagnosed disabilities in a particular area and about which of these services a child and family are likely to need immediately after birth; contact information for a parent-group representative; and contact information for a member of a disability rights group or independent living center. In addition, the parents should be offered a visit with both a family with a child and an adult living with the diagnosed disability.

Although some prospective parents will reject parts or all of this information and these contacts, responsible practice that is concerned with genuine informed decision making and true reproductive choice must include access to this information; it should be timed so that prospective parents can assimilate general ideas about life with disability before testing and obtain particular disability-relevant information if they discover that their fetus carries a disabling trait. These ideas may appear unrealistic or unfeasible, but a growing number of diverse voices support similar versions of these reforms to encourage wise decision making. Statements by groups with interests in women's issues, disability, family issues, and bioethics all urge versions of these proposals for change in the reproductive counseling process (Rothenberg and

Thomson, 1994, appendix; Little People of America, 1996; National Down Syndrome Congress, 1994; Parens and Asch, 1999; Disabled Peoples International Europe, 2000).

These proposals may be startling in the context of counseling for genetically transmitted or prenatally diagnosable disability, but they resonate with the recent discussion about childbearing for women infected with the HIV virus:

> The primary task of the provider would be to engage the client in a meaningful discussion of the implications of having a child and of not having a child for herself, for the client's family and for the child who would be born. . . . Providers would assist clients in examining what childbearing means to them. Providers also would assist clients in gaining an understanding of the factual information relevant to decisions about childbearing. . . . However, the conversation would cover a range of topics that go far beyond what can be understood as the relevant *medical* facts, and the direction of the conversation would vary depending on each person's life circumstances and priorities. (Faden et al., 1996, pp. 453–54 [emphasis added])

This counseling process for women with HIV who are considering motherhood demonstrates that information in itself is not sufficient. As Mary White, Arthur Caplan, and other commentators on genetic counseling have noted, the norm of nondirectiveness, even when followed, may leave people who are seeking help with difficult decisions feeling bewildered and abandoned (Caplan, 1993; White, 1999). Along with others who have expressed growing concern about needed reforms in the conduct of prenatal testing and counseling, I urge a serious conversation between prospective parents and clinicians about what the parents seek in childrearing and how a disabling condition in general or a specific type of impairment would affect their hopes and expectations for the rewards of parenthood. For some people, any impairment may indeed lead to disappointment of parental hopes; for others, it may be far easier to imagine incorporating disability into family life without believing that the rest of their lives will be blighted.

As Beeson and Duster point out in Chapter 7 in this volume, attitudes toward raising a child who would have an impairment are influenced by a host of factors that can include ethnicity, culture, socioeconomic status, the rest of a woman's (or couple's) life circumstances, and, especially, an emotional relationship with someone who has a particular impairment. It also must be pointed out that there is no single, unanimous attitude toward prenatal testing and selective abortion based on ethnicity, social class, or any other factor. Yet the views that dominate professional and media discussion of prenatal testing until now have been shaped by white elites without experiences of disability, rather than including voices of ethnic or racial minorities or people with disability experience (Kaplan, 1994; Rapp, 1999). Alan Stockdale and Sharon Terry (Chapter 4 in this volume) recount how difficult it was for even one person with cystic fibrosis to participate in a national consensus conference on testing policy for cystic fibrosis. Aware of their absence from most professional conversation, Disabled Peoples International Europe calls for changes in how society carries on future conversations about genetics as follows:

1. the use of new human genetic discoveries, techniques and practices are strictly regulated to avoid discrimination and protect fully, and in all circumstances, the human rights of disabled people,

2. genetic counselling is non-directive, rights based, widely and freely available and reflects the real experience of disability,

3. parents are not formally or informally pressured to take pre-natal tests or undergo "therapeutic" terminations,

4. all children are welcomed into the world and provided with appropriate levels of social, practical and financial support, . . .

6. organisations of disabled people are represented on all advisory and regulatory bodies dealing with human genetics,

7. legislation is amended to bring an end to discrimination on the grounds of impairment as exceptional legal grounds for abortion,

8. there is a comprehensive program of training for all health and social care professionals from a disability equality perspective.

(Disabled Peoples International Europe, 2000)

Ideally, such discussions will include mention of the fact that every child inevitably differs from parental dreams, and that successful parenting requires a mix of shaping and influencing children and appreciating the ways children pick and choose from what parents offer, sometimes rejecting tastes, activities, or values dear to their parents. If prospective parents cannot envision appreciating the child who will depart in particular, known ways from the parents' fantasy, are they truly ready to raise would-be athletes if they hate sports, classical violinists if they delight in the Grateful Dead? Testing and abortion guarantee little about the child and the life parents create and nurture, and all parents and children could be harmed by inflated notions of what parenting can bring in terms of fulfilled expectations in this age of genetic knowledge.

Public health professionals must do more than they have been doing to change the climate in which prenatal tests are offered. Think about what people would say if prenatal clinics contained pamphlets telling poor women or African American women that they should consider refraining from child-bearing because their children could be similarly poor and could endure discrimination or because they could be less healthy and more likely to find themselves imprisoned than members of the middle class or whites. Public health is committed to ending such inequities, not to endorsing them, tolerating them, or asking prospective parents to live with them. Yet the current promotion of prenatal testing condones just such an approach to life with disability.

Practitioners and policy makers can increase women's and couples' reproductive choice through testing and counseling, and they can expend energy and resources on changing the society in which families consider raising disabled children. If families that include children with disabilities now spend more money and ingenuity on after-school care for those children because they are denied entrance into existing programs attended by their peers and siblings (Freedman, Lichfield, and Warfield, 1995), public health can join with others to ensure that existing programs include *all* children. The principle of education for all, which is improving public education for disabled children, must spread to incorporate those same children into the network of services and supports that parents count on for other children. Such programs, like other institutions, must change to fit the people who exist in the world, not claim that some people should not exist because society is not prepared for them. We can fight to reform insurance practices that deny reimbursement for diabetes test strips, special diets for people with disabilities, household modifications that give disabled children freedom to explore their environment, and modifications of equipment, games, and toys that enable disabled children to participate in activities comparable to those of their peers. Those in public health can fight to end the Catch-22 that removes subsidies for life-sustaining personal assistance services once disabled people enter the workforce, a policy that acts as a powerful disincentive to productivity and needlessly perpetuates poverty and dependence.

Laws such as the Individuals with Disabilities Education Act and the Americans with Disabilities Act chart a course of inclusion for disabled people of all ages. In 1980, Gliedman and Roth, who pioneered the development of the minority-group paradigm that infuses much of the critique of current genetic technology, wrote a blueprint for the inclusive society that public health professionals should strive to create:

> Suppose that somewhere in the world an advanced industrial society genuinely respected the needs and the humanity of handicapped people. What would a visitor from this country make of the position of the disabled individual in American life? . . . To begin with, the traveler would take for granted that a market of millions of children and tens of millions of adults would not be ignored. He would assume that many industries catered to the special needs of the handicapped. Some of these needs would be purely medical . . . but many would not be medical. The visitor would expect to find industries producing everyday household and domestic appliances designed for the use of people with poor motor coordination. . . . He would anticipate a profusion of specialized and sometimes quite simple gadgets designed to enhance control of a handicapped person over his physical world—special hand tools, office supplies, can openers, eating utensils, and the like. . . .
>
> As he examined our newspapers, magazines, journals and books, as he watched our movies, television shows, and went to our theaters, he would look for many reports about handicap . . . cartoon figures on children's TV programs, and many characters in children's stories who are handicapped. He would expect constantly to come across advertisements aimed at handicapped people. He would expect to find many handicapped people appearing in advertisements not specifically aimed at them.
>
> The traveler would explore our factories, believing that handicapped people were employed in proportion to their vast numbers. . . . He would walk the streets of our towns and cities. And everywhere he went he would expect to see multitudes of handicapped people going about their business, taking a holiday, passing an hour with able bodied or handicapped friends, or simply being alone. . . .
>
> He would explore our manmade environment, anticipating that provision was made for the handicapped in our cities and towns. . . . He would expect the tiniest minutiae of our dwellings to reflect the vast numbers of disabled people. . . .
>
> He would assume that disabled individuals had their share of elected and appointive offices. He would expect to find that the role played by the disabled as

a special interest group at the local and national levels was fully commensurate with their great numbers. (Gliedman and Roth, 1980, pp. 13–15)

Despite the strides of the past few decades, our current society is far from the ideal described by Gliedman and Roth, an ideal toward which the disability community strives. Professionals in medicine, bioethics, and public health can put their efforts toward promoting such a society; with such efforts, disability could become nearly as easy to incorporate into the familial and social landscape as the other differences these professions respect and affirm as ordinary parts of the human condition. Given that more than 50 million people in the U.S. population have disabling traits and that prenatal tests may become increasingly available to detect more of them, we are confronting the fact that tests may soon be available for characteristics that we have until now considered inevitable facts of human life, such as heart disease.

To make testing and selecting for or against disability consonant with improving life for those who will inevitably be born with or acquire disabilities, our clinical and policy establishments must communicate that it is as acceptable to live with a disability as it is to live without one and that society will support and appreciate everyone with the inevitable variety of traits. We can assure prospective parents that they and their future child will be welcomed whether or not the child has a disability. If that professional message is conveyed, more prospective parents may envision that their lives can be rewarding, whatever the characteristics of the child they are raising. Once our professions can realize such communication and make the incorporation and appreciation of people with disabilities a reality, prenatal technology can help people to make decisions without implying that only one decision is right. If the child with a disability is not a problem for the world, and the world is not a problem for the child, perhaps we can diminish our desire for prenatal testing and selective abortion and can comfortably welcome and support children of all characteristics.

REFERENCES

Americans with Disabilities Act. 1990. Pub L No. 101 336, §2.
Asch, A. 1989. "Reproductive Technology and Disability." Pp. 69–124 in *Reproductive Laws for the 1990s*, ed. S. Cohen and N. Taub. Clifton, N.J.: Humana Press.

Asch, A., and G. Geller. 1996. "Feminism, Bioethics and Genetics." Pp. 318–50 in *Feminism and Bioethics: Beyond Reproduction,* ed. S. Wolf. New York: Oxford University Press.

Beaudet, A. L. 1990. "Carrier Screening for Cystic Fibrosis." *American Journal of Human Genetics* 47:603–5.

Beck, M. 1999. *Expecting Adam: A True Story of Birth, Rebirth and Everyday Magic.* New York: Random House.

Berube, M. 1996. *Life As We Know It: A Father, a Family, and an Exceptional Child.* New York: Pantheon.

Bickenbach, J. E. 1993. *Physical Disability and Social Policy.* Toronto: University of Toronto Press.

Boorse, C. 1987. "Concepts of Health." Pp. 359–93 in *Health Care Ethics,* ed. D. Van de Veer and T. Regan. Philadelphia: Temple University Press.

Botkin, J. 1995. "Fetal Privacy and Confidentiality." *Hastings Center Report* 25 (3):32–39.

Brightman, A. J. 1984. *Ordinary Moments: The Disabled Experience.* Baltimore: Paul H. Brookes Publishing Co.

Caplan, A. L. 1993. "Neutrality Is Not Morality." Pp. 149–65 in *Prescribing Our Futures: Ethical Challenges in Genetic Counseling,* ed. D. Bartels, B. Leroy, and A. L. Caplan. New York: Aldine De Gruyter.

Cooley, W. C., E. S. Graham, J. B. Moeschler, and J. M. Graham, Jr. 1990. "Reactions of Mothers and Medical Professionals to a Film about Down Syndrome." *American Journal of Diseases of Children* 144:1112–16.

Daniels, N. J. 1985. *Just Health Care: Studies in Philosophy and Health Policy.* Cambridge: Cambridge University Press.

Davis, D. S. 1997. "Genetic Dilemmas and the Child's Right to an Open Future." *Hastings Center Report* 27 (2):7–15.

Disabled Peoples International Europe. 2000. "Disabled People Speak on the New Genetics." http://www.dpieurope.org/htm/bioethics/dpsng10demands.htm.

Dunne, C., and C. Warren. 1998. "Lethal Autonomy: The Malfunction of the Consent Mechanism within the Context of Prenatal Diagnosis of Genetic Variants." *Issues in Law and Medicine* 14 (2):165.

Duster, T., and D. Beeson. 1997. *Pathways and Barriers to Genetic Testing and Screening: Molecular Genetics Meets the "High Risk" Family.* Final report. Washington, D.C.: U.S. Department of Energy.

Evers-Kiebooms, G., L. Denayer, and H. Van den Berghe. 1990. "A Child with Cystic Fibrosis, II: Subsequent Family Planning Decisions, Reproduction and Use of Prenatal Diagnosis." *Clinical Genetics* 37:207–15.

Faden, R. R., N. E. Kass, K. L. Acuff, A. Allen, J. Anderson, T. L. Banks, M. G. Bloche, R. Chaisson, S. Cohn, N. Hutton, P. A. King, M. Lillie-Blanton, M. E. McCaul, M. Powers, K. H. Rothenberg, A. Saah, L. Solomon, and L. Wissow. 1996. "HIV Infection and Childbearing: A Proposal for Public Policy and Clinical Practice." Pp. 447–61 in *HIV, Aids and Childbearing: Public Policy, Private Lives,* ed. R. Faden and N. Kass. New York: Oxford University Press.

Feinberg, J. 1980. "The Child's Right to an Open Future." Pp. 124–53 in *Whose Child? Children's Rights, Parental Authority, and State Power,* ed. W. Aiken and H. LaFollette. Totowa, N.J.: Rowman & Littlefield.

Ferguson, P. M., A. Gartner, and D. K. Lipsky. 2000. "Experience of Disabilities in Families: A Synthesis of Research and Parent Narratives." Pp. 72–94 in *Prenatal Testing and Disability Rights,* ed. E. Parens and A. Asch. Washington, D.C.: Georgetown University Press.

Field, M. A. 1993. "Killing 'The Handicapped'—Before and After Birth." *Harvard Women's Law Journal* 16: 79–138.

Fine, M., and A. Asch. 1982. "The Question of Disability: No Easy Answers for the Women's Movement." *Reproductive Rights Newsletter* 4 (3):19–20.

.Finger, A. 1987. *Past Due: Disability Pregnancy and Birth.* Seattle: Seal Press.

Freedman, R. I., L. Lichfield, and M. E. Warfield. 1995. "Balancing Work and Family: Perspectives of Parents of the Children with Developmental Disabilities." *Family in Societies: Journal of Contemporary Human Services* 76 (October): 507–14.

Gartner, A., and T. Joe. 1987. *Images of the Disabled, Disabling Images.* New York: Praeger.

Gliedman, J., and W. Roth. 1980. *The Unexpected Minority: Handicapped Children in America.* New York: Harcourt Brace Jovanovich.

Goffman, E. 1963. *Stigma: Notes on the Management of Spoiled Identity.* Englewood Cliffs, N.J.: Prentice-Hall.

Green, R. 1996. "Prenatal Autonomy and the Obligation Not to Harm One's Child Genetically." *Journal of Law, Medicine and Ethics* 25 (1):5–16.

Hockenberry, J. 1996. *Moving Violations: War Zones, Wheelchairs, and Declarations of Independence.* New York: Hyperion.

Hubbard, R. 1990. *The Politics of Women's Biology.* New Brunswick, N.J.: Rutgers University Press, esp. chap. 12–14.

Kaplan, D. 1994. "Prenatal Screening and Diagnosis: The Impact on Persons with Disabilities." Pp. 49–61 in *Women and Prenatal Testing: Facing the Challenges of Genetic Technology,* ed. K. H. Rothenberg and E. J. Thompson. Columbus: Ohio State University Press.

Kuppermann, M., J. D. Goldberg, R. F. Nease Jr., and A. E. Washington. 1999. "Who Should Be Offered Prenatal Diagnosis? The Thirty-Five-Year-Old Question." *American Journal of Public Health* 89: 160–63.

Lippman, A. 1991. "Prenatal Genetic Testing and Screening: Constructing Needs and Reinforcing Inequities." *American Journal of Law and Medicine* 17 (1–2):15–50.

Lippman, A., and B. Wilfond. 1992. "Twice-Told Tales: Stories about Genetic Disorders." *American Journal of Human Genetics* 51 :936–37.

Lipsky, D. K. 1985. "A Parental Perspective on Stress and Coping." *American Journal of Orthopsychiatry* 55: 614–17.

Little People of America. 1996. Position Statement on Genetic Discoveries in Dwarfism. http://www2.shore.net/~dkennedy/dwarfism_genetics.html.

Massie, R., and S. Massie. 1975. *Journey.* New York: Alfred A. Knopf.

Miringoff, M.-L. 1991. *The Social Costs of Genetic Welfare.* New Brunswick, N.J.: Rutgers University Press.

National Down Syndrome Congress. 1994. *Position Statement on Prenatal Testing and Eugenics: Families' Rights and Needs.* Prepared for and approved by the Professional Advisory Committee. http://www.altonweb.com/cs/downsyndrome/index .htm?page=eugenicsndsc.html.

National Organization on Disability. 1999. "1998 Harris Survey of Americans with Disabilities." http://www.nod.org.

Parens, E., and A. Asch. 1999. "The Disability Rights Critique of Prenatal Genetic Testing: Reflections and Recommendations." Supplement, *Hastings Center Report* 29 (5): S1–22.

Purdy, L. 1995. "Loving Future People." Pp. 300–327 in *Reproduction, Ethics and the Law*, ed. J. Callahan. Bloomington: Indiana University Press.

Rapp, R. 1999. *Testing Women, Testing the Fetus: The Social Impact of Amniocentesis in America.* New York: Routledge.

Ray, C., and J. West. 1984. "Social, Sexual and Personal Implications of Paraplegia." *Paraplegia* 22: 75–86.

Retsinas, J. 1991. "Impact of Prenatal Technology on Attitudes toward Disabled Infants." Pp. 75–102 in *Research in the Sociology of Healthcare*, ed. D. Wertz. Westport, Conn.: JAI Press.

Rothenberg, K. H., and E. J. Thomson, eds. 1994. *Women and Prenatal Testing: Facing the Challenges of Genetic Technology.* Columbus: Ohio State University Press.

Russel, M. 1998. *Beyond Ramps: Disability at the End of the Social Contract.* Monroe, Maine: Common Courage Press.

Saigal, S., D. Feeny, P. Rosenbaum, W. Furlong, E. Burrows, and B. Stoskopf. 1996. "Self-perceived Health Status and Health-Related Quality of Life of Extremely Low-Birth-Weight Infants at Adolescence." *Journal of the American Medical Association* 276 (6):453–59.

Saxton, M. 1984. "Born and Unborn: The Implications of Reproductive Technologies for People with Disabilities." Pp. 298–312 in *Test-Tube Women: What Future for Motherhood?*, ed. R. Arditti, R. Duelli-Klein, and S. Mindin. Boston: Pandora Press.

Schneider, J., and P. Conrad. 1983. *Having Epilepsy: The Experience and Control of Illness.* Philadelphia: Temple University Press.

Schuklenk, U., E. Stein, J. Kerin, and W. Byne. 1997. "The Ethics of Genetic Research on Sexual Orientation." *Hastings Center Report* 27 (4):6–13.

Shaw, M. W. 1984. "Presidential Address: To Be or Not to Be, That Is the Question." *American Journal of Human Genetics* 36:1–9.

Shakespeare, T. 1995. "Back to the Future? New Genetics and Disabled People." *Critical Social Policy* 15:22–35.

———. 1998. "Choices and Rights: Eugenics, Genetics and Disability Equality." *Disability and Society* 13:665–81.

Stein, E. 1998. "Choosing the Sexual Orientation of Children." *Bioethics* 12 (1):1–24.

Taanila, A., J. Kokkonen, and M.-R. Jarvelin. 1996. "The Long-Term Effects of Children's Early-Onset Disability on Marital Relationships." *Developmental Medicine and Child Neurology* 38:567–77.

Turnbull A. P., J. M. Patterson, S. K. Behr, D. L. Murphy, J. G. Marquis, and M. J. Blue-Banning, eds. 1993. *Cognitive Coping, Families, and Disability.* Baltimore: Paul H. Brookes Publishing Co.

Turnbull, H. R., and A. P. Turnbull, eds. *Parents Speak Out: Then and Now.* Columbus, Ohio: Charles L. Merrill Publishing Co.

Tyson, J. E., and R. S. Broyles. 1996. "Progress in Assessing the Long-term Outcome of

Extremely Low-Birth-Weight Infants." *Journal of the American Medical Association* 276 (6):492–93.

U.S. Congress, Office of Technology Assessment. 1988. *Mapping Our Genes.* Washington, D.C.: U.S. Congress.

Van Riper, M., C. Ryff, and K. Pridham. 1992. "Parental and Family Well-Being in Families of Children with Down Syndrome: A Comparative Study. *Research in Nursing and Health* 15:227–35.

Walker, L. S., M. B. Ford, and W. D. Donald. 1987. "Cystic Fibrosis and Family Stress: Effects of Age and Severity of Illness." *Pediatrics* 79:239–46.

Watson, J. D. 1996. "President's Essay: Genes and Politics." *Annual Report Cold Springs Harbor*, 1–20.

Wertz, D. C. 1992. "How Parents of Affected Children View Selective Abortion." Pp. 161–89 in *Issues in Reproductive Technology*, ed. H. B. Holmes. New York: New York University Press.

Wertz, D. C., and J. C. Fletcher. 1992. "Sex Selection through Prenatal Diagnosis." Pp. 240–53 in *Feminist Perspectives in Medical Ethics*, ed. H. B. Holmes and L. M. Purdy. Bloomington: Indiana University Press.

———. 1993. "A Critique of Some Feminist Challenges to Prenatal Diagnosis." *Journal of Women's Health* 2:173–88.

White, M. T. 1999. "Making Responsible Decisions: An Interpretive Ethic for Genetic Decisionmaking." *Hastings Center Report* 29:14–21.

Winner, E. 1996. *Gifted Children: Myths and Realities.* New York: Basic Books.

Wright, B. A. 1983. *Physical Disability: A Pyscho-Social Approach.* New York: Harper & Row.

———. 1988. "Attitudes and the Fundamental Negative Bias: Conditions and Correlates." Pp. 3–21 in *Attitudes toward Persons with Disabilities*, ed. H. E. Yuker. New York: Springer.

CHAPTER SEVEN

African American Perspectives on Genetic Testing

Diane Beeson and Troy Duster

Genetic testing is one of the most rapidly proliferating classes of biomedical technologies to emerge from human genome research. From a biomedical perspective, carrier testing and prenatal diagnosis provide welcome opportunities to reduce sharply the risk of bearing children with genetic disorders. These tests are central elements in a strategy to "reduce morbidity and mortality, and alleviate the suffering associated with many serious genetic/congenital disorders" (Council of Regional Networks, 1997, p. 1). However, a number of studies indicate that lay persons often view prenatal diagnosis and issues of genetic risk in ways that differ from biomedical perspectives

This chapter is based on research supported by the director of the Office of Energy Research, Office of Health and Environmental Research of the United States Department of Energy under contract DE-FG03–92ER61393. The authors are indebted to Duana Fullwiley, Nadine Gartrell, Ron Jordan, Arona Ragins, Robert Yamashita, David Minkus, Janice Tanagawa, Jackie Barnett, Christine Ogu, and other members of UC Berkeley's Institute for the Study of Social Change who contributed to this research. We also wish to thank Bert Lubin, Elliot Vichinsky, Herman Pugh, and the men and women who so generously shared their perspectives with us in interviews. The editors of this volume and other colleagues who commented on earlier drafts, including Maxine Craig, Benjamin Bowser, Duana Fullwiley, Terry Lunsford, and Terry Jones, were particularly helpful.

(Lippman-Hand and Fraser, 1979; Beeson, 1984; Saxton, 1984; Rothman, 1986; Rapp, 1994, 1999; Beeson and Doksum, 2001).

Diversity of responses to genetic testing is widely acknowledged, but few studies have focused directly on how cultural perspectives inform the action of members of specific ethnic groups with regard to this issue. Anthropologist Rayna Rapp (1994), while cautioning against stereotypes, has emphasized the need to know more about how stories of genetic testing and its consequences are produced and consumed among various ethnic groups. The voices of African Americans, in spite of their relatively long history with genetic testing for sickle cell disease (SCD), have had little resonance among policy makers (Duster, 1990; Bowman, 1998). In this chapter we report the findings of an exploratory study of responses to genetic testing among African Americans. By adding the perspectives of members of this racial-ethnic group to the literature on genetic testing, we hope to contribute to the development of more responsive health care services.

Background

Before turning to our study itself, it is important to place the examination of African American experiences of genetic testing in historical and social context. The prevalence of SCD among African Americans is the basis of their unique relationship to genetic testing.* Sickle cell disease has a longer and more contentious testing history than any other genetic condition. Sickle cell screening programs were developed during the late 1960s and early 1970s and prompted the first federal legislation on genetic testing—the National Sickle-Cell Anemia Control Act of 1972. This law provided funding for the establishment of comprehensive sickle cell centers across the country and for research, counseling, and testing for sickle cell disease (SCD). The funds made available through this legislation triggered demands for a "fair share" of resources by

*Sickle cell disease (SCD) is a term for a group of genetic disorders characterized by anemia and acute and chronic tissue and organ damage caused by blockage of blood flow owing to abnormally shaped red cells. The main variant is sickle cell anemia (Hb SS), which is estimated to affect more than fifty thousand Americans, making it the country's most common life-threatening genetic disorder. Estimated prevalence of Hb SS in African American live births is approximately 1 in 375. Other common variants among African Americans include SC disease (Hb SC), affecting 1 in 883, and sickle beta-thalassemia (S Beta-thalassemia), with an estimated prevalence of 1 in 1,667. In the United States, sickle cell disease is most commonly found in persons of African ancestry, but it also affects persons of Mediterranean, Caribbean, South and Central American, Arabian, and East Indian ancestry (Sickle Cell Disease Guideline Panel, 1993).

other ethnic and racial minorities, and by 1976 this legislation was rewritten to become an omnibus law covering other genetic conditions as well (Duster, 1990, p. 59). This legislation helped to institutionalize newborn screening in most states and alerted many African Americans to the presence of the sickle cell gene in their families by identifying both affected infants and carriers.

Genetic testing for many other conditions has followed the developments in sickle cell testing, with an increasingly wide range of new prenatal and carrier tests becoming available over the past three decades. Today, genetic testing has become accepted and even welcomed by large segments of the U.S. population as a viable strategy to reduce genetic risk. In the early 1990s, a Gallup poll of attitudes toward prenatal testing for "genetic defects" found attitudes "overwhelmingly favorable," with about two-thirds of respondents saying that they believed the tests would do more good than harm. Young and better-educated people were most favorable to the new technology, suggesting that positive attitudes are likely to increase over time (Singer, 1991). Another indication of increasingly widespread use of genetic testing is a substantial reduction in Down syndrome births (Drugen et al., 1990; Centers for Disease Control and Prevention, 1994; Bishop et al., 1997). The most dramatic example of the potential of genetic testing to avert risk is the more than 90 percent reduction in the incidence of Tay-Sachs disease in Ashkenazic Jewish populations in the United States and Canada between 1970 and 1993 (Kaback et al., 1993, p. 2309). This reduction is a result of the combined use of carrier testing and prenatal diagnosis, in conjunction with the sympathetic response of the Jewish community, under whose auspices the tests were given.

While the proliferation of genetic testing has been welcomed in many quarters, this has not been the case among all groups. In a recent analysis of African American responses to new developments in reproduction, Dorothy Roberts argues, with some supporting notes, that there is a tendency among African Americans to express "an aversion to the genetic marketing aspect of the new reproduction" and that they have "understandably resisted defining personal identity in biological terms." She contends that "a Black parent's essential contribution to his or her children is not passing down genetic information but sharing lessons needed to survive in a racist society" (1997, p. 262).

Roberts's contention that African Americans may be more critical of genetic testing than other racial-ethnic or cultural groups is not surprising. As she points out, the early years of sickle cell testing have been referred to as "the sickle cell screening disaster" (1997, p. 256). Her view is supported by noted geneticist and former member of the Ethical, Legal, and Social Issues Working Group of the Human Genome Project, James Bowman, who characterizes these early programs as discriminating and stigmatizing. Their consequences included "discrimination of carriers for sickle hemoglobin . . . in health and life insurance, in employment, in the Armed Forces, in school athletics, not to mention psychological harm to participants, their families, and the African American community" (Bowman, 1998, p. 145). In contrasting the sickle cell experience with the more successful Tay-Sachs screening programs, a central factor in their disparity was "the relative structural location of Jews and Blacks, their relative educational and economic positions, and the comparative level of trust and confidence one might therefore expect these programs to generate" (Duster, 1990, p. 46–47).

It was not until 1978, on the heels of the controversy over carrier testing, that prenatal diagnosis for SCD became available in U.S. centers. It was apparent from the beginning that few African Americans sought to take advantage of this new technology, but the precise reasons for their reluctance were not clear. At the same, time families from Greece and other Mediterranean countries at risk for a similar (but more lethal) hemoglobinopathy, thalassemia major, began to travel great distances to the U.S. seeking access to virtually the same procedures.

Screening newborns for SCD has been less controversial than prenatal diagnosis because it does not raise the specter of selective abortion. While newborn screening entails risks of misdiagnosis, stigmatization, diminished self-esteem, and potential discrimination, these risks can be minimized. At the same time, there is "indisputable evidence that rates of morbidity and mortality can be significantly reduced by programs that screen newborns for sickle cell disease" providing they are linked to appropriate medical and health education services (National Institutes of Health, 1987, p. 2). By 1990, California and most other states had instituted mandatory newborn screening for sickle cell disease, often as part of programs that test for other genetic conditions as well (Lane, 1994). These programs also identify and notify family members if infants are found to carry sickle cell trait (one of several mutations that contribute to SCD in offspring when combined with a similar gene from the other parent), and, as a result, they have contributed to awareness of the issue even in families where no one has the disease itself.

The extent to which Roberts's analysis accurately characterizes the perspective of a large and heterogeneous racial-ethnic group merits further empirical investigation. However, the existence of substantial racial and ethnic differences in test utilization has been documented in clinic-based studies. For example, significantly lower rates of utilization of genetic services have been reported among nonwhite women (Adams et al., 1981; Sokal et al., 1980; Krivchenia et al., 1993). When significant differences in utilization rates among various groups first became apparent, analysts raised the issue of differential access as a possible explanation. Many forms of genetic testing—including prenatal diagnosis—are expensive, and while programs exist to subsidize costs to patients, economic barriers still exist. Timing is also an issue, since prenatal diagnosis is only available to those who receive care early in their pregnancies.

The fact that African American and Latina women are less likely than white and Asian American women to use prenatal diagnosis has been confirmed in a recent study by M. Kupperman, E. Gates, and E. A. Washington (1996). Their work shows that low rates persist even when controlling for access and education. In interpreting their findings, the authors ask whether minority women are receiving adequate, clearly understandable, and culturally sensitive information regarding the possible outcomes of testing or not testing. They also question whether the lower rates of utilization of genetic testing (including prenatal diagnosis) by minority women reflect accurately their underlying preferences with regard to having a child without a genetic disorder.

The idea that genetic disorders might be regarded differently by different cultural groups has been explored to some extent by Rayna Rapp (1999). She has provided many examples of how women of different racial-ethnic, national, class, and religious backgrounds experience the offer of genetic testing during their pregnancies. She has given particular attention to cases in which genetic services such as amniocentesis are refused and points out that these refusals are associated with certain social and cultural conditions. These include potent religious affiliations, strong kinship or other community social support, and individual reproductive histories. At the same time, Rapp points out that patterns of amniocentesis use and rejection are also highly class structured. Access to information and respectful health care can facilitate acceptance of prenatal diagnosis. Gender relations and male dominance affect patterns of use as well; many women's refusals reflect their partners' opinion.

Rapp's sensitivity to the unique aspects of each woman's reproductive history and personal situation makes her reluctant to generalize about ethnic group patterns. Nevertheless, her general argument is consistent with the work of another anthropologist, Shirley Hill, who has looked very closely at low-income African American mothers of children with SCD (Hill, 1994a, 1994b). Hill emphasizes the fact that these young women's social position fosters a distinctive reality, one that differs from that of healthcare providers. She found that even after having a child with SCD, few mothers embraced the medical model of the disease. *Medical model* is the term she uses to refer to the set of meanings medicine provides for coping with sickle cell disease. For some mothers, a genetic explanation for the cause of the disorder represented an advance because it mitigated self-blame. But, in general, the medical model did not provide satisfying answers to the pain and suffering these mothers experienced, and it often did not alleviate the stress or enhance coping. Hill also found that mothers who rejected the medical model of SCD and drew on nonmedical resources to interpret their experience were much better able to reconcile themselves to the disorder. Furthermore, all the mothers in her study said they would not have had an abortion to avoid the birth of a child with SCD. The ideology of motherhood was a key factor in their position; but Hill points out that, for these women, the reality of the abortion question never arose. Family secrecy about the disease, denial, the indifference of their partners, and the lack of access to early prenatal care all contributed to their taking the risk of having a child with sickle cell disease.

Most important for these mothers was not to grasp the genetic explanation of the disease but to know that SCD could be controlled through effective home care and management. Other strategies included normalizing and focusing on their child's other abilities. Without money, power, education, or spouses, these mothers tended to rely on intrafamilial sources of support and on religion. In other words, as Hill emphasizes, they responded to having a child with SCD in a manner consistent with their own race- and class-based values and resources and with the realities that emerged from their social position. The medical model of SCD did not resonate with their own family and SCD experiences, and so it failed to provide workable strategies for caring for children who have the disease.

Hill further asserts that young women often perceive accurate SCD medical knowledge as a threat to their reproductive autonomy and respond by obfuscating medical knowledge. Her study is an excellent contribution, focusing specifically on unmarried mothers with low levels of education and low economic status. Our study is an effort to build on and extend these findings.

Methods

This study, conducted by a multiethnic research team, began with fieldwork and observations in clinical settings, support groups, and advocacy organizations serving individuals and families with SCD and cystic fibrosis (CF). We selected SCD and CF because they are the two most common inherited, potentially lethal, single-gene disorders in the United States (McKusick et al., 1994). Cystic fibrosis occurs primarily among Americans of northern European descent, and sickle cell disease occurs primarily among Americans of West African descent (Bowman and Murray, 1990). With the recent identification of the gene for cystic fibrosis, we recognized a unique opportunity to compare the variable penetration and meaning of genetic testing in two populations differentiated by socially designated categories of race while also looking at social meanings attendant to racial stratification in the United States.

Between 1992 and 1996, we conducted individual interviews with 369 men and women who have, or have had, a relative with one of these conditions (or in some cases a known carrier). We expected that these people would have concerns about genetic testing. Most respondents were living in California, but we included individuals and families in ten states. We conducted semistructured, open-ended interviews designed to elicit narratives related to disease, genetic testing, health, and reproductive issues.

Sampling

Our initial individual interviews in each family were conducted with a person affected by sickle cell disease or cystic fibrosis or a parent of an affected individual, usually the mother. This respondent was asked to refer us to other family members. In those cases in which the initial respondent agreed and was successful in recruiting other family members, we were able to move more deeply into the family system. Where family members were located within about fifty miles, interviews were conducted in person. When necessary, usually because of distance, we conducted interviews by telephone (34% were telephone interviews).

We employed three sampling strategies. First, we used opportunity sampling to identify families in medical settings and advocacy organizations; second, we used referrals from one family member to another; and finally, where possible we sought individuals and families who would diversify our sample by including those with a wide range of education, income levels, religions, and types and stages of relationships with affected persons. Our sample, therefore, is not random, but it enables us to identify recurrent patterns and ranges of responses to the issues across a wide band of social life.

We interviewed 189 adults in the SCD sample and 180 in the CF sample. Fifty-two (28%) of the SCD respondents were male, compared to sixty-seven (38%) of the CF sample. The ages of the SCD respondents ranged from a 17-year-old emancipated minor and mother of a child with SCD to an 87-year-old grandparent. The CF respondents ranged from age 18 to 84. The median ages were 39 and 43, respectively. The differences seem to reflect patterns of younger childbearing among African Americans as well as greater participation by grandparents in the CF sample.

We were successful in moving beyond the nuclear family with both groups, but significantly more so in the CF families. Of the CF respondents, 61 percent were extended family members, compared to 33 percent of SCD family members. (The recruitment process was facilitated by the payment of a twenty-dollar honorarium to interviewees in both populations.) Although there are several other factors that help explain the greater ease with which our staff members gained access to extended family members among the CF families, the most apparent was the greater mistrust among African Americans of research and researchers. We had much more success in recruiting interviewees in African American families when the interviewers were perceived as African American as well. In all but two of the African American families from which we were able to interview four or more members, interviewers were of African descent. Racial categories, particularly "black" and "white," hold such power in the United States that, had we employed an all-white research team, we would have been much less successful in our recruitment efforts among these families. African American interviewees frequently indicated their greater willingness to be open and candid with interviewers perceived to belong to the same racial-ethnic group.

The greatest difference between the two groups of interviewees was in income level. Our lowest income category was under $10,000 per year. This was the modal category for African Americans. Our highest income category, $50,000 or more, was the modal income category for the predominantly white CF sample. This sharp disparity in income levels was not correlated with significant differences in educational levels; the modal educational level for both groups was "some college." We were successful in our effort to see that interviewees from the highest as well as lowest income categories in both groups were included in the study.

Analysis

We began our analysis with typed verbatim transcripts of tape-recorded interviews. We used these transcripts and field notes to generate quantitative and qualitative coding categories. We coded each interview to provide a demographic description of our sample and, using the statistical package for the social sciences (SPSS), catalogued each respondent's basic relationship to genetic testing. For example, we coded for relationship to affected person, experience with testing, carrier status, attitudes toward abortion, and other basic themes, as well as education, income, and so on. Our primary focus in interviews was always to elicit narratives rather than to move the interviewee through a rigidly structured interview guide. This made quantitative coding difficult and sometimes resulted in gaps, but the stories our interviewees provided revealed processes and concerns that we could not possibly have anticipated.

As we began to see certain themes repeated, we used them to generate theoretical notes and memos. We used what Barney Glaser and Anselm Strauss (1967) call "the constant comparative method" to compare cases with one another and determine which types of concerns and responses constituted recurring patterns. This process also helped us to clarify the conditions under which each type of response occurred. We looked for both similarities and differences among those who were related to individuals with CF or SCD, noting how they responded to issues of genetic disease and genetic testing.

Findings

There are two sets of findings that we wish to report. The first set is labeled "General Findings Regarding Genetic Disease" because it applies to the overall data set for both SCD and CF. The second set is labeled "Findings Regarding SC" because it highlights issues prevalent among African American families affected by this condition, issues that are the main focus of this chapter.

General Findings Regarding Genetic Disease

The manner in which participants viewed and responded to genetic disorders in their families can be seen as forming a continuum, ranging from what

can be described as *vigilance* to *avoidance*. On the vigilant end of the continuum, family members and individuals diagnosed with the genetic disorder
(i.e., SCD or CF) accepted the diagnosis and often became absorbed with
reading as much as possible about the disease. They would contact the relevant
organizations, spend time with others in similar situations, and in many cases
become politically active, advocating more research and secondary care funding. The vigilant were also more likely to challenge their health care providers
with their knowledge of the latest research results, experimental protocols, and
experimental drugs. They used the Internet to access the National Institutes of
Health or other relevant websites. The vigilant were often, but not exclusively,
middle or upper-middle class. Avoiders were found in all social classes. These
individuals and family members used a variety of strategies to play down, or
even hide, the presence of the disorder in their family. Their goal was to
normalize their situation. The behavior of avoidance ranged from an initial
denial that their side of the family could possibly be implicated to emotional
retreat and divorce.

Two subsidiary findings are pertinent. First, distribution of responses was
bimodal. That is, there was not a uniform distribution from vigilance to
avoidance. Rather, interviewees tended to cluster toward one end or the other
of the continuum. Second, there was an unmistakable gender difference: men
tended toward avoidance, women toward vigilance. These responses to genetic
disorders have many parallels in responses to genetic testing. However, some
issues of particular concern to African Americans tempered their responses to
carrier testing and prenatal diagnosis as means of preventing SCD. We discuss
theses issues in the next section of this chapter.

Findings Regarding SC Testing

The demographics of our sample reveal something about the differences in
the social context in which families encounter genetic disease and genetic
testing. While educational levels are similar, income levels differ dramatically.
The markedly lower average income levels among African Americans reflect
not only racial-ethnic disparities in the general population but also the toll
SCD often takes on families. Those who were precariously situated in the
middle class often found that the care required for a child with SCD caused
them to descend significantly in socioeconomic status. This was particularly
true of single parents, usually mothers, who were unable to maintain secure
employment while responding to the often frequent crises children with SCD

go through. On the other hand, some were able to make use of support from extended family and the public health sector to avoid abject poverty.

While our sampling procedures were not designed to produce results that would meet the traditional tests applied to large-scale quantitative surveys, the number of cases (369) is sufficient to reveal some socially patterned differences in responses of the two groups. While discussing these patterns it is important to keep in mind that African Americans are extremely heterogeneous. Identifying an individual as African American does not enable us to confidently predict his or her response to genetic testing. Indeed, as we move up the socioeconomic ladder, the differences between African Americans' and European Americans' responses to genetic testing become less clear (see Beeson and Doksum, 2001). At the same time, the power of racial categories in the United States has created a shared history and sensibility among African Americans that often transcends social class and other social categories. This shared history and collective memory is sufficiently salient that persistent themes can be identified.

Not surprisingly, given the longer history of testing for sickle cell trait, a much higher percentage of African Americans had been tested and knew their own carrier status (61% as opposed to 25% for CF). For those who had reason to suspect CF, prenatal diagnosis had not been an option until the 1990s, so it is no surprise that more women from the sickle cell group (fifteen) underwent amniocentesis than CF respondents (seven). What is most notable and, we hope, most illuminated by the following analysis is that selective abortion was not used by anyone in our sickle cell sample, even though in at least twenty pregnancies the risk was known by the mothers to exist. Three respondents acknowledged that they received positive amniocentesis results but rejected the idea of abortion for sickle cell disease. Two reported receiving false negative results. In sharp contrast, out of the four pregnancies in which genetic disorders were identified as a result of amniocentesis in the CF group, two couples chose selective abortion.

Some women reported they simply accepted the diagnostic procedure because their physician recommended it, or because they hoped to relieve themselves of worry. While acceptance of amniocentesis by African Americans does not imply receptivity to selective abortion, two women who had negative results did report that they would have aborted had their results been positive. Our sense that the SCD and CF groups differ in their perception of the value and appropriateness of genetic testing for the purpose of reducing genetic disorders is consistent with these figures. This difference was made clearer as the respondents expressed their thoughts and feelings in interviews.

Most significantly, we found that those African Americans who accepted genetic testing often still minimized or ignored the information garnered from such tests when it came to selection of a partner and reproductive planning. Four themes stand out in our data that, while not necessarily unique to African Americans, were expressed with distinctly greater frequency and intensity by members of this group and help to explain their responses to genetic testing. These themes are: (1) mistrust of the motives of genetic medicine; (2) fear of stigmatized "risk" identity; (3) perceived irrelevance of genetic threat; and (4) aversion to selective abortion.

Mistrust of the Motives of Genetic Medicine

In general, African Americans express a greater degree of mistrust concerning the motives of medical practitioners. When our African American interviewers, as opposed to white interviewers, made contact and interviewed African Americans with sickle-cell disease and their family members, they achieved greater access to a wider range of discussions about social and political issues than was typical with white interviewers. African American interviewers were also more successful in getting referrals to other family members. But even with white interviewers, African American respondents gave many indications that they mistrust the so-called neutrality of the U.S. public health system and that of public or private medical providers. This mistrust goes far beyond occasional references to the Tuskegee syphilis study.* Their narratives are saturated with references to medicine as an instrument of domination and control. This is particularly striking in comparison to the narratives of the predominantly white members of families at risk for CF. African American parents are much more likely to have had health care providers suspect their child's symptoms to be the effects of child abuse or to have relatives or friends who have experienced what they consider to be medical abuse. The widespread discourse of mistrust is often confirmed through personal experience. A woman with sickle cell reports that an army doctor who diagnosed her as a

---

*The Tuskegee Syphilis Study, conducted by the U.S. Public Health Service from 1932 to 1972, is a well-known example of unethical research. Even after penicillin became the drug of choice in 1947, the researches withheld adequate treatment from 399 poor black men who had the disease. The study participants were deliberately deceived and therefore unable to give informed consent. President Clinton officially apologized on behalf of the United States government on May 16, 1997. The president's apology is at http://clinton4.nara.gov/textonly/New/Remarks/Fri/19970516–898.html.

child warned her mother, " 'They like to do a lot of tests on sickle cell patients.' And he told my mother, 'Don't let them do that to your kids because they don't have a cure. They'll promise you that they have one and they don't have one.' And so she was worried about letting them do anything to us. . . . So she just told us, if you're getting medical attention, make sure . . . you're not just being a run-of-the-mill guinea pig."

This concern about being used as "guinea pigs" arises frequently among African Americans and goes much deeper than the Tuskegee study, which was mentioned by several respondents. The field of genetic medicine is a particularly sensitive area in this regard. One father of a child with sickle cell disease told us:

> I don't have a whole lot of trust around the way the whole medical field operates, and there may be some very well-intended people out there . . . but, you know, the problem is now that things are becoming very polarized around issues that are coming up. . . . If you don't know your history, you are doomed to repeat it. . . . They had folks during WWII and before who were trying to create a super race and people who view genetic weakness—and what does this mean for the country. . . . I think all that comes into play. . . . We get used as cannon fodder sometimes you know, we're throwaways. I think there's always been doctors who tried to prove that black folks were inferior.

Among those closer to the bottom of the economic range, and particularly among black men, we find a very explicit belief that medical advances are unlikely to benefit anyone in their community. A man with sickle cell disease told us:

> I sincerely do believe that a lot of the diseases that are out right now . . . the government does have cures for them. I know the power does. . . . I believe they've got a cure for it. . . . If that happens, the FDA is gonna lose a lot of money, the pharmaceutical companies is gonna lose a lot of money, doctors . . . because they wouldn't need Motrin, Ibuprofen, and a lot of other transfusions and things. They wouldn't need a lot of that stuff. . . . People with sickle cell anemia, they do pop a certain amount of money into, I mean, I've spent my share to get those forms of help. If I have sickle cell anemia and I have a cure, I don't need those things no more. That's gonna be a couple thousand dollars lost by me alone. Imagine the other people. I don't know what the percentage rate is, as far as finances. It's up there. It's up there. It's in the millions.

This distrust is sometimes associated with personal values of providers, but generally African Americans understand racism in medicine as a result of larger social and political processes. Often those in our study saw problems with science as extending beyond race to values associated with power in general. As one woman explained:

> If I were confident that genetic testing would be used for the proper and righteous reasons, I probably would not have a problem with it. But I know that is not the case. . . . I know people will be discriminated against. . . . I can see people even being divided up into groups—dictating to people what they can and cannot do. And I think that is just wrong. I'm not comfortable with it because I don't think our society is mentally capable of handling it properly. . . . This is difficult because almost like yesterday, you could say you had a baby, it had a problem and you dealt with it. What is all this "you got to know what sex it is, you gotta know if it's going to be blond hair and blue eyes or brown eyes and curly hair?" People start picking and choosing their kids as if they are going to K-mart! I don't like it!

Both men and women across the class spectrum gave evidence in these interviews of mistrust of the motives of genetic medicine. However, the women were more likely to focus on and speak about individual providers, while the men generalized more readily. It is not clear whether this is a cause or a consequence of women's greater likelihood of actually negotiating the world of biomedicine, but women frequently seemed more able than men to forge personal relationships of trust in clinical settings.

Fear of Stigmatized "Risk" Identity

When medical professionals offer counseling for genetic testing or other services, they usually do so using the language of risk. The meaning of the term *risk* is a function of context, and the context is quite different for biomedical experts than it is for laypersons in the African American community, particularly those caught in poverty. Identifying risk is most useful for those who have managed to eliminate constant danger and unpredictability from their lives. For those with significant resources (such as money and expertise) at their disposal, identifying a risk can increase their control. Today, however, from the point of view of many African Americans, particularly those at the lower end of the economic spectrum, risk is merely another source of blame, stigma, and exclusion.

This is apparent in the accounts of our respondents who do not describe statistical risks but instead speak of individuals as "being" risks. For example, "They told me I was a risk." This usage, describing individuals rather than probabilities as risks, strongly suggests that in the experience of these people the term is used to negatively label a person rather than to empower him or her. Exclusion based on genetic vulnerabilities has become a new social practice. Instead of creating mutual support and solidarity, as the concept of risk historically has done among the middle class, it is now used to create and isolate the "at-risk individual."

Regina Kenen (1996) placed the emergence of the concept of "at-risk health status" in historical context, pointing out that once acute illnesses were under control, the medical community expressed more interest in chronic illnesses and extended its control over formerly nonmedicalized conditions such as pregnancy and childbirth. She suggests that the new at-risk status appeals particularly to the upper-middle class, who expect to exert a high level of control over their lives and have the means to implement precautions, and to the corporations and medical institutions that cater to this class.

In contrast, when we looked at how members of families with SCD typically speak of risk, we found that typically the term is used neither as a quantitative nor as a mathematical one but is simply another word for danger. When *risk* is used to refer to an undesirable possibility, the "risk" of genetic disease is no more likely to be a central concern than are many other potential problems, such as loss of employment, health insurance, or a relationship. In our attempts to elicit narratives, the word rarely was used. When the interviewee introduced the concept, he or she was often quoting a provider, using a statement such as, "I was told that if we both were carriers there would be a 25 percent risk that our baby would have sickle cell disease." However, even the most well-educated interviewees indicated that they thought their own precise risk figures were not especially relevant to them.

Among the poor, risk also means a "stigmatized identity." For example, one woman told us, "The insurance companies don't want to cover you because you are a risk." Or as another woman explained, "I can't even get burial insurance . . . no kind of insurance . . . because you are too much of a high risk." In this quote, as in a number of others that refer to people as risks, interviewees indicate their aversion to the term by using it only in the second person rather than the first, even if they have to switch midsentence.

A woman in her thirties with SCD told us that her fiancé's family describes her as "a risk." She talks about the difficulty she had telling people she had SCD and how this resulted in them thinking she is a risk. In her experience, people have called her "a risk" when they wanted to discourage her from becoming a wife or mother. Her response to this situation was to have four children, two of whom have SCD. She takes pride in her ability to prevent and respond to her children's crises without having to resort to hospitalization. In this context, her experience with SCD is valuable. She no longer sees herself as stigmatized as a threat or potentially dangerous. She is now seen as useful and productive by the people who matter most to her because she knows how to prevent and overcome the crises of the disease. Contrary to the "preventive" measures that defined her social role as a "risk" not only to her personal family but also to the public health in general, mothering actually provided a way to triumph over the perception of herself as a risk. Her family and her two children with SCD can appreciate her expertise in dealing with their situation.

Like this woman, most of our respondents rejected prenatal diagnosis and selective abortion. If there is one clear finding to emphasize in this regard, it is that our respondents had no objection to abortion per se, but they rejected selective abortion specifically.

The association of risk with stigma may be related to the fact that since 1987 the courts have increasingly used medical testimony to prosecute women labeled "high risk" for failure to comply with medical advice when their fetuses or babies have died (Handwerker, 1994). She suggests that attempts to prosecute such women discourage other women from seeking medical care. Even though the assessment and management of risk for many conditions is neither standardized nor consistently applied, health care providers and the legal system unfortunately make decisions as if risk were objective fact. By contrast, patients understand risk as part of their complex and ambiguous social world. They are well aware that the label of risk itself has a negative connotation with weighty implications, while any possible benefit it could confer is both obscure and remote, particularly for those with fewer resources.

Perceived Irrelevance of Genetic Threat

Closely related to the concept of risk is the issue of relevance. In talking with our respondents we observed that it rarely occurred to many of them to give SCD the attention a health care provider might expect it to demand. Except for crisis situations, the danger of SCD may be perceived as less serious than many other problems. This is most obvious in situations of severe poverty, when people are struggling to meet their own and their children's basic needs of shelter, transportation, food, and clothing. We observed many people who had difficulty even keeping their families together due to the economic distress they were experiencing. One father in our study made this particularly clear. Besides his own children, he had taken in two of his brother's sons, ages 10 and 13, whom he describes as "needing some structure." He had been unemployed for the last year and was constantly trying to create work for himself, while his own sons were both entering "manhood" and facing confusion about their own futures. His oldest son's SCD was just only one of many problems. He explains: "There's an old proverb that [says] when your house is on fire you don't think about broken windows. In a lot of communities where sickle cell is [present], they're struggling. People are very poor and they have a lot of problems so they don't look at this particular problem [SCD] as being one that's overwhelming in relation to other problems that they have."

It is not surprising that preventing SCD is not a priority in his life, particularly when one observes that his son's health crisis is one of the few problems for which assistance is readily available. It is not unusual for a child with SCD to receive better medical care than other family members when they are located in urban areas near sickle cell centers staffed by specialists in the disorder.

For African Americans living in poverty, as many of our interviewees were, questioning or "testing" the genetic status of a potential partner, or considering the health of unborn, or yet-to-be-conceived children, is not a high priority. When an uneducated young woman fails to remember her precise risk figures, or doesn't appear to be taking them as seriously as clinical geneticists or genetic counselors think she should, she may be engaging in a much more complex calculus of multiple risks. One of those risks is her assessment of the probability of finding an enduring love relationship, marital partner, or of bearing children at all. As one woman told us, "Lots of kids have problems. . . . I wouldn't let that [the risk of SCD] be an issue."

Those who experience life as an endless series of challenges are particularly resistant to integrating medical constructions of risk into partner selection. Doing so threatens one area of life that offers happiness—the possibility of romantic love. Respondents frequently indicated that they felt calculating risk was incompatible with emotional commitment. One woman asked incredulously, "I'm supposed to ask what are your genes, and then do I love you?" She answered the question herself, saying, "That's like breeding dogs." We found very few women who were willing to adopt a "scientific" or "instrumental rational" approach to their own pregnancies. This is partly because pregnancy represents a commitment to a relationship that is recognized to have multiple dimensions of vulnerability, risks, and more immediate perils.

Aversion to Selective Abortion

Selective abortion was found to be acceptable to only a minority of the parents of children with cystic fibrosis surveyed by Wertz and colleagues. (1991). We also found significant indications of disapproval of selective abortion among both the CF and SCD groups. Of those interviewees who expressed a clear position on this issue, African Americans were significantly more disapproving of selective abortion for SCD (62%) than were whites for CF (46%). African Americans also distinguished more sharply than whites between the concept of selective abortion and abortion based on a more general desire not to become a parent at all. The dominant pattern was to explicitly reject selective abortion while simultaneously making a point of being "pro-choice." Respondents thus affirmed the right to reproductive control while making it clear that to abort on the basis of specific characteristics of the fetus was much less acceptable.

The aversion to selective abortion for SCD was strongest among individuals who were closest to someone with SCD. A good example of how such a relationship may alter one's view is the case of a college-educated woman we interviewed who actively sought prenatal diagnosis for the purpose of preventing the birth of an affected child. She was erroneously informed that the fetus was free of the disease and thus carried the pregnancy to term. Several years later, and after a wrongful-life lawsuit, she now believes it is wrong to use selective abortion for this condition. She feels the value of her child's life and the joy and meaning he brings into her life far outweigh the problems of his disease. This case illustrates both the greater receptivity to selective abortion among college-educated women and the tension between this receptivity and the strong emotional bond that develops when one is close to a family member with SCD. It should also be noted that the severity of the condition and the perception of how much the affected person suffers is a factor. Those who see the most severe manifestations of sickle cell often develop different responses to selective abortion than those who are exposed to more mild cases.

We found many African American parents who were aware of the risk of SCD before and during pregnancy yet would not even consider selective abortion. This option was routinely dismissed with statements such as "I'm not that kind of person." However, this does not mean they would not consider amniocentesis. As reported above, fifteen women in our sample who were aware of a risk of SCD did undergo prenatal diagnosis. But the refusal of selective abortion by all three of the women who received a positive result is testimony to the seriousness of this aversion. While rejection of selective abortion is often embedded in larger discourses about racism and genocide or mistrust of medicine, many cited an existing relationship with an affected person as a major factor in rejecting this possibility.

When it was suggested by health care professionals, African Americans implicitly (and often explicitly) considered selective abortion to be analogous to, or a surrogate form of, racial discrimination. Some respondents justified their position by saying, "Sickle cell is not so grave," or that a cure could come during the child's lifetime. But most of those who rejected selective abortion made it clear that it was more acceptable to choose not to be a parent, even after conception, than it would be to choose not to have a particular child on the basis of its physical characteristics, imperfect or not. One male respondent said, "I would not be with someone who thought aborting an imperfect fetus was okay." This is consistent with Dorothy Roberts's contention that "blacks have understandably resisted defining personal identity in genetic terms" (1997, p. 261).

Conclusion

We began this research with a desire to understand more fully how culture mediates responses to genetic testing. In this chapter we focused primarily on how genetic testing fits into the lived experience of African Americans. By interviewing members of families in which the disease or trait had been identified, we hoped to elicit narratives that would provide us with a deeper appreciation of the social processes behind African Americans' responses to genetic testing.

Not surprisingly, in many respects the responses of African Americans were similar to those of whites at risk for CF. Both groups include a wide range of subcultures, social classes, religions, and political perspectives. In both groups some interviewees had been exposed to only mild forms of genetic disorder, while others had seen more debilitating cases and fatalities. Both black and white respondents tended to regard genetic testing as an inappropriate concern when making an emotional commitment to a member of the opposite sex. They found the calculatedness of testing a potential partner incompatible with their concept of personal commitment and, of course, romantic love (Beeson and Doksum, 2001). Another similarity was that those in both ethnic groups often gave indications that there was stigma associated with being a carrier of a genetic disorder, maintaining that the label did not apply to them or that their side of the family was not, should not be, or did not want to be implicated. Members of both groups also often found that the experience of loving a person with SCD or CF made it more difficult to decide that such a condition merited selective abortion.

The greater prevalence of sickle cell disease and longer testing history for that disorder among African Americans meant that many more members of families at risk for SCD than CF had undergone carrier testing. It also meant that more individuals in that group knew they could have an affected child, yet this knowledge did not often lead them to ascertain a potential partner's genetic status prior to pregnancy. We found no African American families in which selective abortion had been used to prevent the birth of a baby with SCD, although certainly many such families exist—and some of our respondents did report that they would consider it.

While all of the perspectives on genetic testing we found among white families could also be found among African Americans, the critical narratives, or narratives of resistance, of African Americans were more elaborated, more developed, and more complex. They reflect a community memory that is sometimes only vaguely invoked and at other times sharply articulated; inevitably, this memory calls forth both a history and a present that distinguishes African Americans from their European American counterparts regardless of their social class.

The first theme we identified was the mistrust surrounding motives of genetic medicine. References made by African Americans to genetics indicate they see it as the basis of a new potential twist on discrimination, experimentation, and manipulation of groups. While many of these comments by our interviewees related specifically to genetic medicine, there is evidence that such mistrust transcends this specialty. For example, recent research on organ donation has shown African Americans to be significantly less likely than whites or Hispanics to trust the medical system with their organs (Yuen et al., 1998); and a study of eighty females who were initially nonresponsive to a recent Women's Health Initiative clinical trial found that black women are much more likely to agree that scientists cannot be trusted (Mouton et al., 1997). Whether or not interviewees personally had negative experiences, our data strongly suggest that they were likely to identify with the history and shared knowledge of other African Americans who did not fare well in their encounters with medical science.

The second theme that we identified, the association of the concept of genetic risk with stigma, was present among white as well as black respondents. However, the link between risk and stigma becomes highly intensified in contexts of racism and poverty. The use of medical risk to justify various forms of social control such as incarcerating pregnant women or removing babies from their mother's custody are practices disproportionately experienced by people of color (Handwerker, 1994). The themes of stigma and mistrust of medicine often coexist and reinforce each other in the narratives of African Americans, and these themes intensify as we move down the socioeconomic scale.

The third theme, the perceived irrelevance of a genetic threat, only makes sense when we recognize the greater vulnerability to poverty, the myriad other health problems, and the stresses of everyday life our respondents faced. This is a theme that has a particularly strong inverse relationship to social class within this racial-ethnic group. A specialized focus on genetic issues, whether in biomedical or social science research, makes it difficult to understand the importance of social context in priority-setting. Nevertheless, when many of the elements of daily life are problematic, they inevitably take precedence over a more abstract concept such as genetic risk.

Aversion to selective abortion, the final theme we describe, is distinctly stronger among African Americans than among other interviewees. The fact that respondents voiced this position in close association with a pro-choice stance seems at first counterintuitive. Only by recognizing African American women's unique struggle for reproductive autonomy, from slavery through the eugenics and birth-control movements, does their insistence on choice *and* the determination to protect all pregnancies from devaluation become fully understandable. This finding is consistent with Roberts's contention that African Americans recognize that "a focus on genetics will more likely be used to justify limiting black reproduction rather than encouraging it" (1997, p. 261).

All of these themes speak directly to the context in which many African American families live, a context that extends several hundred years back into American history because it persists in a community memory with varying degrees of clarity and intensity. Although this collective memory is constructed using concepts of race and ethnicity, present-day economic resources and opportunity structures also shape it. The African Americans who are least mistrustful of what genetics might offer, as we have emphasized, are those who are most successful. But even their receptivity is tempered by awareness of historical evidence that power is easily abused.

We believe these themes help to explain racial-ethnic differences in rates of utilizing prenatal diagnosis and other forms of genetic testing. They reveal key issues of concern to African Americans, many of whom find themselves at the lower end of the social hierarchy. They tell us how the social and cultural contexts in which genetic testing is offered affect its appeal.

The divergence between the narratives within the African American community and the dominant discourse regarding genetic testing cannot be ignored. Avoidance and denial of past betrayals perpetuates a cycle of mistrust. Efforts to resolve these tensions are consistent with the expressed goal of more consumer involvement in genetic services policy making (Holtzman and Watson, 1997, p. 15). However, the dialogue between African Americans and those who advocate genetic intervention has barely begun. Both policy makers and genetic service providers must do much more to acknowledge the abuses of the past if they are to gain the trust of African Americans. Just as important, African Americans have a lot to teach those whose focus has been limited to the laboratory or the clinic or who have failed to heed the lessons of history as they break new ground in genetic testing policy. We hope this chapter contributes to such a dialogue.

REFERENCES

Adams, M. M., S. Finley, H. Hansen, R. I. Janiel, G. P. Oakley, W. Sanger, G. Wells, and W. Wertelecki. 1981. "Utilization of Prenatal Genetic Diagnosis in Women Thirty-Five Years of Age and Older in the United States, 1977–1978." *American Journal of Obstetrics and Gynecology* 139: 673–77.

Beeson, D. 1984. "Technological Rhythms in Pregnancy: The Case of Prenatal Diagnosis by Amniocentesis." Pp. 145–81 in *Cultural Perspectives on Biological Knowledge*, ed. Troy Duster and Karen Garrett. Norwood, N.J.: Alex Publishing Co.

Beeson, D., and T. Doksum. 2001. "Family Values and Resistance to Genetic Testing." Pp. 153–79 in *Bioethics in Social Context*, ed. Barry Hoffmaster. Philadelphia: Temple University Press.

Bishop, J., C. A. Huether, C. Gorfs, F. Lorey, and J. Deddens. 1997. "Epidemiologic

Study of Down Syndrome in a Racially Diverse California Population, 1989–91." *American Journal of Epidemiology* 145 (2):134–47.

Bowman, J. E. 1998. "Minority Health Issues and Genetics." *Community Genetics* 1:142–44.

———, and R. F. Murray. 1990. *Genetic Variation and Disorders in Peoples of African Origin*. Baltimore: Johns Hopkins University Press.

Centers for Disease Control and Prevention. 1994. "Down Syndrome Prevalence at Birth—United States, 1993–1990." *MMWR Morbidity and Mortality Weekly*, August 26, 43 (33):617–22.

Council of Regional Networks for Genetic Services. 1997. *Guidelines for Clinical Genetic Services for the Public's Health*. Vienna, Va.: National Maternal and Child Health Clearinghouse.

Drugen, A., A. Greb, M. P. Johnson, E. L. Krivchenia, W. R. Uhlman, K. S. Moghissi, and M. I. Evans. 1990. "Determinants of Parental Decisions to Abort for Chromosome Abnormalities." *Prenatal Diagnosis* 10:483–90.

Duster, T. 1990. *Backdoor to Eugenics*. New York: Routledge.

Glaser, B., and A. Strauss. 1967. *The Discovery of Grounded Theory*. Chicago: Aldine.

Handwerker, L. 1994. "Medical Risk: Implicating Poor Pregnant Women." *Social Science and Medicine* 38 (5):665–75.

Hill, S. A. 1994a. *Managing Sickle Cell Disease in Low-Income Families*. Philadelphia: Temple University Press.

———. 1994b. "Motherhood and the Obfuscation of Medical Knowledge: The Case of Sickle Cell Disease." *Gender and Society* 8, no. 1 (March):29–47.

Holtzman, N. A., and M. S. Watson. 1997. *Promoting Safe and Effective Genetic Testing in the United States: Final Report of the Task Force on Genetic Testing*. Washington, D.C.: National Institutes of Health and the Department of Energy.

Kaback, M., J.-L. Steele, D. Dabholkar, D. Brown, N. Levy, and K. Zeiger. 1993. "International TSD Data Collection Network." *JAMA* 270, no. 19 (November 17):2307–15.

Kenen, R. H. 1996. "The At-Risk Health Status and Technology: A Diagnostic Invitation and the 'Gift' of Knowing." *Social Science and Medicine* 42 (11): 1545–53.

Krivchenia, E., C. A. Huether, L. D. Edmonds, D. S. May, and S. Guckenberger. 1993. "Comparative Epidemiology of Down Syndrome in Two United States Populations." *American Journal of Epidemiology* 137:815–28.

Kupperman, M., E. Gates, and E. A. Washington. 1996. "Racial-Ethnic Differences in Prenatal Diagnostic Test Use and Outcomes: Preferences, Socio-economics or Patient Knowledge?" *Obstetrics and Gynecology* 87 (5): 675–82.

Lane, P. A. 1994. "Targeted vs. Universal Screening." Pp. 157–60 in *Newborn Screening for Sickle Cell Disease: Issues and Implications*, ed. Karin Seastone Stern and Jessica G. Davis. New York: Council of Regional Networks for Genetic Services, Cornell University Medical College.

Lippman-Hand, A., and F. C. Fraser. 1979. "Genetic Counseling: Parents' Responses to Uncertainty." *Birth Defects: Original Article Series* XV 5C:325–39.

McKusick, V. A., with C. A. Francomano, S. E. Antonarakis, and P. L. Pearson. 1994. *Mendelian Inheritance in Man: A Catalog of Human Genes and Genetic Disorders*. 11th ed. Baltimore: Johns Hopkins University Press.

Mouton, C. P., S. Harris, S. Rovi, P. Solorzano, and M. S. Johnson. 1997. "Barriers to

Black Women's Participation in Cancer Clinical Trials." *Journal of the National Medical Association* 89 (11):721–27.

National Institutes of Health. 1987. "Consensus Development Conference Statement." *Newborn Screening for Sickle Cell Disease and Other Hemoglobinopathies* 6, no. 9 (April 6–8).

Rapp, R. 1994. "Women's Responses to Prenatal Diagnosis: A Sociocultural Perspective on Diversity." Pp. 219–33 in *Women and Prenatal Testing: Facing the Challenges of Genetic Technology*, ed. K. Rothenberg and E. Thompson. Columbus, Ohio: Ohio State University Press.

Rapp, R. 1999. *Testing Women, Testing the Fetus: The Social Impact of Amniocentesis in America*. New York: Routledge.

Roberts, D. 1997. *Killing the Black Body: Race, Reproduction, and the Meaning of Liberty*. New York: Pantheon Books.

Rothman, B. K. 1986. *The Tentative Pregnancy, Prenatal Diagnosis and the Future of Motherhood*. New York: Norton.

Saxton, M. 1984. "Born and Unborn: The Implications of Reproductive Technologies for People with Disabilities." Pp. 298–312 in *Test-tube Women: What Future for Motherhood?*, ed. R. Arditti, R. D. Klein, and S. Minden. Boston: Pandora Press.

Sickle Cell Disease Guideline Panel. 1993. *Sickle Cell Disease: Screening, Diagnosis, Management, and Counseling in Newborns and Infants*. Clinical Practice Guideline No. 6. AHCPR Pub. No. 93–0562. Rockville, Md.: Agency for Health Care Policy and Research.

Singer, E. 1991. "Public Attitudes toward Genetic Testing." *Population Research and Policy Review* 10:235–55.

Sokal, D. C., J. R. Bryd, A. T. L. Chen, M. F. Goldberg, and G. P. Oakley. 1980. "Prenatal Chromosomal Diagnosis: Racial and Geographic Variation for Older Women in Georgia." *JAMA* 244:1355–57.

Wertz, D. C., J. M. Rosenfield, S. R. Janes, and R. W. Erbe. 1991. "Attitudes toward Abortion among Parents of Children with Cystic Fibrosis." *American Journal of Public Health* 81:992–96.

Yuen, C. C., W. Burson, P. Chiraseveenuprapund, E. Elmore, S. Wong, P. Ozuah, and M. Mulvihill. 1998. "Attitudes and Beliefs about Organ Donation among Different Racial Groups." *Journal of the National Medical Association* 90 (1):13–18.

CHAPTER EIGHT

Genetics, Race, and Ethnicity

Searching for Differences

Joseph S. Alper and Jon Beckwith

Throughout recorded history, people have sought to define differences between members of their own self-identified groups and people in other groups. For instance, at the height of the Roman Empire, the historian Tacitus described those characteristics he observed among northern Europeans: "Their physical type is everywhere the same—wild, blue-eyes, reddish hair and huge frames that excel only in violent effort. They have no corresponding power to endure hard work. . . . When not engaged in warfare, they spend some little time in hunting, but more in idling abandoned to sleep and gluttony" (Tacitus, 1960).

But it was not until the mid–nineteenth century that the rise of modern science appeared to provide more solid approaches to analyzing differences between human populations. Biologists, anthropologists, and scientist-physicians applied their expertise to categorizing the peoples of the world into groups based on supposed biological differences (Gould, 1981). While scientists often disagreed on the exact number of distinct groups constituting the human species, they did agree that their efforts would lead to a scientific definition of "race." Such a definition would provide a rigorous scientific basis for the classifying and ranking of peoples. This scientific program had broader goals than simply an increased understanding of the human species. It also provided an explanation and a justification for racial discrimination and for the unequal distribution of resources among groups. Scientific researchers were among the first to propose these presumed social implications of their findings.

Today, scientists, with a few notable exceptions, believe that racial and ethnic categorizations have no scientific meaning or value (Marks, 1996; Ehrlich, 2000). Nevertheless, using techniques developed since Watson and Crick's discovery of the molecular basis of heredity in 1953, geneticists can now examine genetic differences between one individual and another as well as search for genetic markers that might distinguish groups. Such techniques have been employed to reveal the genetic basis of many traits and diseases. The success of this approach has encouraged some scientists to apply these molecular genetics–based approaches to the old problem of identifying genetic differences among populations that are thought to represent distinct ethnic and racial groups.

These new attempts to search for differences between groups may have social consequences for the members of those groups. Already, some have questioned the impact of genetic screening programs on certain ethnic groups in the United States. Others have expressed concerns about the possible adverse effects on ethnic groups throughout the world resulting from the Human Genome Diversity Project. We suggest that if care is not taken, the application of molecular genetics to the study of group differences could be used to support racist attitudes. We conclude that geneticists have an obligation to anticipate the possible harmful social consequences of research that explores differences and to take steps to prevent this misuse of their research.

Definition of Race

A scientific discussion of genetic characterization of groups requires definitions of the terms *race* and *ethnicity*. Ideally, such a definition would provide an unambiguous classification of any individual as belonging to one race or another. Today, most scientists agree that no such definition is possible (Marks, 1996; Cavalli-Sforza, 1997; Ehrlich, 2000). Those of us living in a racially diverse country can see that skin color, facial features, and body structure vary continuously across a wide spectrum. Furthermore, if we were to choose one physical or physiological characteristic (e.g., skin color or blood type) to define a racial group, the members of each group would still differ among themselves in other physical and physiological characteristics. Although it is not widely known, for many years researchers in genetics have accumulated evidence that physical and physiological characteristics are not suitable categories for defining races.

How much genetic difference is there between peoples of any two populations labeled as racial or ethnic groups (e.g., black Africans or white Europeans)? Human geneticists have learned that the vast majority of corresponding genes in any two people in the world are likely to be identical. Some genes, however, exhibit forms that differ significantly among peoples. These different forms of the same gene are called alleles. Since each person has two copies of each gene (with the exception of the genes on the sex chromosomes in men), a person can carry different alleles of the same gene. However, particular alleles are not specific to one population; any given allele can be found in most populations in the world.

Beginning with the work of Richard Lewontin a few decades ago (1974), geneticists have repeatedly confirmed that about 85 percent of the total genetic variation among the entire human species is found within single groups (e.g., within a race) (Cavalli-Sforza, 1997; Ehrlich, 2000). This finding means that only a relatively small number of genetic differences are responsible for the traits that distinguish groups—and, at the present time, we do not know which genes are involved. We do not even know which genes are responsible for such characteristics as skin color, hair type, and facial features. It seems clear that, at least for the foreseeable future, genetics will be of no use for categorizing the human species into the type of subgroups that we call races.

Nevertheless, to quote the title of Cornel West's book, *Race Matters* (1993). While race has no scientific basis, it is of enormous cultural, sociological, psychological, and even legal importance. People identify themselves as belonging to particular racial groups, and they mentally assign the people they encounter to racial groups. Race matters significantly to a black person having difficulty getting a taxi in New York City or being stopped by the police as a result of racial profiling while driving down the New Jersey Turnpike. Debates rage over the controversial use of racial categories in census forms, for affirmative action, and in correlating race and criminality.

Because race matters socially, some scientists still pursue the study of genetic differences among groups even though they realize that these groups are not scientifically well defined. These scientists explore issues such as whether different groups differ in their athletic ability, in their intelligence, or in their susceptibility to disease. For example, on average, African Americans have more severe medical problems than do white Americans. Are these differences genetic, or are they manifestations of social inequities and racism in our society? And, if these differences are genetic, does it matter?

Determining Genetic Differences among Groups

One source of information about genetic differences among groups comes from the detection of human genes correlated with specific diseases. Some genetic diseases are more common in certain ethnic populations than in others. Sickle cell anemia occurs most frequently among African Americans and other peoples of Mediterranean descent. Tay-Sachs disease is most common in Ashkenazic Jewish and French Canadian populations. In the United States and Europe, cystic fibrosis is primarily a disease of the white population. The blood disease ß-thalassemia occurs with high frequency in Mediterranean islands such as Cyprus, Crete, and Sardinia. Yet, for each of these genetic diseases, only a small fraction of the population in question is affected. Furthermore, individuals from any ethnic group can develop the disease. Therefore, one could not tell with certainty anything about the ethnic origins of a person from the finding of a particular disease-causing mutation.

Not only does the frequency of particular genetic diseases vary among different groups, but two groups subject to the same disease also may differ in the specific genetic mutation that causes the disease. For example, although cystic fibrosis is always caused by a mutation in the CFTR gene, the most common disease-causing mutation, deltaF508, occurs in 87 percent of Danish patients but only 27 percent of Turkish patients (Casals et al., 1992). As a result of the variations in specific mutations, genetic diagnostic tests for diseases must be tailored to the particular population being tested.

Genome-wide screening of a geographically diverse set of populations provides another source of information about genetic differences among groups (Pennisi, 1997; Enserink, 1998; Billings, 1999; Rosenberg et al., 2001). These screening programs are designed to distinguish groups by the frequency and type of their polymorphisms. Polymorphisms are differences between one person and another in DNA sequences at specific sites. Some polymorphisms are due to different alleles within a gene; others are due to alterations of portions of human chromosomes that do not contain any genes. Polymorphisms are detected by comparing the sequences of small regions of DNA among a large number of people. With the exception of identical twins, each individual has a pattern of polymorphisms that is distinct from every other individual in the world. For this reason, the criminal justice system has used the characterization of polymorphisms to identify perpetrators of crimes. This approach, called "DNA fingerprinting," involves the analysis of the DNA found in bodily fluids or tissues left at a crime scene.

The study of variations in polymorphisms among groups provides information about historical migration patterns and also lends insight into the relationships among languages. Groups closely related to each other are likely to share a higher proportion of polymorphisms than unrelated groups. Information gained by genetic comparisons of groups complements anthropological and archaeological data in the effort to understand the earliest history of Homo sapiens. In addition, scientists may be able to correlate distinctive polymorphisms in particular groups with specific diseases that are relatively more common in these groups. This approach would provide another avenue leading to the detection of disease genes.

The Historical Background

Why should we be concerned about advances in our understanding of genetic differences among people? These research efforts promise to provide new insights into genetic disease, offer the public genetic tests for many of these diseases, and expand our knowledge of early human history. The searches for the genetic basis of group differences have worthy goals. Nevertheless, history teaches us that, despite the worthiness of these goals, research on real or imagined genetic differences between groups has been used to justify racial and ethnic discrimination.

We have already mentioned how, in the nineteenth century, many respected scientists argued that the (presumed) behavioral attributes of racial groups could be correlated with physical features. Some focused on brain size, others on cranial structure, and still others on facial characteristics. Cesare Lombroso, for example, believed that criminals could be identified by merely observing their physiognomy (Gould, 1981).

The use of physical attributes to predict and explain behavior continued well into the twentieth century. Harvard Professor William H. Sheldon argued that body type provides important information about an individual's abilities, personality, and talents (Sheldon, Stevens, and Tucker, 1942). He defined three body types, which he called mesomorph, endomorph, and ectomorph, and described the type of personality associated with each type. William Shockley, a Nobel prize–winning physicist who turned his attention to eugenics, once stated that people were color-coded according to their intelligence (Shockley, 1972). Black skin, according to Shockley, was associated with the lowest intelligence. Even to this day, J. Phillippe Rushton of the University of Western Ontario argues that large penis size is correlated with small head size, which in turn is correlated with low IQ (Rushton, 1994). Since Rushton believes that men of African descent have larger than average penises, he argues for the biological basis for what he presumes is low intelligence in blacks. Needless to say, most modern scientists regard such pronouncements as ridiculous as well as racist.

The use of hereditary arguments to categorize human racial and ethnic groups predates the founding of modern genetics in 1900, the year Mendel's laws were rediscovered. Even before individual genes could be identified, scientists relied on family studies in their search for the genetic basis of such characteristics as intelligence, criminality, and even seafaringness, the tendency to "run away to sea" (Kevles, 1985; see Chapter 2 in this volume). In the first decade of the twentieth century, those who proffered a genetic theory of intelligence transformed Alfred Binet's newly developed psychological test from one designed to detect children who needed remedial skills to one that measured the supposedly genetically fixed trait now known as IQ. Almost immediately thereafter, the IQ test was used by American psychologists to determine the relative intelligence of groups. In 1917 Henry Goddard and his coworkers gave IQ tests to members of different ethnic groups immigrating into the United States and found that 83 percent of the Jews, 80 percent of the Hungarians, 79 percent of the Italians, and 86 percent of the Russians were "feeble-minded" (Kamin, 1974).

Although tests to "measure" the presumed innate basis of other personality traits were never developed, early-twentieth-century scientists felt free to draw conclusions about the origins of group differences in temperament, mental illness, and antisocial behavior. In a succession of articles in *Popular Science Magazine,* most of which were published between 1910 and 1920, scientists argued that a wide variety of personality traits had a genetic basis. In "A Study in Jewish Psychopathology," Dr. J. G. Wilson argued that "Jews are a highly inbred and psychopathically inclined race" (Wilson, 1913). David Starr Jordan, evolutionist and president of Stanford University, in "Biological Effects of Race Movements" spoke of the "lower races" that were immigrating into the United States from Europe and Asia and lowering "our own average" (Jordan, 1915). Dr. H. E. Jordan, of the University of Virginia, in "The Biological Status and Social Worth of the Mulatto," cites geneticist Davenport and statistician Karl Pearson in concluding that "negro traits (e.g. cheerful temperament, vivid imagination . . .) are of the nature of unit characteristics [i.e., mendelian traits]" (Jordan, 1913). Elsewhere in this volume we cite similar examples from the widely used German genetics textbook written by scientists Erwin Baur, Eugen Fischer, and Fritz Lenz (Baur, Fischer, and Lenz, 1931; see Chapter 2).

In the United States, these claims of racial inferiority and superiority from the scientific community, together with the analyses of the IQ tests, were used by state and federal legislators to garner sufficient support to pass eugenic laws (Kevles, 1985). These laws authorized the sterilization of men and women with supposedly bad genes, banned miscegenation (interracial marriages), and restricted immigration to the United States from those countries whose populations were considered inferior. Adolf Hitler, who had read the human genetics text of Baur, Fischer, and Lenz, used many of the same racialist views in his manifesto *Mein Kampf* (Müller-Hill, 1998). It is not unreasonable to speculate that this genetics textbook may well have contributed to the ideology that led to the Holocaust, in which millions of Jews, Slavs, Gypsies, homosexuals, and mentally ill people were killed. The belief in the genetic inferiority of these groups—and thus their threat to the purity of the so-called Aryan race—was considered sufficient reason to eliminate them.

For a considerable period of time after World War II, genetic explanations of human behavior fell into disrepute. But by the 1960s scientists were again arguing that genetically based differences in capabilities existed between supposed races. In 1962, Harvard anthropologist Carleton Coon, in his book *The Origin of Races*, suggested that "the step from the ancestral *Homo erectus* was taken by Caucasoid man in Europe no less than 200,000 years before the same step was taken by Negro man in Africa" (Coon, 1962). These scientifically invalid arguments were publicized by the Ku Klux Klan in support of their calls for continued racial segregation (Armstrong, 1976).

In a 1969 article in the *Harvard Educational Review* entitled "How Much Can We Boost IQ and Scholastic Achievement?" (Jensen, 1969), Arthur Jensen stated that identical twin studies had established the genetic basis of intelligence. Therefore, he argued, mean differences in intelligence between whites and blacks were largely due to genetic differences. He suggested that compensatory education programs as a means of creating equality were doomed to failure. Jensen's article was widely publicized, read into the *Congressional Record* several times, and used during the Nixon Administration to justify reduced funding for compensatory education programs (Allen, 1974). In their book *The Bell Curve* (1994), Richard Herrnstein and Charles Murray updated Jensen's claims. They argued, based on evidence that few other researchers accept as valid, that because African Americans were innately less intelligent than whites, welfare programs were doomed to failure. Glayde Whitney, in his speech as outgoing president of the Behavior Genetics Association in 1995, stated, "Like it or not, it is reasonable scientific hypothesis that some, perhaps much, of the race difference in murder rate is caused by genetic differences in contributory variables such as low intelligence, lack of empathy, aggressive acting out and impulsive lack of foresight" (Carlier, 1999).

While the claims for genetic differences in intelligence among races or ethnic groups have continued to this day, there are as yet no confirmed reports of genes that are responsible for the variation in normal intelligence among individuals. (There are, of course, genes that cause diseases that result in various forms of mental retardation.) Nor are there any confirmed genes that would enable a geneticist to distinguish groups based on the genomes of individuals belonging to these racial or ethnic groups.

Contemporary Concerns about the Search for Group Differences

In view of this historical background, minority communities are justifiably concerned about of the impact of genetic discoveries that bear on group differences. African American academics, in particular, have issued warnings about the misuse of genetic information.

Patricia King, law professor at Georgetown University, states: "Information in this case is going to fall into a society where racism is pervasive, where ethnic stereotyping and economic inequalities are rampant. Our problem is: how can we talk about our differences and not have our differences used against us— because historically that is how differences have been used" (King, 1997). Fatima Jackson, professor of anthropology at the University of Maryland, worried: "However, it is also recognized that these same data, in the wrong hands and with the wrong motivations, can concretize current socioeconomically rooted inequities under a thin veneer of 'science' " (Jackson, 1997). Physicians James Bowman of the University of Chicago and Robert Murray of Howard University, in their volume on genetic variation in peoples of African origin, hoped that their review will eliminate "common prejudices that are frequently associated with biological population variation" (Bowman and Murray, 1990). And University of California sociologist Troy Duster, in his book *Backdoor to Eugenics* (1990), warns of the potential negative impact of the new genetics on minorities.

These academics are all concerned about the use of genetic information to reinforce traditional racial stereotypes. They and others worry that reports will propose that some polymorphic differences are correlated with traits claimed to characterize African Americans, such as lower intelligence, aggression, sports ability, or talent for music and dance. These academics are also concerned that molecular genetics will lead to new forms of discrimination based on discoveries that certain groups are more susceptible to certain genetic diseases.

In the 1970s, several genetic screening programs that focused on particular racial and ethnic groups were introduced. These efforts resulted from the finding that certain genetic diseases appear more commonly in one group than another. The best-known and most successful program is the screening of individuals of Ashkenazic Jewish descent for the mutations causing Tay-Sachs disease (Kaback et al., 1993). Owing to a biochemical screening test, it was possible to implement this program before the Tay-Sachs gene was sequenced. The screening program was introduced in Jewish communities because of the relatively high frequency of the disease among Ashkenazic Jews.

Tay-Sachs is a fatal genetic metabolic disease for which there is no treatment. Affected infants usually live only a few years and suffer severe physical problems for most of their short lives. The disease is recessive; it can be inherited only if both parents are carriers of a Tay-Sachs mutation (see Chapter 1). The carrier parents exhibit no symptoms of the disease and are perfectly healthy. In families where both parents are carriers, the probability that each newborn child will inherit the condition is one in four.

In the Tay-Sachs screening programs, married couples were tested for the mutations. If both spouses were found to be carriers, they were so advised, and any pregnancies could be monitored. If the prospective parents agreed, the woman could undergo amniocentesis, and, if the fetus were found to carry both parents' mutations, the mother could obtain an abortion. The participants in the Tay-Sachs screening programs received detailed information about the nature of the disease, its genetics, and the alternative courses of action available if the fetus was found to be homozygous for the mutation—that is, affected with the disease. This education was for the most part administered by the local Jewish community and its religious institutions. Most carrier parents chose to abort a fetus found to be homozygous for the Tay-Sachs mutation. As with the use of a genetic test for any serious or fatal disease, some individuals experienced psychological stress. However, on balance, the genetic screening programs for Tay-Sachs disease have been, and still are, extremely well received by the Jewish community. In addition, there have been no reported instances of anti-Semitism arising from the publicity concerning the prevalence of Tay-Sachs disease among Jews.

Within the past few years, Ashkenazic Jewish women have learned that they are more likely to carry a mutation conferring high susceptibility to breast cancer (the BRCA1 mutation) than women in other groups in the United States (Struewing et al., 1995). Some leaders of the Jewish community feared that publicizing this fact could lead to increased discrimination against Jews. When a researcher from Johns Hopkins University, Ann Pulver, herself a Jew, began working with the Jewish community to implement a project designed to find new disease genes, she met considerable resistance and public criticism. Michael Grodin, a physician and ethicist at Boston University Medical School, worried that "Jews could become stigmatized as having high-risk gene pools" (Wen, 2000). However, despite these reactions, a recent survey suggests that most Jewish women are not concerned about such discrimination and worry much more about breast cancer itself (Lehmann et al., forthcoming).

This diversity of opinion within the Jewish community concerning BRCA1, in contrast to the strong support for of Tay-Sachs screening programs, probably reflects the growing awareness of the possibility of genetic discrimination. Within the past few years, the public has learned that information about the genes they carry could be used to deny them a job, health insurance, or life insurance (Beckwith and Alper, 1998; see Chapters 12 and 13 in this volume). It is not surprising that Jews, who have suffered discrimination for thousands of years, would be extremely sensitive to the possibility of a new type of anti-Semitism, one based on their genes.

Although introduced at the same time as the original Tay-Sachs screening program, the sickle cell disease screening program targeting African Americans was not nearly so successful (Bowman and Murray, 1990; Duster, 1990).

Sickle cell disease is a genetic disease that affects red blood cells. Like Tay-Sachs, it is a recessive disease, and, like Tay-Sachs, an accurate test for the disease preceded the sequencing of the gene. The sickle cell disease screening program was developed in response to pressure from the African American community, who argued that the health needs of African Americans were being ignored. Widespread screening, carried out through government initiatives, tested populations ranging from schoolchildren to married couples.

Unfortunately, the sickle cell program was much less thought out than the corresponding Tay-Sachs program. The accompanying education was often of such poor quality that healthy individuals who carried a single copy of the sickle cell mutation were told that they had the disease and would develop symptoms. In some cases, these individuals suffered psychological problems as a result of this misinformation, and some carriers experienced employment discrimination. The Air Force, for example, decided not to allow sickle cell carriers to become pilots. This decision was based on the theory, supported by only very weak evidence and subsequently refuted, that carriers produced some red blood cells that were defective in the transport of oxygen and so would have physical problems flying at high altitudes.

Despite these negative consequences of the sickle cell genetic screening program, there is little evidence that knowledge of sickle cell carrier status was ever used for overtly racist purposes. There is no doubt that racism, especially the belief that African Americans are not worth as much as white Americans, contributed to the poor design and implementation of the sickle cell screening program. Nevertheless, no one has pointed to the high frequency of sickle cell carriers (approximately 15%) in the African American population to suggest that the sickle cell gene be used to discriminate against that population as a whole.

More recently, researchers have begun to explore the unusually high frequency of diseases such as diabetes and hypertension (high blood pressure) among African Americans (Cooper, Rotimi, and Ward, 1999). Since it is known that genes can play a role in these diseases, some scientists argue that genetic differences between African Americans and white Americans are responsible for the disparity in the incidence of these diseases. These proposals are problematic. Other researchers point out that African Americans are among the most genetically diverse peoples in the world. This genetic diversity results from two factors: First, since the earliest Homo sapiens came from Africa, Africans have the longest history of all human geographical groups, allowing more time for genetic diversity to have developed. Second, during the slavery era in the United States, there was a very high incidence of interbreeding between black slaves and their white masters. It is known that genetic diseases are most common in relatively isolated and inbred populations. (Sickle cell disease is an exception. It is common in African Americans because carrier status also provides protection against malaria, which is endemic to many regions in Africa, so this gene no doubt has been selected for over time.) Considering the genetic diversity among African Americans, it is hard to explain, on a genetic basis, the high incidence of diabetes and hypertension among African Americans.

In view of these observations, many researchers have focused on environmental causes of diseases like hypertension and diabetes among African Americans. Several of their studies lead to the conclusion that the major contributor to high blood pressure among African Americans is the stress and other psychological pressures resulting from their daily confrontations with the various manifestations of racism. In one study, the researchers found that African Americans think about their race several times a day, compared to white Americans, who seldom think about their race (Jones, 2000). In another study, African American college students did more poorly than their white American fellow students on a test they were told would measure their ability, but they did as well as the white students if they were told that the test was simply a psychological one (Steele and Aronson, 1995). Studies of the psychological consequences of racism on African Americans do not prove that racism causes hypertension, but they do suggest that racism and thoughts about race play an important part in the lives and probably the health of African Americans.

Some scientists still appear to ignore environmental factors and focus instead on genetic explanations for all types of disparities that exist between African Americans and white Americans. This stance may reflect ignorance or willful dismissal of the reality and effects of racism as determining factors for some illnesses. This bias in itself is yet another manifestation of the pervasiveness of racism in our society.

The Human Genome Diversity Project

The Human Genome Diversity Project (HGDP) is an undertaking of great scientific interest (Gillis, 1994). It aims to "arrive at a much more precise definition of the origins of different world populations" (Report of the International Planning Workshop, 1993) by cataloging the genetic similarities and differences among populations. These populations are chosen for their relative genetic homogeneity. Thus, a geographically isolated group that has been living in a remote area for centuries might be studied, but a genetically hetero-geneous racial group like African Americans would not.

The HGDP is expected to provide detailed information about the frequency distribution of different genetic markers in different groups and contribute to the drawing of a family tree detailing the genetic relationships among popula-tion groups. This information will illuminate our understanding of the "his-tory and geography of populations," to quote from the title of the book on this subject by Dr. Luca Cavalli-Sforza, the leader of the project (Cavalli-Sforza, Menozzi, and Piazza, 1994).

Anthropologists will use this information to increase our knowledge about prehistoric migrations. Linguists will learn more about the relationships among languages by studying the genetic relationships among the groups that speak these languages. Population geneticists will be provided with a vast amount of new data for their research. If successful, the HGDP will reflect some our highest aspirations, reinforcing our humanity by continuing the age-old quest for human self-knowledge.

Some proponents of the HGDP have argued that the project will be of particular help to those indigenous populations being studied. They suggest that this benefit would arise from the knowledge gained about the genetics of various diseases in different populations (Resnik, 1999). We question this ex-pectation. The HGDP concentrates on genome-wide comparisons among population groups in order to achieve its goals of understanding the histories of peoples and their migrations. This methodology is not efficient if the goal is knowledge about the specifics of different disease patterns or etiologies among these groups. Any information about diseases acquired using the HGDP meth-odology would arise more by chance than by design. If a major goal were really to improve the health of ethnic minorities and indigenous populations, then a *direct* attempt to define the genetic and, probably more importantly, the en-vironmental factors associated with the particular diseases plaguing these peo-ples would be required.

Moreover, even if genetic information about specific diseases associated with an indigenous population were obtained from the HGDP, it is not clear that this knowledge would be of significant benefit to that population. It is widely recognized that, despite the public promises of imminent cures and treatments derived from new genetic knowledge, surprisingly little progress has been made in turning this information into improved treatments for genetic diseases. Tay-Sachs disease remains incurable, and the treatments for sickle cell disease, while improving, still show only limited success. We have no doubt that future genetic research will lead to cures and treatments for many diseases, but by that time many of the indigenous populations may no longer exist, at least not as homogenous entities. Furthermore, the history of transferring health advances to the poorer peoples of the world does not give cause for optimism. The grossly inadequate treatment of AIDS in Africa compared with treatment of the disease in the United States and Europe provides an especially stark example.

Despite its potential benefits, the HGDP has been controversial. Commentators have discussed several potential difficulties with, and negative consequences that might arise from, the program. These include monopolistic control over genetic information through gene patenting, economic exploitation of the genes of third world peoples, interference in traditional cultural patterns of indigenous peoples, and the ethical issues involved in obtaining informed consent from peoples to whom the concept of such consent is foreign.

We argue that racism is the central problem facing the HGDP. Because the aim of the HGDP is to define genetic differences (as well as similarities) among peoples, the potential for racism is *inherent* in the study design of the project. In view of genetics' sorry history of racist uses, we believe that it will require unprecedented efforts on the part of all researchers involved in the HGDP to prevent racism from negating the expected achievements of the project.

The HGDP, the Genetics of Groups, and Racism

Concerns about the Human Genome Project, in some ways the parent of the HGDP, have centered primarily on the possible harm to *individuals*. This harm might result from the loss of privacy concerning one's genetic information and the use of this information by others for discriminatory purposes. The controversy about the HGDP arises because of the fear that *entire groups* of people may be adversely affected by the project.

The HGDP employs a methodology common in science; it exploits differences in some observable phenomenon in order to understand the mechanism underlying that phenomenon. For example, geneticists generate or select for mutations in a gene associated with a particular trait. They then study the phenotypic (observable) differences in that trait arising from the mutations as a means of understanding the genetics and biology of that trait. For genetic studies of disease, the researcher will look at genetic differences between individuals who have the disease and those who do not, with the goal of understanding the genetic contribution to the disease itself.

However, unlike this sort of study, the HGDP is not concerned with the genetics of any particular trait or even with the genetic variation of that trait among individuals. Instead its focus is on the aggregate genetic variation among groups. This focus has the obvious danger of providing fodder for those who promote racist politics and ideology. Racists use information about group differences, whether real or imagined, to explain and justify social hierarchies and discrimination. The intent of HGDP is not racist; the researchers involved in the project, including its leader, Dr. Cavalli-Sforza, are known for their antiracist views. In fact, the founders of the project suggest that the information obtained "will make a significant contribution to the elimination of racism" (Cavalli-Sforza, 1997). Nevertheless, if a single-mindedly racist group of scientists were to design a study to provide evidence to support their ideology, it would not be surprising to find that their methodology closely resembled that employed by the HGDP.

If this analysis is correct, the HGDP is quite different from other scientific projects that have had unintended social consequences. In most of these projects, the consequences are what might be called by-products of the primary purpose of the study. The Human Genome Project, for example, has supported research that has facilitated the development of genetic tests for a wide variety of human illnesses. While the incentive for support of such project has been to improve human health and to provide aid in reproductive decisions, these tests can also be used for discriminatory purposes. After widespread reports of individuals unable to obtain health insurance or even jobs because of such tests (Beckwith and Alper, 1998; see Chapters 12 and 13 in this volume), some women at high risk for breast cancer refused genetic tests that might have been beneficial (Kolata, 1997). Such adverse consequences of the Human Genome Project can, to some extent, be separated from the desired applications of the research by means of antidiscrimination policies and legislation. However, because the focus of the HGDP is on the ethnic groups themselves, it seems to us that many of the possible deleterious applications of the HGDP's genetic information cannot be so easily isolated or controlled.

Racists concentrate on those differences among groups that they believe reflect essential characteristics of people, such as their behavior and aptitudes. Today, this essentialist perspective is bolstered by the perception, promoted both by the popular media and even by some scientists, that these characteristics are substantially explained by people's genetic makeup (Nelkin and Lindee, 1995; Beckwith, 1997). Thus, those making racist arguments often use the fact that there exist genetic differences among different racial and ethnic groups to explain, for example, differential performance by these groups on IQ tests. There is even a hint of this perspective in the National Research Council report *Exploring Human Genetic Diversity* (National Research Council, 1997). According to the authors of this report, "cultural differences between Mayans and U.S.-situated plains Indians are striking, and it would be of interest to know whether these differences are reflected in genetic differences" (p. 18). The expectation here appears to be that an explanation for the contrast in cultural accomplishments of the two groups (e.g., the elaborate Mayan temples and religious artifacts versus the less "advanced" nature of the plains Indians) may well be found in their genes. The social assumptions behind this statement are striking.

We do not fear the finding of genetic markers that correlate with differences in such characteristics among groups. Given the complexity of genetic and environmental factors that shape behavioral traits such as intelligence, any findings of genetic factors will contribute little to explaining the differences in those traits among groups. Rather, our concern is based on a long history of flawed scientific studies of the genetics of human behavior and on the misrepresentation of the genetic knowledge we have acquired about human behavior (Kevles, 1985; Billings, Beckwith, and Alper, 1992; Alper and Beckwith, 1993). Contemporary scholars making racist genetic arguments have repeatedly cited these flawed studies, ignored their refutations, and perpetuated the fundamental mistake of genetic determinism, namely, that a heritable trait is impervious to changes in the social or physical environment (Lewontin, 1976; Alper and Beckwith, 1993).

In view of this history, we worry that discoveries arising from the HGDP will be misinterpreted and misused to bolster racist theories of group differences. The HGDP will be searching for both the genetic similarities and genetic differences among groups, but, clearly, the project will be of little interest if no differences are found. Consequently, we argue that the major factor distinguishing the HGDP from a racist project is how its founders propose to make use of this knowledge. HGDP researchers can use the information to

learn about human history and geography; scientific racists can use this information to justify their theories that certain groups are superior to others.
Some scientific racists might even conduct further research in an attempt to
correlate the specific genetic differences found by the HGDP with group differences in those traits they believe to be important for ranking the races.

Is a Racist-Free HGDP Possible?

A promising avenue of research should not be abandoned solely because the
results can be misused (Beckwith, 1997). In the case of the HGDP, the knowledge that will be obtained promises to be fascinating and of significant potential intellectual interest. However, as we have argued, it is unlikely that this
knowledge will be of material benefit to the indigenous peoples who will be
studied. We are strongly in favor of research whose major impetus is an intellectual one. Nevertheless, because the only certain benefits are purely abstract,
any likely negative consequences of such a project require extremely careful
scrutiny and a firm societal commitment to prevent such consequences. The
potential danger that information from the HGDP will be used to fuel racism,
arguably one of the most pernicious evils facing the world today, mandates
such scrutiny.

The historic role of geneticists in confronting misuse of their science does
not inspire confidence that they will act to prevent the racist uses of the HGDP
(Ludmerer, 1972; Allen, 1975; Beckwith, 1993, 1997). It is true that for many
years a small number of geneticists, including Dr. Cavalli-Sforza himself,
have used already existing genetic knowledge to argue against racist ideas. In
Cavalli-Sforza's words: "Races do not exist. There is such a remarkable continuity in the variation from place to place that it is practically impossible to
define races, except in very approximate ways" (Cavalli-Sforza, 1997). The
realization that the construct of race has no biological meaning is just beginning to reach beyond the narrow academic community. A major article in the
New York Times was entitled "Do Races Differ? Not Really, Genes Show." In it,
geneticist Aravinda Chakravarti states: "The differences that we see in skin
color do not translate into widespread biological differences that are unique to
groups" (Angier, 2000). In the same article, the head of the Genome Project at
MIT, Eric Lander, points out: "There's no scientific evidence to support substantial differences between groups, and the tremendous burden of proof goes
to anyone who wants to assert those differences." Other geneticists have ex-

posed the flaws and misrepresentations of studies claiming a genetic basis for IQ score differences among groups (Beckwith, 1999).

Some proponents of the HGDP have argued that the genetic knowledge obtained by the project will only strengthen these antiracist arguments. We are not so optimistic. Since the antiracist arguments, already based on substantial scientific evidence, have not yet carried the day, why should we expect that the same arguments, strengthened with the new information generated by the HGDP, will be more effective? What will prevent racists from using that same genetic information?

If geneticists are to prevent the HGDP from becoming a goldmine of genetic information for racist ideologies, those involved in the project will need to become much more active in countering racist claims. Only a few geneticists have succeeded in bringing the antiracist argument before the public, and, all too often, it appears that their argument has not been sufficiently persuasive to overcome deeply ingrained racism. There are indeed genetic differences among groups, and, no matter how insignificant these might be, racists can always justify their hierarchical ranking of the races on the basis of these genetic differences.

We suggest that the relative ineffectiveness of geneticists' efforts to eliminate "scientific racism" arises from the lack of a social activism tradition among these scientists. As a result, today's generation of geneticists have largely failed to speak out to the public in sufficient numbers and with sufficient force to counter racist claims.

In several other scientific fields, scientists have, to different degrees, recognized the potential impact of their work and attempted, often successfully, to mitigate any harmful consequences. This recognition of the social responsibility of scientists dates primarily from the last half of the twentieth century. As a result of examining their activities during the colonial period in the third world, anthropologists have become extremely sensitive to the harm they can cause the societies they study. Physicists became concerned about the destructive power of nuclear weapons after seeing the devastating effects of their use in Japan in the final days of World War II. In this way, a heightened social conscience in both anthropology and physics arose out of an awareness of the harm caused by the activities of researchers themselves.

Unlike the situation in anthropology and physics, there has been a noticeable lack of concern among the vast majority of geneticists about the social consequences of their work. Throughout most of its early history, human genetics had been primarily an ivory-towered discipline with ideological but no technological impact on people's lives. Genetics began to move into the public spotlight only in the mid-1970s, with the application of molecular genetics to the study of human diseases. Furthermore, since the end of the Nazi era, there have been no dramatic cases of genetics' harmful effects analogous to nuclear weapons in physics or the negative impact on indigenous peoples in anthropology.

One might have thought that the use of genetic arguments and genetic studies by the eugenics movement of the early twentieth century and later by the Nazis would have caused geneticists to be more aware of the potential destructive uses of their field (Kevles, 1985; Müller-Hill, 1988). Unfortunately, most geneticists now teaching in colleges and universities rarely discuss this history with their students, perhaps believing it to be irrelevant to the new genetics, with its focus on the molecular basis of heredity. This absence of a historical consciousness has made it difficult for the younger generations of geneticists to integrate ethical concerns into their everyday work.

An intensive effort will be required to educate both those working on the HGDP and the genetics community in general. Such education would include a far broader range of issues than we have discussed here. At a minimum, the education of geneticists should include a history of the use of genetics in racist arguments and the social impact of these arguments. An important component of these studies would be an analysis of the role played by geneticists in making these arguments themselves, countering them, or failing to respond to them. The activities of scientists in other disciplines, most notably anthropology, in confronting the social impact of their research could provide models for study. Organizations such as the Human Genome Project and the various genetics professional societies should provide financial support in order to encourage the genetics community to embark on these educational efforts. These efforts would help to ensure that projects such as the HGDP will enrich rather then diminish our humanity.

REFERENCES

Allen, G. 1974. "A History of Eugenics in the Class Struggle." *Science for the People* 6 (2):32–39.
———. 1975. "Genetics, Eugenics and Class Struggle." *Genetics* 79:29–45.

Alper, J. S., and J. Beckwith. 1993. "Genetic Fatalism and Social Policy: The Implications of Behavior Genetics Research." *Yale Journal of Biology and Medicine* 66:511–24.

Angier, N. 2000. "Do Races Differ? Not Really, Genes Show." *New York Times,* August 23, pp. D1, D6.

Armstrong, R. A. 1976. "Science Exposes the Equality Hoax." *Crusader* (January/February):4.

Baur, E., E. Fischer, and F. Lenz. 1931. *Human Heredity.* New York: Macmillan.

Beckwith, J. 1993. "A Historical View of Social Responsibility in Genetics." *BioScience* 43 (5):327–33.

———. 1997. "The responsibilities of scientists in the genetics and race controversies." Pp. 83–94 in *Plain Talk about the Human Genome Project,* edited by E. Smith and W. Sapp. Tuskegee: Tuskegee University Press.

———. 1999. "Simplicity and Complexity: Is IQ Ready for Genetics?" *Current Psychology of Cognition* 18:161–69.

———, and J. S. Alper. 1998. "Reconsidering Genetic Antidiscrimination Legislation." *Journal of Law, Medicine and Ethics* 26:205–10.

Billings, P. 1999. "Iceland, Blood and Science." *American Scientist* 87:199–200.

———, J. Beckwith, and J. S. Alper. 1992. "The Genetic Analysis of Human Behavior: A New Era?" *Social Science and Medicine* 35:227–38.

Bowman, J. E., and R. F. Murray. 1990. *Genetic Variation and Disorders of Peoples of African Origin.* Baltimore: Johns Hopkins University Press.

Carlier, M. 1999. "Le contexte actuel des controverses sur les différences entre races: analyse de quelques évènements récents." *Psychologie Française* 44:107–11.

Casals, T., C. Vasquez, C. Lazaro, E. Girbau, F. J. Gimenez, and X. Estivill. 1992. "Cystic Fibrosis in the Basque Country: High Frequency of deltaF508 in Patients of Basque Origin." *American Journal of Human Genetics* 50:404–10.

Cavalli-Sforza, L. L. 1997. "Race Differences: Genetic Evidence." Pp. 51–58 in *Plain Talk about the Human Genome,* ed. E. Smith and W. Sapp. Tuskegee: Tuskegee University Press.

———, P. Menozzi, and A. Piazza. 1994. *The History and Geography of Human Genes.* Princeton, N.J.: Princeton University Press.

Coon, C. 1962. *The Origin of Races.* New York: Knopf.

Cooper, R. S., C. N. Rotimi, and R. Ward. 1999. "The Puzzle of Hypertension in African-Americans." *Scientific American,* February, 56–63.

Duster, T. 1990. *Backdoor to Eugenics.* New York: Routledge.

Ehrlich, P. 2000. *Human Natures: Genes, Cultures and the Human Prospect.* Washington, D.C.: Island Press.

Enserink, M. 1998. "Physicians Wary of Scheme to Pool Icelanders' Genetic Data." *Science* 281:890–91.

Gillis, A. M. 1994. "Getting a Picture of Human Diversity." *BioScience* 44:8–11.

Gould, S. J. 1981. *The Mismeasure of Man.* New York: W.W. Norton & Co.

Herrnstein, R. J., and Murray, C. 1994. *The Bell Curve.* New York: Free Press.

Jackson, F. 1997. "Assessing the Human Genome Project: An African American and Bioanthropological Critique." Pp. 95–104 in *Plain Talk about the Human Genome Project,* ed. E. Smith and W. Sapp. Tuskegee: Tuskegee University Press.

Jensen, A. R. 1969. "How Much Can We Boost IQ in Scholastic Achievement?" *Harvard Educational Review* 33:1–123.

Jones, C. P. 2000. "'Race'-Consciousness and Experiences of Racism: Data from the Black Women's Health Study." Paper presented at the American Public Health Association annual meeting, Boston, November 12–16.

Jordan, D. S. 1915. "Biological Effects of Race Movements." *Popular Science Monthly* 87:267–70.

Jordan, H. E. 1913. "The Biological Status and Social Worth of the Mulatto." *Popular Science Monthly* 82:573–82.

Kaback, M., J. Lim-Steele, D. Dabholkar, D. Brown, N. Levy, and K. Zeiger. 1993. "Tay-Sachs Disease: Carrier Screening, Prenatal Diagnosis, and the Molecular Era: An International Perspective, 1970 to 1993." *Journal of the American Medical Association* 270:2307–15.

Kamin, L. 1974. *The Science and Politics of I.Q.* Potomac: Earlbaum Associates.

Kevles, D. 1985. *In the Name of Eugenics: Genetics and the Uses of Human Heredity.* Berkeley: University of California Press.

King, P. 1997. "The Dilemma of Difference." Pp. 75–81 in *Plain Talk about the Human Genome Project*, ed. E. Smith and W. Sapp. Tuskegee: Tuskegee University Press.

Kolata, G. 1997. "Advent of Testing for Breast Cancer Leads to Fears of Disclosure and Discrimination." *New York Times*, February 4, pp. C1-C3.

Lehmann, L. S., J. C. Weeks, N. Klar, L. Biener, and J. E. Garber. Forthcoming. "A Population-Based Study of Ashkenazi Jewish Women's Attitudes toward Genetic Discrimination and BRCA1/2 Testing."

Lewontin, R. C. 1974. *The Genetic Basis of Evolutionary Change.* New York: Columbia University Press.

———. 1976. "The Fallacy of Biological Determinism." *The Sciences* 16 (2):6–10.

Ludmerer, K. 1972. *Genetics and American Society.* Baltimore: Johns Hopkins University Press.

Marks, J. 1996. "Science and Race." *American Behavioral Scientist* 40:123–33.

Müller-Hill, B. 1988. *Murderous Science: Elimination by Scientific Selection of Jews, Gypsies and Others, Germany, 1933–1945.* Oxford: Oxford University Press.

———. 1998. "Human Genetics and the Mass Murder of Jews, Gypsies, and Others." Pp. 103–14 in *The Holocaust and History: The Known, the Unknown and the Reexamined*, ed. M. Berenbaum and A. J. Peck. Bloomington: Indiana University Press.

National Research Council, Committee on Human Genome Diversity. 1997. *Evaluating Genetic Diversity.* Washington, D.C.: National Academy of Sciences.

Nelkin, D., and M. S. Lindee. 1995. *The DNA Mystique: The Gene as a Cultural Icon.* New York: W. H. Freeman.

Pennisi, E. 1997. "NRC OKs Long-Delayed Survey of Human Genome Diversity." *Science* 278:568.

Report of the International Planning Workshop of hte Human Genome Diversity Project. 1993. Porto Conte, Sardinia, September 9–12. Available at http://www.stanford.edu/group/morrinst/hgdp/summary93.html.

Resnik, D. B. 1999. "The Human Genome Diversity Project: Ethical Problems and Solutions." *Politics and the Life Sciences* 18:15–23.

Rosenberg, N. A., E. Woolf, J. K. Pritchard, T. Schaap, D. Gefel, I. Shpirer, U. Pavi, B. Bonné-Tamir, J. Hillel, and M. W. Feldman. 2001. "Distinctive Genetic Signatures in the Libyan Jews." *Proceedings of the National Academy of Sciences, USA* 98:858–63.

Rushton, J. P. 1994. *Race, Evolution and Behavior.* New Brunswick: Transaction Publishers.

Sheldon, W. H., S. S. Stevens, and W. B. Tucker. 1942. *The Varieties of Human Physique: An Introduction to Constitutional Psychology.* New York: Harper.

Shockley, W. 1972. "Dysgenics, Geneticity, and Raceology." *Phi Delta Kappan,* January, 307.

Steele, C. M., and J. Aronson. 1995. "Stereotype Threat and the Intellectual Test Performance of African Americans." *Journal of Personality and Social Psychology* 69:797–811.

Struewing, J. P., D. Abeliovich, T. Peretz, N. Avishai, M. M. Kaback, F. S. Collins, and L. C. Brody. 1995. "The Carrier Frequency of the *BRCA1* 185delAG Mutation Is Approximately 1 Percent in Ashkenazi Jewish Individuals." *Nature Genetics* 11:198–200.

Tacitus, 1960. *Tacitus on Britain and Germany.* New York: Penguin Books.

Wen, P. 2000. "Jews Fear Stigma of Genetic Studies." *Boston Globe,* August 15, pp. F1,F5.

West, C. 1993. *Race Matters.* Boston: Beacon Press.

Wilson, J. G. 1913. "A Study in Jewish Psychopathology." *Popular Science Monthly* 82:264–71.

CHAPTER NINE

The Origins of Homosexuality

No Genetic Link to Social Change

William Byne, Udo Schuklenk, Mitchell Lasco,
and Jack Drescher

During the early 1990s homosexuality was reported to be moderately heritable in both men and women. In men it was reported to be linked to the tip of the X chromosome in some families. The sizes of three different brain structures were reported to vary with sexual orientation in men, and the size of a fourth was reported to vary as a function of gender identity (Byne and Stein, 1997). These studies garnered a great deal of positive attention from the news media; however, reaction from the scientific community was, and continues to be, mixed. Some researchers concluded that "science is converging on the conclusion that sexual orientation is innate" (Bailey and Pillard, 1991a). More cautiously, others warned not only that reports of simple and direct links between biological factors and sexual orientation were founded on questionable assumptions about the nature of sexual orientation but that such reports also had a poor track record of reliability (Byne and Parsons, 1993).

Reaction to these reports has also been mixed among gay men and women. Some gay activists have maintained that, by bolstering the argument that sexual orientation is innate rather than chosen, the biological evidence will enhance society's tolerance of homosexuality. Increased tolerance would then make a variety of social and political goals more easily attainable. According to Gregory J. King, a spokesman for the Human Rights Campaign Fund, the largest gay lobbying group in the United States: "Fundamentally, [this research] increases our understanding of the origins of sexual orientation, and at the same time we believe it will help increase public support for lesbian and gay rights" (Angier, 1993). On the other hand, some have suggested that the very motivation for seeking the origins of sexual orientation may be symptomatic of homophobia at the societal level (Schuklenk et al., 1997). For example, Darrell Yates Rist of the Gay and Lesbian Alliance against Defamation countered: "Intellectually, what do we gain by finding out there's a homosexual gene? Nothing, except an attempt to identify those people who have it and then to open them up to all sorts of experimentation to. change them" (Angier, 1993).

It is difficult to conduct representative surveys of gay people's opinions about sexual orientation research, because it is impossible to know if subjects are gay or lesbian unless they choose to reveal themselves as such. As a consequence, surveys will potentially be biased in a variety of ways. In the United States, a survey was undertaken on a gay website (Barillas, 1998). Of the several hundred respondents, nearly 80 percent assumed that a genetic tag denoting a predisposition for homosexuality will be found. However, respondents seemed ambivalent about the implications of the finding. More than 70 percent assumed that if laws were passed to prevent abortions on the basis of a homosexual genetic marker, they would be ignored. Nevertheless, nearly 65 percent believed that a biological cause of homosexuality would prove vital to the struggle for gay equality. While these findings may reveal something about American attitudes, it is more likely than not that sexual minorities in different cultures will tend toward different views on the potential benefits and harms that could result from sexual orientation research.

What follows is a brief review of the current status of genetic research into sexual orientation and a consideration of the ethical and social implications of the quest for a biological explanation. Most of this research has been premised on a variety of questionable assumptions. These assumptions have been analyzed extensively elsewhere (Byne and Parsons, 1993; Banks and Gartrell, 1995; Gooren, 1995; Herrn, 1995; McGuire, 1995; Swaab, Gooren, and Hofman, 1995) and will not be examined in detail here. It should further be noted that problems in defining the phenotypes in question (homosexual, heterosexual, bisexual) are particularly problematic and have been addressed at length by Terry McGuire (1995).

The Status of Current Research

Neuroendocrinological Research

The neuroendocrinological approach assumes that the brains of heterosexual men and women differ from each other both structurally and functionally and that those differences result from early hormonal influences on the developing fetus. From this perspective, sexual orientation is viewed as derivative of a hormonally mediated developmental process that alters the normal course of sexual differentiation of the brain. Consequently, the brains and/or endocrine systems of homosexual individuals are expected to exhibit characteristics that would be considered more typical of the other sex. The hypothesis that the constitution of homosexual individuals is somehow intermediate between that of their heterosexual male and female counterparts is sometimes referred to as the "intersex hypothesis of homosexuality" (Byne and Parsons, 1993). A non-scientific prototype of this model was put forward in the nineteenth century by Carl Heinrich Ulrichs (1864), who defined a male homosexual as having a woman's spirit trapped in a man's body.

A number of studies have been interpreted as support for that hypothesis. Some of those are now widely regarded as theoretically untenable (e.g., Dörner et al., 1975; Gladue, Green, and Hellman, 1984). Some have not been subjected to replication attempts (e.g., LeVay, 1991), others have failed replication, and to date none has been adequately corroborated. In some cases, the very attribute in homosexual men that was hypothesized to be female-typical was subsequently shown not to differ between heterosexual men and women (Gooren, 1995).

Genetic Research

As in the neuroendocrinological research, some genetic studies have also been premised on the intersex hypothesis. These include attempts to show that homosexuals have opposite sex chromatin (chromosomal material) in their cells (Money and Ehrhardt, 1972) and studies seeking to link homosexuality with genetically controlled aberrations in the process of sexual differentiation (Macke et al., 1993). None of those studies met with success. More recent genetic studies (discussed below) are not necessarily based upon the intersex assumption and are compatible with a variety of more diverse and complex pathways to sexual orientations.

Heritability Studies: Although studies have suggested that homosexuality runs in families (Pillard and Weinrich, 1986; Bailey and Pillard, 1991b), such studies are not helpful in distinguishing between genetic and environmental influences because most related individuals share environmental influences as well as genes. Disentangling genetic and environmental influences often involves comparisons between identical and fraternal twins. The most thorough study of this sort was conducted by Bailey and Pillard (1991b). This study assessed sexual orientation in identical and fraternal twins, nontwin biological brothers, and unrelated adopted brothers of gay men. The concordance rate for identical twins (52 %) in that study was much higher than the rate for the fraternal twins (22 %). The higher concordance rate in the identical twins is consistent with a genetic effect because identical twins share all of their genes, while fraternal twins, on average, share only half of their genes. These studies assume that environmental influences would be the same for all brothers.

It would be a mistake, however, to attribute the increased concordance rate in identical twins to genes alone. If there were no environmental effect on sexual orientation, then the rate of homosexuality among the adopted brothers should have equaled the rate of homosexuality in the general population. Recent studies place the rate of homosexuality in men between two and five percent (Hamer et al., 1993; Michael et al., 1994). The fact that the concordance rate in adopted brothers was 11 percent (two to five times higher than in the general population) suggests a major environmental contribution. The rate for homosexuality among nontwin biological brothers was only 9 percent, a figure statistically indistinguishable from the 11 percent rate recorded for adopted brothers. Since the concordance rate for homosexuality among nontwin brothers is the same whether or not the brothers are genetically related, the concordance rate cannot be explained exclusively by genetics.

When considered together, the data from the twins and from the adopted brothers suggest that the increased concordance in the identical twins may be due to a combination of both genetic and environmental influences. Perhaps the most interesting finding to emerge from twin studies is that approximately 50 percent of identical twins are discordant for sexual orientation even when they are reared together. This finding, which has been consistent across studies, underscores just how little we actually know about the origins of sexual orientation. For further discussion, see McGuire (1995) and Stein (1994).

Linkage Studies: Of all the biological studies on sexual orientation, a genetic linkage study by Dean H. Hamer and his colleagues (1993) is perhaps the most conceptually complex—and the most likely to be misinterpreted, especially by those unfamiliar with the rationale of genetic linkage studies. Briefly, that study presented statistical evidence that genes influencing sexual orientation reside on a portion of the X chromosome known as the q28 region. Contrary to some media reports and popular belief, that study did not claim to discover any particular genetic sequence associated with homosexuality. It is important to understand that the statistical significance of genetic linkage studies depends on assumptions about the rate of homosexuality in the population (Risch, Squires-Wheeler, and Keats, 1993). Problems involved in calculating this rate have been reviewed elsewhere (Lautmann, 1993). Hamer's conclusions rest on the assumption that the rate of male homosexuality in the population at large is 2 percent; however, if the base rate is actually 4 percent or higher, the results he reported are not statistically significant. One leading geneticist argues that Hamer's own data support the 4 percent estimate (Risch, Squires-Wheeler, and Keats, 1993), and a Canadian team has been unable to duplicate the Xq28 finding in men using a comparable experimental design (Rice et al., 1999). Hamer's team subsequently found no evidence that Xq28 is linked to sexual orientation in women (Hu et al., 1995).

"Gay Genes": While many authors have recently speculated about the existence of "genes for homosexuality," genes alone cannot directly determine any behavior or psychological phenomenon. Genes merely direct a particular pattern of RNA synthesis that, in turn, specifies the production of a particular protein that then may influence behavior. There are necessarily many intervening pathways between a gene and a specific behavior and even more intervening variables between a gene and a pattern that involves both thinking and behaving. The term *gay gene* is, therefore, without meaning, unless one is proposing that a particular gene, perhaps through a hormonal mechanism it acts on, directs the brain to develop in such a way that an individual can be erotically attracted only to others of the same gender. Evidence in support of such a simple and direct link between genes and sexual orientation is lacking. Indeed, we do not know enough about how sexual orientation is encoded in the brain to even know if such a link is possible.

It is worth underscoring that "gay genes" are not required for homosexuality to run in families or for researchers to determine that it is heritable. That is because, to geneticists, *heritability* has a precise technical meaning and is defined as the ratio between genotypic variation (genetic variation) and phenotypic variation (observable expressed variation in a trait). Thus, heritability reflects only the *degree* to which a given trait is *associated* with genetic factors. It says nothing about the specific genetic factors involved or about the mechanisms through which they exert their influence. Furthermore, heritability gives no information about how a particular trait might change under different environmental conditions. Therefore, as described in the next section, homosexuality could be highly heritable even if genes influenced sexual orientation entirely through very indirect pathways.

How Might Genes Influence Sexual Orientation?

Since humans are biological beings, everything we do, think, or feel has a biological substrate at some fundamental level. From this perspective, the answer to the often-asked question, "Is sexual orientation biological?" can be only "yes." However, this answer is not very illuminating. It would be more productive to ask, "How might genes (or other biological factors) influence sexual orientation?" The possibilities can be considered from the perspective of three models (Byne, 1996).

The first is the *permissive effects model,* in which biology is viewed as providing the neural substrate on which sexual orientation is inscribed by formative experience (i.e., at birth the brain would be viewed as a blank slate). In this model, genes or other biological factors could also delimit the period during which the formative experiences that shape sexual orientation must occur. For example, some song birds can learn their species' song only if they hear it during a relatively restricted period of early development. If they hear the song of another species during that time, they may learn it instead. Once a song has been learned, that is the bird's song for life. The bird can neither unlearn that song nor learn another. While the song is clearly acquired through experience, it is biology that determines exactly when in development that experience must occur. (This example only illustrates how the impact of a particular experience may depend in part upon the developmental period in which it occurs—by no means does it imply that sexual orientation is acquired through simple mimicry.)

Formative experience is a subjective internalization of one's interactions with the environment and should not be equated with the environment itself. Internalization involves the biological processes of perception and the neural activity involved in interpreting and integrating ongoing experience in the context of the moment as well as in the context of one's life history. Because different individuals have different subjectivities, the same external environment would generate unique formative experiences for different individuals. From the perspective of this model, it is not surprising that attempts to find the origins of sexual orientation in parental relationships and other external environmental and social factors have been unsuccessful (Bell, Weinberg, and Hammersmith, 1981). The subjective internal representation of these variables would be of greater importance than the variables themselves.

In the second model, the *direct effects model,* biological factors are seen as exerting their influence through the organization of hypothetical brain circuits that mediate sexual orientation. This model is called direct because the arrow of causation points directly from discrete biological factors such as genes or hormones to sexual orientation. For example, it is possible that prenatal exposure to atypically large amounts of androgens (i.e., the so-called male hormones) organizes particular brain circuits in female fetuses so that they will subsequently be sexually attracted to other females. The direct effects model, nevertheless, allows for the possibility that direct biological effects could be subsequently modified by experience. Sexologist John Money speculated that the majority of women who were exposed as fetuses to masculinizing hormones become heterosexual because "social factors override their biological predisposition toward lesbianism" (Money, Schwartz, and Lewis, 1984). Thus *direct model* effects could either determine sexual orientation or produce a predisposition toward the development of a particular sexual orientation.

In the third model, the *indirect effects model,* the arrow of causation does not lead from biological factors directly to sexual orientation. Instead, biological factors would directly influence some other trait that in turn influences how sexual orientation develops. For example, rather than directly organizing the brain for one sexual orientation or another, genetic factors might instead influence temperament or other personality traits. These characteristics would then influence not only how the environment is experienced internally but also how one interacts with and modifies the environment in shaping the relationships and experiences that influence the development of sexual orientation. This model is similar to the *permissive effects model* but goes beyond it by including the possibility that the relevant formative experiences may, themselves, be strongly affected by hormonally or genetically influenced personality variables. To put it another way, individual differences, present from the moment of birth, influence how one perceives, interacts with, and modifies one's environment. That environment, which an individual has modified, becomes the substrate for the formative experiences that shape many aspects of that individual's psychological development, including sexual orientation. In contrast to direct model effects (which can be either determinative or predisposing), indirect model effects can only be predisposing, they can never be determinative.

Both the direct and indirect models are compatible with the existing neuroanatomical, endocrinological, and genetic data. The two models lead to different interpretations of three of the more commonly cited findings in the biological literature on sexual orientation. The first of these findings is that the propensity to engage in rough-and-tumble play appears to be influenced by prenatal exposure to androgens, the so-called male sex hormones. While this finding is controversial (Bleier, 1984), it has been described in several species, including humans (Goy and McEwen, 1980). Of course, the secretion of androgens and the expression of the brain receptors through which their effects are mediated are genetically influenced. The second finding is that, compared to heterosexual men, more, but not all, homosexual men recall a childhood aversion to competitive rough-and-tumble play (Bell et al., 1981). The third finding is that, compared to heterosexual men, more, but again not all, homosexual men recall their fathers as having been distant or rejecting (Bell, Weinberg, and Hammersmith, 1981; Isay, 1989).

In a direct model interpretation of these data, an aversion to rough-and-tumble play is the childhood expression of a brain that has been prewired for homosexuality in adulthood. This is the position adopted in the developmental theory of psychoanalyst Richard Isay. He explains a finding involving distant fathering by suggesting that biological factors wire the brain for sexual orientation and determine the polarity of the Oedipus complex. In Freud's positive resolution of the Oedipus complex, a boy's heterosexual instincts predominate and he identifies with his father while desiring a woman like his mother. In the negative Oedipus complex, a boy's identification with his mother and desire for his father are seen as the expression of homosexual instincts (Freud, 1924). Consequently, during the Oedipal period, prehomosexual boys would be erotically interested in their fathers. The father would recoil from the son's sexual interest, and, subsequently, "Gay men would distance themselves from their father in their memory in order to avoid recognition of this erotic attachment" (Isay, 1989).

Alternatively, an indirect model interpretation postulates that the biologically influenced aversion to rough-and-tumble play does not imply prewiring for homosexuality at all. Instead, this aversion would become a potent factor predisposing to homosexual development only in particular environments, perhaps where such an aversion is stigmatized as "sissy" behavior and causes a boy to see himself as being different from his father and male peers. This early sense of difference from other males might contribute to the subsequent consolidation of a homosexual identity (Bem, 1996). In an indirect model scenario, homosexuality would result from, rather than cause, the father's withdrawal from his son. This temperamental variant would arguably have different consequences in environments where a boy's aversion to rough-and-tumble play is socially acceptable, perhaps making no contribution to the development of sexual orientation at all.

The above example should not be taken to imply that either an aversion to sports or a rejecting father is a feature of all or even the majority of pathways to male homosexuality (Bell, Weinberg, and Hammersmith, 1981). Using the indirect model, one could conjecture how any number of temperamental variants might have an impact upon the development of sexual orientation. A given variant might predispose to homosexuality in one environment, to heterosexuality in another, and have no contribution to sexual orientation in others (Byne and Parsons, 1993). If the indirect model approximates reality, focusing on only genetic or other biological factors will result in incomplete and misleading findings. The interactions between biological and environmental factors need to be taken into account and controlled for in adequate longitudinal studies.

Social and Ethical Issues Raised by Genetic Research

Potential Benefits of Genetic Research to Sexual Minorities

Vigorous defenses of etiologic research on sexual orientation have been mounted by scientists defending their research and by T. F. Murphy, a U.S.-based bioethicist (Hamer and Copeland, 1994; LeVay, 1996; Murphy, 1997). Despite some differences in their respective approaches, common themes in their arguments can be outlined as follows:

1. Finding a biological cause would demonstrate that homosexuality is a natural occurrence, and it would put to rest claims that homosexuality is abnormal or unnatural. People who believe that homosexuality is natural are less likely to discriminate against sexual minorities.

2. Finding a biological cause is likely to result in a better public under-
    standing of homosexuality. People are likely to discriminate less
    against gays when it is realized that one does not choose his or her sex-
    ual orientation.

3. Finding a biological cause might allow gays to receive similar civil pro-
    tections under the U. S. Constitution as minority ethnic groups.

Doubts about the Potential Benefits of Genetic Research to Sexual Minorities

Normativeness of Naturalness and Normality. It is often assumed that nature
has a prescriptive normative force such that what is deemed natural or normal
is necessarily good and, therefore, ought to be. Historically, Western culture
has believed that homosexuality did not occur in nature (Boswell, 1980), and
traditionally scientists, religious figures, and philosophers have argued that
this constitutes sufficient reason to consider homosexuality worth avoiding
(Levin, 1984). Positions that homosexuality is unnatural and, therefore, wrong
are inherently problematic. Not only do they fail to explicate the basis upon
which the line between natural and unnatural is drawn, but they also do not
explain why we should consider all human-made or artificial things immoral
or wrong. Consequently, those holding such a position must define arbitrarily
what is natural and import other normative assumptions and premises to
build a basis for their conclusions. For example, they may rely on a spiritual
view of the world that considers man's activities as immoral or wrong when
they stray from nature's design. Inevitably, those holding such a "natural
order" position will employ the normative assumptions and premises of the
culture in which they live to rationalize their conclusions.

Normality can be defined in a number of ways, but none of them should
direct us in the making of moral judgments. First, "normality" may be defined
in a functional sense, where what is normal has served an adaptive function
from an evolutionary perspective. But even if we could establish that certain
behavioral traits were the direct result of biological evolution, no moral assessment of these traits would follow. Suppose that any trait that can reasonably be
believed to have served an adaptive function at some evolutionary stage is
"normal." Some questions arise that exemplify the problems with deriving
normative conclusions from descriptive science. For example, are traits that
are perpetuated simply because they are linked to selectively advantageous loci
less "normal" than those for which selection was direct? These could be traits
that, on their own, have no selective advantage at all. And, given that social

contexts now exert selective pressure in a way that nature once did, how are we to decide which traits are to be intentionally fostered?

"Normality" can also be defined in a descriptive sense as a statistical average. Appeals to what is usual, regular, or conforming to existing standards ultimately collapse into statistical statements. For an ethical evaluation, it is irrelevant whether homosexuality is normal or abnormal in this sense. Many human traits and behaviors are abnormal in a statistical sense (e.g., celibacy, vegetarianism), but this is not a sufficient justification for a negative ethical judgement about them.

The Issue of Choice. Historically, many advocates for sexual minorities have supported their cause by noting that people do not choose their sexual orientations. They reason, sometimes only implicitly, that people should not be punished or discriminated against because of feelings or behaviors that are beyond their control. This "lack of choice argument" is not restricted to gay-rights activists. According to a 1993 poll (Schmalz, 1993), compared with people who believe that homosexual individuals could change their orientation if they really wanted to, people who believe homosexuality cannot be changed are more likely to believe that social and criminal sanctions against homosexuality and homosexual behavior should be eliminated. Because the phrase "cannot be changed" is usually (but mistakenly) interpreted as being synonymous with "biologically determined," the results of this and similar surveys may be used to support the conclusion that belief in a biological cause leads to acceptance of homosexuality. However, such survey results do not establish that etiologic research changes attitudes. They are equally compatible with the interpretation that individuals who are more accepting of homosexuality are also more likely to believe it is immutable.

The lack of choice argument is flawed in several ways. Just because a trait is "not chosen," does not necessarily mean that it is genetically determined. The fact that we do not choose our native language does not suggest that the language we speak is innate. Furthermore, animal research (e.g., song acquisition in some birds as discussed above) has shown that behaviors that are socially acquired can, nonetheless, be immutable (Nottebohm, 1972). Thus, sexual orientation need not be biologically determined in order to be resistant to change. It could be equally impervious to change whether it is determined by genes or by experiential factors. The case that sexual orientation is not consciously chosen or freely mutable can be made without appealing to biology. The enduring nature of sexual orientation is shown clearly in critical reviews of the psychological literature reporting the low success rates of therapies aimed at converting individuals from homosexuality to heterosexuality (Drescher, 1998a). Very few, if any, of even the most highly motivated individuals have been able to change their sexual orientation, despite subjecting themselves to dehumanizing aversion therapies or investing tremendous emotional and financial resources in years of more conventional psychotherapy or psychoanalysis (Isay, 1989; Silverstein, 1991). Yet these results do not prove that homosexuality is biological, they only illustrate that, regardless of its cause, it is difficult to change.

Civil Rights and Legal Protections. It is worth asking why gay men and women should need to seek political cover behind the lack of choice argument. The rights of other kinds of minorities are not contingent on the issues of choice and immutability. For example, members of religious minorities are not asked to demonstrate that their religious affiliations or practices are innate or immutable. In fact, in the United States, one can change one's religion without suffering any loss of rights. The same can be said of the rights of political minorities in Western democracies. Edward Stein (1994) pointed out that, at best, the lack of choice argument can lead to only an impoverished form of gay and lesbian rights. Arguments for more genuine rights of gay men and women, like the rights for religious minorities, should be cast in terms of justice, privacy, equality, and liberty, rather than in moral terms about lack of choice or genetic determinism. That is, even if sexual orientation were entirely a matter of conscious choice (which is clearly not the case), homosexual individuals should be afforded full legal civil rights protections against discrimination on the basis of their orientation.

Another difficulty with the lack of choice argument is that, while sexual orientation is not consciously chosen, choice is involved in decisions to participate in sexual behavior and to publicly acknowledge one's homosexuality. Even if we agree that individuals should not be penalized for matters over which they have no control, proof that sexual orientation is genetically determined would not preclude legislating against all conscious expressions of homosexuality. For example, the "Don't Ask, Don't Tell" policy of the U.S. military penalizes the choice to express or to acknowledge one's homosexuality, not homosexuality per se.

Some advocates of civil rights for gay men and women have made (implicitly if not explicitly) what has been referred to as "the pragmatic argument" in support of biologically deterministic theories (Stein, 1994). This argument asserts that genetic and other biologically deterministic theories of sexual orientation should be embraced because they are persuasive and seem to have a desirable political effect. Stein argues that it is a risky strategy to link one's rights to the vicissitudes of such research. Biological research into sexual orientation has an extremely poor track record in regard to reliability (Byne and Parsons, 1993). What are touted as valid results today could turn out to be mistaken in the future. Making any set of fundamental civil rights contingent on a particular unproven scientific finding is, therefore, precarious. That people are persuaded by biologically deterministic arguments may offer a public relations strategy that will be successful in the short term, but it does not suggest a strategy suited for solidly grounding the civil rights of gay men and women.

Finally, using the biological thesis to argue for rights has proved to be as ineffective as it is flawed (Halley, 1994). The genetic basis and immutability of skin color, for example, do not seem to have a mitigating influence on racism. The legal efficacy of the biological argument was called into question by the highly publicized court battle over Colorado's Amendment 2, which sought to prevent any municipality from specifically offering civil rights protections to gay men and women. The appeal to immutability presented by civil rights advocates is conspicuously absent from the opinion written by Justice Kennedy of the U.S. Supreme Court. The courts determined that Amendment 2 was unconstitutional because it made gay men and women a separate class of citizens who were then denied access to the political process (Greenhouse, 1996; Schuklenk and Brookey, 1998). That is, the Supreme Court's ruling suggests that homosexuals deserve the same protection afforded other citizens not because they are gay but because they are citizens.

Potential Dangers of Genetic Research

In the absence of social tolerance, history suggests that any theory (biological, psychological, or social) for the origins of sexual orientation can be turned against sexual minorities. For example, in the late nineteenth and early twentieth centuries, medical sexologists like Richard von Krafft-Ebing (Schuklenk and Brookey, 1998) and the German homophile movement, led by Magnus Hirschfeld, sought legal protections for homosexuals on the grounds that they constitute a biologically defined "third sex." Before his death, Hirschfeld conceded that not only had he failed to prove his biological thesis, but he had also unwittingly contributed to the Nazis' persecution of homosexuals by stigmatizing them as biologically defective (Plant, 1988). It is highly unlikely that Nazi attitudes toward homosexuality were shaped by Hirshfeld. After all, the Nazis also simultaneously espoused contradictory environmental theories of homosexuality. Thus, while some homosexuals were imprisoned to prevent contamination of the German youth by exposure to adult homosexuals, others were castrated or sent to death camps to remove them from the breeding stock (Plant, 1988).

Some have argued that evidence of a genetic basis for homosexuality not only will make the case for rights but also will discourage psychotherapists from trying to "cure" homosexuality. Although in this chapter we argue against the relevance of genetic evidence to ethical and political questions, it is nevertheless possible that such evidence (even if it is ultimately discredited) may have some positive short-term impact on how the mental health profession views homosexuality. The long-term strength of this impact, however, remains to be seen.

It has been argued among those who find homosexuality morally unacceptable that, like alcoholism, it should be regarded as undesirable even if it does have a biological basis. A genetic predisposition to alcoholism might encourage affected individuals to abstain from using alcohol at all. By analogy, even if a therapist is convinced that sexual orientation is substantially influenced by genetic factors, he or she might encourage homosexual patients to change behaviors and sexual relationships or discourage them from publicly disclosing their sexual orientation. Alternatively, the therapist might view homosexuality as less desirable than heterosexuality and continue to accept a variety of mistaken and potentially harmful stereotypes about gay men and women. Thus, the therapist might set lower therapeutic goals for homosexual patients as opposed to heterosexual patients. More troubling is the possibility that those who think that homosexuality is undesirable will, in the face of seemingly credible biological research, abandon conversion or reparative psychotherapies and instead support medical or genetic treatments and preventative strategies.

The very language of the biologically deterministic theories may itself contribute to the stigmatization of homosexuality. Within the neuropsychiatric literature, biologically deterministic theories are frequently framed in pejorative terms such as *hormonal abnormality, deficiency, aberration* and "gene-controlled disarrangement of psychosexual maturation patterns" (Byne and Parsons, 1993). The danger here is that states perceived as undesirable and of biological origin are often assumed to be amenable to medical remedy or prevention. Within the past thirty years, physicians have used a variety of biological approaches in attempts to "cure" homosexuality. These included various hormonal therapies, castration, and brain surgery. The rationale of the brain surgery was to destroy the hypothetical "female mating center" in homosexual sex offenders. As recently as 1974, the *Journal of the American Medical Association* reviewed the results of this surgical approach and glibly concluded, without moral commentary, that the brain surgery was more effective than chemical castration (JAMA, 1974). Concerns have also been raised about the use of amniocentesis to detect genes for homosexuality so that it might be prevented in one's offspring (Hamer and Copeland, 1994). One researcher studying prenatal hormonal levels was initially preoccupied with the possibility of using his results to prevent homosexuality (Dörner, 1989), although he later repudiated his early enthusiasm for such an application.

If prospective parents believe that they are able to predict the future sexual orientation of a fetus with a prenatal screening technique, perhaps they would choose to abort a fetus that would not be heterosexual. If employed, such techniques, even if theoretically unsound, might appear to prevent homosexuality merely because the vast majority of individuals become heterosexual anyway. Abortion of "prehomosexual" fetuses would be most likely to occur in regions that continue to consider homosexuality pathological and provide no legal protections for sexual minorities. For example, in India homosexuality continues to be viewed as a mental illness and professional journals offer articles on its treatment. Furthermore, the World Islamic Mental Health Association also views homosexuality as a mental illness requiring management by mental health professionals (Schuklenk and Brookey, 1998). As recently as 1995, medical journals in Singapore debated whether a potential prenatal test for a "gay gene" should be offered to the public, given a lack of treatment for this "condition" (Lim, 1995).

Conclusion

When proponents of genetic research argue that finding a genetic basis of homosexuality will lead to improvements in the legal and social status of homosexual people, their argument is of a consequentialist nature. It is, therefore, open to ethical counterarguments of a similar nature. A consequentialist type of ethical analysis would require us to balance the likelihood and magnitude of potential benefits against the likelihood and magnitude of potential harms. Should the benefits of etiological research outweigh the potential harms, that research should proceed. Should the harms outweigh the benefits, it should cease. Our analysis suggests that defending this line of research because of its presumed political benefits is shortsighted and misguided. Such benefits could just as well be achieved by other means. Our analysis also suggests that the potential for misuse of this research by societal elements opposed to gay and lesbian civil rights is a real possibility.

Various scholars have appealed to the value of the truth in defending research on sexual orientation in the face of such ethical concerns. Even granting that, in general, knowledge is better than ignorance, we must ask whether all risks for the sake of knowledge are worth taking. Historically, hypotheses about the causes of homosexuality have led to attempts to "cure" what we would argue were perfectly healthy people—sometimes with disastrous physical as well as psychological consequences (Lautmann, 1993; Drescher, 1998b). As long as laws or cultural attitudes exist anywhere on the globe that discriminate against homosexual individuals, researchers who study the genetics of sexual orientation have an ethical obligation to consider the potentially negative impact of their work. Rather than dismissing these concerns, we believe that it is morally and ethically incumbent on those who support or conduct such research to work toward making the world a safer place to receive it.

REFERENCES

Angier, N. 1993. "Link of Homosexuality to Gene Splits Activists." *International Herald Tribune*, July 17–18, p. 5.
Bailey, J. M., and R. C. Pillard. 1991a. "Are Some People Born Gay?" *New York Times*, December 17, p. A19.
———. 1991b. "A Genetic Study of Male Sexual Orientation." *Archives of General Psychiatry* 48:1089–96.
Banks, A., and N. K. Gartrell. 1995. "Hormones and Sexual Orientation: A Questionable Link." *Journal of Homosexuality* 28:247–68
Barillas, C. 1998. "Gene Wars." *The Data Lounge*, March 3. http:/www.datalounge.com/cgi-bin/datalounge/survey/record?record=1252.
Bell, A. P., M. S. Weinberg, and S. K. Hammersmith. 1981. *Sexual Preference: Its Development in Men and Women*. Bloomington: Indiana University Press.
Bem, D. J. 1996. "Exotic Becomes Erotic: A Developmental Theory of Sexual Orientation." *Psychological Review* 103:320–35.

Bleier, R. 1984. *Science and Gender: A Critique of Biology and Its Theories on Women.* New York: Pergamon Press.

Boswell, J. 1980. *Christianity, Social Tolerance, and Homosexuality.* Chicago: University of Chicago Press.

Byne, W. 1996. "Biology and Homosexuality: Implications of Neuroendocrinological and Neuroanatomical Studies." Pp. 129–46 in *Comprehensive Textbook of Homosexuality,* ed. T. S. Stein and R. Cabaj. New York: American Psychiatric Press.

——, and B. Parsons. 1993. "Human Sexual Orientation: The Biologic Theories Reappraised." *Archives of General Psychiatry* 50:228–39.

——, and E. Stein. 1997. "Ethical Implications of Scientific Research on the Causes of Sexual Orientation." *Health Care Analysis* 5:136–44.

Dörner, G. 1989. "Hormone-Dependent Brain Development and Neuroendocrine Prophylaxis." *Experimental and Clinical Endocrinology* 94:4–22.

——, W. Rhode, F. Stahl, L. Krell, and W.G. Masius. 1975. "A Neuroendocrine Predisposition for Homosexuality in Men." *Archives of Sexual Behavior* 4:1–8.

Drescher, J. 1998a. "I'm Your Handyman: A History of Reparative Therapies." *Journal of Homosexuality* 36:19–42.

——. 1998b. *Psychoanalytic Therapy and the Gay Man.* Hillsdale, N.J.: Analytic Press.

Freud, S. 1924. *The Dissolution of the Oedipus Complex,* standard ed. Vol. 19. London: Hogarth Press.

Gladue, B. A., R. Green, and R. E. Hellman. 1984. "Neuroendocrine Response to Estrogen and Sexual Orientation." *Science* 225:1496–99.

Gooren, L. J. 1995. "Biomedical Concepts of Homosexuality: Folk Belief in a White Coat." *Journal of Homosexuality* 28:237–46.

Goy, R. W., and B. S. McEwen. 1980. *Sexual Differentiation of the Brain.* Cambridge: MIT Press.

Greenhouse, L. 1996. "Gay Rights Laws Can't Be Banned, High Court Rules: Colorado Law Void." *New York Times,* May 21, p.1.

Halley, J. 1994. "Sexual Orientation and the Politics of Biology: A Critique of the New Argument from Immutability." *Stanford Law Review* 46:503–68.

Hamer, D. H., and P. Copeland. 1994. *The Science of Desire: The Search for the Gay Gene and the Biology of Behavior.* New York: Simon and Schuster.

Hamer, D. H., S. Hu, V. L. Magnuson, N. Hu, and A. M. Pattatucci. 1993. "A Linkage between DNA Markers on the X Chromosome and Male Sexual Orientation." *Science* 261:321–27.

Herrn, R. 1995. "On the History of Biological Theories of Homosexuality." *Journal of Homosexuality* 28:31–56.

Hu, S., A. M. Pattatucci, C. Patterson, L. Li, D. W. Fulker, S. S. Cherny, L. Kruglyak, and D. Hamer. 1995. "Linkage between Sexual Orientation and Chromosome Xq28 in Males but Not in Females." *Nature Genetics* 11:248–56.

Isay, R. 1989. *Being Homosexual: Gay Men and Their Development.* New York: Avon Press.

Journal of the American Medical Association. 1974. [Medical News] "Stereotaxic Surgery Results in 'Cures' of German Sex Offenders." *JAMA* 229:718.

Lautmann, R., ed. 1993. *Homosexualitat: Handbuch der Theorie und Forschungsgeschichte.* Frankfurt am Main: Campus Verlag.

LeVay, S. 1991. "A Difference in Hypothalamus Structure between Heterosexual and Homosexual Men," *Science* 253: 1034–1037.

——. 1996. *Queer Science: The Use and Abuse of Research into Homosexuality.* Cambridge: MIT Press.

Levin, M. 1984. "Why Homosexuality Is Abnormal." *Monist* 76:251–83.

Lim, L. C. 1995. "Present Controversies in the Genetics of Male Homosexuality." *Annals of the Academy of Medicine Singapore* 24:759–62.

Macke, J. P., N. Hu, S. Hu, M. Bailey, V. L. King, T. Brown, D. Hamer, and J. Nathans. 1993. "Sequence Variation in the Androgen Receptor Gene Is Not a Common Determinant of Male Sexual Orientation." *American Journal of Human Genetics* 53:844–52.

McGuire, T. R. 1995. "Is Homosexuality Genetic?: A Critical Review and Some Suggestions." *Journal of Homosexuality* 28:115–45.

Michael, R. T., J. H. Ganon, E. O. Laumann, and G. Kolata. 1994. *Sex in America.* New York: Little, Brown & Co.

Money, J., and A. A. Ehrhardt. 1972. *Man and Woman, Boy and Girl.* Baltimore: Johns Hopkins University Press.

Money, J., M. Schwartz, and V. G. Lewis. 1984. "Adult Erotosexual Status and Fetal Hormonal Masculinization and Demasculinization: 46,XX Congenital Virilizing Adrenal Hyperplasia and 46,XY Androgen-Insensitivity Syndrome Compared. *Psychoneuroendocrinology* 9:405–14.

Murphy, T. F. 1997. *Gay Science: The Ethics of Sexual Orientation Research.* New York: Columbia University Press.

Nottebohm, F. 1972. "The Origins of Vocal Learning." *American Naturalist* 105:116–40.

Pillard, R. C., and J. D. Weinrich. 1986. "Evidence of Familial Nature of Male Homosexuality." *Archives of General Psychiatry* 43:808–12.

Plant, R. 1988. *The Pink Triangle.* New York: Henry Holt.

Rice, G., C. Anderson, N. Risch, and G. Ebers. 1999. "Male Homosexuality: Absence of Linkage to Microsatellite Markers at Xq28." *Science* 284:665–67.

Risch, N., E. Squires-Wheeler, and B. J. Keats. 1993. "Male Sexual Orientation and Genetic Evidence." *Science* 262:2063–65.

Schmalz, J. 1993. "Poll Finds an Even Split on Homosexuality's Cause." *New York Times,* March 5, pp. A 14.

Schuklenk, U., and R. A. Brookey. 1998. "Biomedical Research on Sexual Orientation: Researchers Taking Chances on Homophobic Societies. *Journal of the Gay/Lesbian Medical Association* 2:79–84.

Schuklenk, U., E. Stein, J. Kerin, and W. Byne. 1997. "The Ethics of Genetic Research on Sexual Orientation. *Hastings Center Report* 27:6–13.

Silverstein, C. 1991. "Psychological and Medical Treatments of Homosexuality." Pp. 101–4 in *Homosexuality: Research Implications for Public Policy,* ed. J. C. Gonsiorek and J. D. Weinrich. Newbery Park, Calif.: Sage.

Stein, E. 1994. "The Relevance of Scientific Research about Sexual Orientation to Lesbian and Gay Rights." *Journal of Homosexuality* 27:269–308.

Swaab, D. F., L. J. Gooren, and M. A. Hofman. 1995. "Brain Research, Gender and Sexual Orientation." *Journal of Homosexuality* 28:283–301.

Ulrichs, K. 1984. *The Riddle of "Man-Manly" Love,* trans. M. Lombardi-Nash. Buffalo, N.Y.: Prometheus Books.

CHAPTER TEN

Diversity and Complexity in Gay/Lesbian/Bisexual/Transsexual Responses to the "Gay-Gene" Debates

C. Phoebe Lostroh and Amanda Udis-Kessler

Toward an Inclusive Approach to the "Gay-Gene" Debates

What causes Republicanism? Is it God? Genetics? Poor socialization? Over-socialization? Abnormal psychological development because of poor parenting? Would learning the cause of Republicanism help us prevent Republicans from recruiting more Republicans? Have societies always had Republicans even if they weren't called that? If Republicans can't help being Republican, should we even try to prevent people from showing their Republican tendencies? Shouldn't their lived experience as Republicans be just as valued as that of people who are not Republicans? No matter what causes it, isn't Republicanism just another example of human variation, no stranger or more harmful than many others? Who benefits from the fact that there are Republicans (and, therefore, non-Republicans)? Is Republicanism even something we should care about in the face of more pressing issues?

Ridiculous? Absolutely. But consider how frequently such questions arise if we substitute the words *gay* and *homosexuality* for the words *Republican* and

We are extremely grateful to the people who responded to our survey and to Angela Bricker and Lisa Geller for their thoughtful suggestions. We also thank the Genetic Screening Study Group for lively discussion of our ideas.

Republicanism throughout. Then it becomes clear that GLBT (a commonly used abbreviation for gay/lesbian/bisexual/transexual/transgendered) identities are awash in controversy.

Part of the controversy revolves around whether there is a genetic component or cause of homosexuality. While such questions of causation are not new, recent work by evolutionary psychologists has increased public awareness of this issue. Evolutionary psychology claims that certain traits are not only "inherited" (as, for example, socioeconomic status often is) but also inherited genetically. Investigation of homosexuality as one such trait resurfaced in the 1990s with advances in molecular genetics (e.g., Hamer and Copeland, 1994). Hereafter, we use the term *gay gene* to refer to any and all genes implicated in the determination of homosexual behaviors or identities, a usage consistent with that of evolutionary psychologists.

GLBT people do not all agree about the gay gene. Consider two hypothetical scenarios. Jack thinks that there could be genetic factors that influence a person's sexuality but that it is immoral to seek those factors. Jack's position is supportive of the notion of a gay gene in that he accepts the idea that sexuality is biologically based and caused by one or several genes. His position is also, however, opposed to research intended to identify such genes. Leslie, on the other hand, thinks that while genetic factors influence her own homosexuality, they cannot account for every GLBT person's sexual identity. Leslie's position does not clearly support or challenge the existence of the gay gene, nor does her position involve any apparent claims about gay-gene research.

While these examples are hypothetical, they are consistent with perspectives that we have encountered. We believe that GLBT perspectives are more complex than those most often portrayed in the general popular press. Although it is common to speak of the "gay and lesbian community" as a unified whole, there is a status hierarchy within the whole. This hierarchy affects who tends to be most visible and whose perspective is taken most seriously. Here, we are particularly interested in the thoughts of those at the bottom of the status hierarchy—bisexuals, transsexuals, and transgendered people (collectively, BT people), the ones most often left out of the debates.

The Importance of the Gay-Gene Debates for GLBT People

While there are several reasons why GLBT people take the gay-gene debates extremely seriously, we mention only two here. First, the gay-gene debates involve questions that are basic to one's very sense of self as a GLBT person. To have one's experiences, desires, and identities be considered such an object of concern—indeed, a social problem—is jarring and discomforting. Second, at the same time, the debates have been seized upon by some GLBT people as a way to finally gain public acceptance of their experiences. In such a situation, it is not surprising that causation is so loaded a question for the GLBT community.

It is also absolutely crucial to understand the social context of homophobia (fear, hatred, and disgust aimed at GLBT people and homosexuality) within which these debates occur. GLBT people are stigmatized and treated as second-class citizens because they are not heterosexual (e.g., Blumenfeld and Raymond, 1993, Chapter 5).* In most places, they cannot hold hands in public without risking verbal or physical abuse. GLBT people can lose jobs, homes, and even children simply because of their sexuality. They are rarely allowed to adopt children, even the biological children of their partners. Except in unusual circumstances, they cannot obtain health insurance benefits for families organized around a same-sex partnership, nor can they collect a pension or social security benefits if a same-sex partner has died, no matter how long-term or monogamous the partnering. Their inability to legally marry deprives them of social status, claims to normalcy, and the great many material and symbolic resources that go with marriage. (Vermont currently offers a domestic partner registry that is functionally equivalent to marriage but does not have much of marriage's status. Moreover, the extensive outrage among conservative Vermonters suggests how much work remains before same-sex coupling is recognized as legitimate.) In a number of states, same-sex sexual activity is explicitly criminal. As a social force that perpetuates and encourages discrimination against GLBT people (Blumenfeld and Raymond, 1993, p. 224), homophobia ensures that it is publicly acceptable to treat GLBT people less humanely than heterosexual people on levels ranging from the interpersonal to the institutional. Even violence against GLBT people remains somewhat acceptable (e.g., Herek and Berrill, 1992).

The presence of homophobia and the GLBT goal of eliminating it underlie the gay-gene debates and give them a special sense of urgency. While all GLBT people identify homophobia as key to the negative experiences we face because of our sexualities, we are divided on whether finding a gay gene would alleviate or exacerbate homophobia. Some GLBT people believe that finding a gay gene

---

*Here, we need to be careful to note that transsexual and transgender people may consider themselves heterosexual and may face social penalties more for their gender identities than for their sexual identities. However, even this distinction does not always come into play, as when cross-dressing men are taken to be gay and treated accordingly.

would provide irrefutable proof that homosexuality is not chosen, which in turn would remove most of the justification for homophobia. Other GLBT people (the authors included) argue that the causes of homophobia are too complex, and homophobia itself too institutionalized, to be eradicated on the basis of scientific evidence alone.

The ways in which the gay-gene debates impact GLBT senses of self, and questions of the relationship between these debates and the eradication of homophobia, appear in GLBT responses to the gay-gene debates, as do a number of other themes and concerns. We now turn to the responses to a survey that we distributed and consider what these responses can tell us about the diversity and complexity in GLBT responses to the gay-gene debates.

A Survey of GLBT Opinion on the Gay-Gene Debates

We used the Internet to send an open-ended survey to sixty individuals and organizations comprised of GLBT people and allies (heterosexual people who support GLBT people). After identifying our sexual identities, feminist commitments, and interest in the gay-gene debates,* we asked:

1. Do you believe that there is a biological cause for homosexuality (same-sex attraction, or whatever word is most comfortable for you)? If so, do you think there is a genetic component? If you don't believe that there is a "gay gene," how do you address the issue of causation (or do you simply not address it)?

2. How do your beliefs on the subject impact your political sensibilities and priorities, religious values and practices, reproductive choices, etc. (if they do at all)?

3. How do you think proof of the presence or absence of a biological/ genetic component of homosexuality would impact homophobia/ heterosexism/social stigma/discrimination, if at all?

4. Finally, we'd like to know a bit about you to help us sort out whether people with different political, religious, social, economic, or other (e.g., racial, bi/trans) affiliations and identities answer the above questions differently in patterned ways.

---

*We share a commitment to feminism but have different sexual identities (bisexual and lesbian) even though our sexual histories are not very different. One of us is a molecular biologist concerned about ethical issues and genetics, and the other is a sociologist with a focus on inequality, sexuality, and religion. Together, we have been "out" for more than thirty-one years and have lived as "out" people in places including Manhattan, Boston, rural New Mexico, the Rust Belt, and the Midwest.

GLBT Responses to the Gay-Gene Debates

Only two people who explicitly identified themselves as gay or lesbian (as opposed to BT, queer, or heterosexual) responded to our survey, and both of them believe that genetics played a causal role in their homosexuality. This corresponds with our personal experience, in which lesbians and gay men are more likely than BT people to support gay-gene research and to be more invested in there being a genetic cause for their sexual desires. Consider this response from Lydia, a lesbian (all names are pseudonyms): "I was married 28 years before I realized that I was gay, but once I did well my whole life made sense. Is gayness genetic? You bet! No question. No doubt. . . . The vast majority of us gay folks grew up in straight families, so nurture could not be the culprit [it has] to be nature." Lydia believes that her gayness is genetic rather than learned and expresses no discomfort in seeking the culprit (her word) for homosexuality. She is also willing to generalize from her own personal experience to that of all "gay folks." Finally, Lydia reports a sexual history with women and men but identifies exclusively as lesbian (which might not be true of all women with her sexual history).

To explain why we think lesbians and gay men are likely to give responses similar to this one, it is helpful to consider briefly the notion of "naturalness." The sexual desire that heterosexuals experience toward people of the opposite sex not only "feels natural" but also is treated as natural by a range of social institutions; that is, heterosexuals are explicitly taught that this desire is natural. Same-sex attraction also feels natural to those of us who experience it, but the social support for its naturalness is missing; indeed, certain social institutions (particularly the church and the medical establishment) have gone out of their way to make sure we know that there is something unnatural and abnormal about same-sex desire. In grasping for support for the naturalness of their sexual desires, lesbians and gay men are likely to rely on whatever language is currently grounding the idea of sexual desire being natural (which, in this cultural moment, is genetics).

Lesbians and gay men, while clearly identified as "other" by heterosexuals and significantly penalized for this, actually seem *more* like heterosexuals in certain ways than do BT people. Lesbian and gay sexual desire is directed at a single gender (unlike bisexual sexual desire) and is experienced by people who tend to have a single gender identity consonant with their biological bodies (which separates them from transgendered/transsexual people). We suspect that BT people, falling farther from the current sexual and gender order than do lesbians and gay men, are more likely to be suspicious of such an order and to find little comfort in claims of genetic naturalness. This may be even more the case given that no one has proposed seeking a gene for bisexuality, transgender identity, or transsexuality. We suspect that homosexuality's resemblance to heterosexuality (as well as its difference from heterosexuality) plays a role in this fact. Other likely reasons for the search for a "gay" gene (rather than a "bi" or "trans" gene) include the greater visibility of homosexuality, the relatively newer presence of bi- and trans-identified people in the GLBT community, and the belief among many that BT people are really just lesbians and gay men who cannot accept their homosexuality.

As noted, the gay man, Cary, who answered our survey was also supportive of the idea of a gay gene: "God created gay genes. God loves variety. God loves play. Though [proof of a gay gene] shouldn't be necessary to end homophobia, I am told that it helps those who don't have personal experience of homosexuality accept it as a 'given.' My fear is that such proof won't enable them to see it as a 'gift' but rather [to] regard it as a 'disability.'" Like Lydia, Cary believes that homosexuality is genetically determined. Unlike Lydia, his answer draws on religious claims, as well as including a (somewhat ambivalent) comment on the potential role that the existence of a gay gene could play in reducing homophobia. We briefly address each of these points in turn.

Homophobia is deeply embedded in religious traditions, particularly the Christian tradition(s) most widely practiced in the United States. Most of the claims grounding both personal disgust with GLBT people and the refusal of various rights to us are based on Biblical passages and religious tradition. At the same time, a growing number of religious GLBT people such as Cary, from various traditions, are seeking to change both the official stances of their religious bodies and the personal sense of welcome to GLBT people from religious communities. Some representative examples of writing on this subject include S. Geis and D. Messer (1994), a series of pros and cons about homosexuality in the church; K. Hartman (1996), a series of stories about congregations struggling over homosexuality; and J. Wood (2000), a scholarly and pastoral study on the struggle within one Christian denomination, the United Methodist Church.

Religion and the gay-gene debates can become interwoven when, for example, GLBT Christians, responding to conservative Christian claims of homosexuality's unnaturalness, claim, "God made us this way." We see a variant of this claim in Cary's answer, which is only unusual in its direct linking of gay genes and the idea that God makes people gay. A bisexual witch (Max) provided another perspective on religion and the causality debates: "I know that many queers feel that their preference was with them from birth. Therefore, we must accept that either there is a biological component to some (or all) sexuality, or that our personalities are shaped by something not biological before we are born. This last possibility leads us to consider the idea of souls." More frequently, GLBT people raise the two ideas of genetics and religion separately. Claims made about the existence of a gay gene are seen as valuable by Christian or Jewish GLBT people in terms of helping to convince their religious institutions to accept them fully, despite what scripture and tradition may say.

Turning from religion to politics, Cary's comment that finding a genetic cause helps heterosexuals accept homosexuality as a given touches on a theme common among GLBT activists. This is the idea that GLBT people will be most effectively able to overcome homophobia by establishing themselves as a pseudoethnic minority equivalent to African Americans or other race-based groups. GLBT people subscribing to this idea tend to favor a civil rights strategy focused on obtaining access to mainstream institutions such as marriage and the military. We believe that GLBT people who favor this approach are more likely to support gay-gene research because there is precedent for (at least some) success in the civil rights movement to outlaw discrimination based on race and in the women's rights movement to end discrimination based on biological sex. It has also been our experience that lesbians and gay men are more likely than BT people to support the pseudoethnic minority–civil rights approach to fighting homophobia. We suspect that our earlier comments about GL versus BT support for the idea of a gay gene could also be applied to this point.

There are, of course, GLBT people who support pursuing civil rights but nevertheless do not support gay-gene research. For example, Beth responded: "Hello! Wake up! We don't care whether there is a gay gene. We don't care about anything beyond doing all that we can to ensure equal treatment and rights in all aspects of life." Similarly, a bisexual man, Brian, included the following in his answer: " 'This is what feels right and works best for me' should be just as valid a reason in a free society as 'I was born this way.' "

Another objection to gay-gene research expressed by several of our respondents is that society should not use genetics to attempt to explain homosexuality. For example, as part of his answer, Ian wrote: "Why do we need to explain homosexuality when no one has successfully explained heterosexuality?" He suggests that using genetics to study homosexuality inevitably exaggerates the "abnormality" of homosexuality, finally emphasizing what he understands as the inappropriate nature of seeking a gay gene by ending his response, "Is there a straight gene?"

Similarly, Darren wrote: "Because our culture tends to focus on the scientific aspects of any discussion, identifying genetic influences on sexuality will probably lead to our rabid fixation on them (how to detect them, whether to alter them, what they imply for us as a protected class, etc.). This is a great shame, because our culture is very sex-phobic and wants to avoid the important emotional/cultural discussions about sexuality by focusing on the medical, which [discovering a gay gene] would play right into."

Traci, a transgendered woman, expressed her belief that there is a physiological cause for homosexuality and transgenderism (carefully avoiding the issue of whether or not the cause is genetic) but cautioned that searches for causation are hurtful to GLBT people: "I believe there is a physiological cause for transgender [based on gestational hormones]. I also believe that homosexuality has a physiological cause. . . . I decided long ago that asking 'why' I am the way I am is a manifestation of nonacceptance. For someone else to ask why I am the way I am is similarly a manifestation of nonacceptance. Those people who hate people based on one's homosexuality or one's transgender will continue to hate, no matter what causative conditions are ultimately proved." This quotation expresses a key view held by those who oppose gay-gene research, which is that explaining the origins of homosexuality or transgenderism will not aid in ending homophobia. GLBT people may react with suspicion to questions of causation for a number of reasons. Our experience has been that more BT people than lesbians and gay men harbor this kind of suspicion, possibly for reasons discussed above. Some GLBT people may also mistrust science more generally, as seen in Ian's and Darren's answers. A number of politically progressive GLBT people believe that "scientific progress" has historically supported many of the privileges accorded to higher-status people simply by virtue of their race, gender, and class, and that higher-status people may in turn invest science with more positive value.

We believe that "causation suspicion" is common in the GLBT community but is underrepresented in the mainstream debates for several reasons. First, this kind of response is harder than others to categorize as either for or against the gay gene, even though it is clearly against gay-gene research. Furthermore, people suspicious of causation arguments may refrain from publicly participating in the debates on the grounds that any involvement would support the debates, which they see as inappropriate to begin with.

An extensive and complex response that incorporates many of these themes came from Anne, a bisexual woman who identifies herself as politically leftist. She wrote:

> I believe for some people [sexuality] is mostly genetic/biological, and for others, it is an environmental response. That is, it seems a lot of people could go "either way" genetically speaking, but some are programmed genetically one way or another. For the "either way" folks (such as myself) it is about preference, experience, etc. (And for some reason, it seems to be more often genetically programmed for men than women.) I do not believe ANYTHING so complex as orientation could ever be ALL genetic. Whether nonstraightness has a genetic component or not is irrelevant, although it does make a useful argument against the "sin against God" folks. If people could detect nonstraightness in [a human embryo], they might abort.

Several contradictory opinions are evident in Anne's complex response, which appears to be a conversation between herself and a devil's advocate. First, she takes the position that sexuality is neither entirely environmental nor biological in origin and, furthermore, that the exact same sexuality (e.g., lesbianism) may be biological for one person but not for another. Then, perhaps in allegiance with political leftists who criticize biological determinism in general, she seemingly contradicts her first statements regarding sexuality as "programmed" by stating that orientation cannot be entirely genetic. Anne continues to wrestle with the possibilities, next stating that the cause of "nonstraightness" is irrelevant, presumably meaning that its cause is irrelevant to the question of whether or not GLBT people should be discriminated against. She ends her commentary by once again stating both sides of an argument, hoping that discovery of a gay gene could help end discrimination but worrying that it could also provide a new tool to further exaggerate discrimination.

Brian's and Kate's responses make some of the same points raised by the other BT respondents. Brian comments: "As far as I know, there is insufficient evidence to meaningfully state whether or not there is a biological cause for same-sex attraction. It seems entirely possible to me that for most people, sexual orientation could be due to some combination of genetics, other biological influences, and social environment, quite possibly in different ratios for different people. I think most people who are unaccepting of same-sex attraction would probably either not accept the results, or would see the biological/genetic differences as 'flaws' rather than as natural variations." Kate, meanwhile, says, "For some people there is a biological component [to their sexuality], for others there isn't. . . . It is a choice for some, perhaps based on life experience or politics, although others may be 'hard wired' to such an extent that they can't not choose it or can't choose it."

Brian and Kate are also unwilling to claim that there is a single cause for same-sex attraction or to generalize from their own experiences to those of other people. Like Anne, they indicate some familiarity with scientific claims made about the genetics of homosexuality but still find them unconvincing. The only two BT respondents who felt their own sexuality might be inborn (Max and Traci) were still unwilling to attribute their sexuality to anything as simple as a gene or genes.

Conclusion

In the preceding sections, we have argued that there is good reason to believe that GLBT responses to the gay-gene debates are not straightforward. Nonetheless, we have remarked upon some likely patterns in responses to the debates. For example, the GLBT people most likely to support gay-gene research in a straightforward manner are those who, for multiple reasons, already have higher social status than other GLBT people. In terms of sexuality, gay men and lesbians have higher status than BT people and, likewise, are more likely to support gay-gene research than BT people. Despite the small number of responses, our survey results support this experiential insight. As noted earlier, the only GLBT people to express more positive than negative feelings about the idea of a gay gene, and about gay-gene research, were a lesbian and a gay man.

In claiming that the more marginal status of BT people, compared to that of lesbians and gay men, impacts their response to the gay-gene debates, we have also raised the possibility that there is a more general link between one's social status and one's perspective on these issues. This possibility can be considered in terms of a broader set of identities (or factors) impacting a person's perceived status in the world. Social scientists and political progressives have identified certain key identities (race, class, gender, and sexuality) that delineate clear status hierarchies in our society—for example, white over nonwhite, rich over poor, male over female, heterosexual over nonheterosexual (Andersen and Collins, 1992; Hurst, 1995). Extrapolating from the case of BT people suggests that the lower a GLBT person is on the status hierarchy scale just described, the more likely he or she is to reject the idea that a gay gene exists, or to reject gay-gene research. GLBT people (and others) with left-leaning political perspectives may also reject both the idea of a gay gene and the value of gay-gene research regardless of their location on the status hierarchy, particularly if they are concerned about science being used more generally in support of inequality, as with the *Bell Curve* controversy (Fischer et al., 1996). More extensive studies are required to test these hypotheses.

Why might bisexuals be predisposed toward repudiating gay-gene research? One possibility, beyond the matter of status described above, involves the definition of sexuality used for the purposes of identifying genes that influence the trait. A trait is more easily explained by genetics when its manifestation (phenotype) is clearly one thing or the other instead of something in between. Genetic researchers know that, to prove a genetic influence on any trait, a scientist must be sure of which people have the trait and which do not. Failing to categorize or measure a trait properly can invalidate an entire study, erasing or decreasing the probability of any linkage between a gene and the trait.

As bisexuals remind us by their very existence, a person's erotic behaviors vary with time and place. Is it accurate to posit that bisexuals have a "homosexual trait" missing in heterosexuals, or a "heterosexual trait" absent from lesbians and gay men? Most bisexuals reject the claim that they are "really" homosexual or "really" heterosexual. At the same time, some bisexuals behave no differently than people with heterosexual or homosexual identities. If such bisexuals are neither heterosexual nor homosexual, how can a researcher tell if anybody at all is really straight or gay? Most recently, gay-gene researchers have tried to circumvent this problem by lumping bisexuals in with homosexuals, thus polarizing human sexuality into "heterosexual" versus "nonheterosexual." This solution is unlikely to result in identification of gay genes because there is no basis for arguing that bisexuals are more like homosexuals than like heterosexuals.

Despite its limited size, our survey produced some unexpected findings. One striking outcome was that none of our respondents (including a biologist) articulated a scientifically based rejection of biological research, genetic or otherwise, into the cause of homosexuality. It is possible that we simply did not hear from GLBT people who use scientific explanations to dismiss the gay-gene theory. We think it more likely, however, that the popular appeal of evolutionary psychology remains a strong challenge to anyone promoting an antideterminist critique of gay-gene research.

Most important, many of our respondents believe that any potentially positive benefits of gay-gene research may be outweighed by negative consequences, whether or not a gene is actually found. Conscientious researchers should take the dissident voices of our respondents seriously and turn their attention to genetic questions other than that of the gay gene. Our respondents' concerns confirm our conviction that the world is not a safe enough place to use institutional power, funds, and the prestige of molecular genetics to ask why some of us are heterosexual and many of us are not.

REFERENCES

Andersen, M. L., and P. H. Collins. 1992. *Race, Class and Gender: An Anthology.* Belmont, Calif.: Wadsworth Books.

Blumenfeld, W. J., and D. Raymond. 1993. *Looking at Gay and Lesbian Life,* updated and expanded ed. Boston: Beacon Press.

Fischer, C. S., M. Hout, M. S. Jankowski, S. R. Lucas, A. Swidler, and K. Vos. 1996. *Inequality by Design: Cracking the Bell Curve Myth.* Princeton: Princeton University Press.

Geis, S. B., and D. E. Messer. 1994. *Caught in the Crossfire: Helping Christians Debate Homosexuality.* Nashville: Abingdon Press.

Hamer, D., and P. Copeland. 1994. *The Science of Desire: The Search for the Gay Gene and the Biology of Behavior.* New York: Simon & Schuster.

Hartman, K. 1996. *Congregations in Conflict: The Battle over Homosexuality.* New Brunswick, N.J.: Rutgers University Press.

Herek, G. M., and K. T. Berrill, eds. 1992. *Hate Crimes: Confronting Violence against Lesbians and Gay Men.* Newbury Park, Calif.: Sage Publications.

Hurst, C. E. 1995. *Social Inequality: Forms, Causes and Consequences,* 2d ed. Needham Heights, Mass.: Allyn & Bacon.

Wood, J. R. 2000. *Where the Spirit Leads: The Evolving Views of United Methodists on Homosexuality.* Nashville: Abingdon Press.

CHAPTER ELEVEN

The Commercialization of Genetic Technologies

Raising Public Awareness

Catherine Ard and Deborah Zucker

The last twenty-five years have witnessed dramatic changes in the fields of molecular biology and genetics. These changes began in the early 1970s with the development of technologies that allowed the manipulation of DNA and have culminated in the announcement of the nearly completed sequencing of the human genome in 2001. Federally funded research once primarily devoted to pursuing a basic knowledge of life processes has been transformed to hold promise for understanding and treating human disease and for commercializing genetic technologies. Many biologists and biomedical researchers who had formerly restricted their focus to basic science became involved in biotechnology companies. Advances in contemporary genetics have raised society's hope for vast improvements in health care. Thousands of biotechnology companies have organized, hoping to reap financial rewards from this promising science. Also, in anticipation of successful diagnostics and therapeutics, many individuals have become investigators in biotechnology companies.

This intersection of science, medicine, and business is beginning to bear fruit in the development of new medications and treatments. Yet, at the same time, these advances have been accompanied by potentially serious conflicts and social problems. The applications of genetics and genetic technologies to address public health issues have raised questions about the role of government, industry, and academic scientists in assuring that the remarkable new developments are used to benefit and not to harm people.

Consider the case of the biotechnology company DeCODE Genetics. Established by a former Harvard Medical School professor, DeCODE has been allowed by the government of Iceland to create a gigantic genetic and health data bank of that country's entire population. The company hopes to discover new disease genes and develop therapies for the diseases. Furthermore, DeCODE has twelve-year exclusive rights to market the data to anyone or any country willing to pay for the information. One critic who originally agreed with the project now argues, "The problem arose when they came up with the database. It ignores the rights of privacy, and patients rights. . . . Society is now so dominated by profit. It's not about science anymore, it's about money" (Specter, 1999, p. 48). Fears have been voiced about whether private health information will be used against Iceland's citizens and whether any health benefits will truly accrue to the population of that country.

In the United States, families with the genetic condition called Canavan disease have joined together in a lawsuit asking that researchers be prevented from commercially offering the prenatal test to diagnose Canavan. The families who donated tissue samples and financial resources for research claimed their rights were violated when researchers patented the gene for financial gain.

Another controversy surrounded the genetically engineered human growth hormone (hGH) developed for use in the treatment of certain genetic forms of dwarfism. Genentech, the manufacturer of the drug, and Caremark, the distributor of the drug, pushed the use of hGH among families with shorter children. Company-sponsored doctors reportedly used unethical tactics to shame parents into purchasing the drug for their children (Kolata, 1994). It was questioned whether some children with normal hormone levels were prescribed the drug simply because they were short. This was done in the absence of any indication that the drug would increase these children's heights.

These examples illustrate that genetic technologies are being applied to diverse populations in ways never before imagined. In addition, the sometimes negative influence of the profit motive on the use of these technologies and their final products has continually raised concerns of trust in the public sphere. While the commercialization of scientific advances is neither new nor unique to the biotechnology industry, the extraordinarily rapid expansion of an industry based on analysis of human genes has taken place with little in the way of guidelines or government regulation. The transfer of technology from the academic setting to industry is an old phenomenon, but nowhere is it taking place faster and in more complex ways than in the field of biotechnology (Orsengio, 1989).

In this chapter we highlight some of the moral and ethical issues surrounding the commercialization of genetic technologies. To illustrate the complexity of the commercialization process, we use four examples of genetic technologies that either have touched on or may someday affect the reader. These cases highlight the intertwined roles of government, academia, and business; various incentives for product development; clinical research ethics; and research-industry conflicts of interest in the commercialization process.

The Basic Science behind the New Products

Case 1: The Human Genome Project

Perhaps the most publicized example of a conflict between the interests of competing parties in the new genetics is found in the history of the Human Genome Project (HGP). In 1989, the United States government, via the National Institutes of Health (NIH) and the Department of Energy, initiated a project to obtain the complete sequence of the human genome within fifteen years. The HGP funded academic, government, and industry-connected researchers. This unique "big science" biology project was supported for its potential for scientific and medical benefits as well as its potential to aid the United States' international competitiveness in the emerging industrial biotechnology sector. The very direct connection between the genome sequence and commercial products was recognized by Congress, researchers, and venture capitalists alike. However, in 1998, Dr. J. Craig Venter, a former NIH researcher, announced that he and the Perkin-Elmer Corporation, an instrument manufacturer, were forming a joint private venture (Celera) to complete the sequence of the human genome. They would fund it with only one-tenth the money being accorded the HGP and complete it sooner (U.S. Congress, 1998).

Celera's announcement led to an ongoing saga that is still not resolved. Initially, the NIH was concerned that they might be publicly humiliated if Celera kept its promises (Wade, 1999). In addition, Celera planned to file for patents on any DNA sequences that had potential commercial value, and their sequence data would only be made available once completed and patented. This private venture could potentially result in substantial limitation of researchers' access to basic genetic information, knowledge that might be essential for studying human disease and development. And yet, to obtain the complete sequence, Celera would have to rely not only on their own accomplishments but also on sequence data that had already been achieved with U.S. government funding. One reason for consternation regarding Celera's proprietary approach was that, even though Celera's venture was private, the company could not have formulated its plan without the bulk of the basic research conducted by NIH and the NIH-funded academic programs (U.S. Congress, House Committee on Science, 1998). All HGP scientists agreed to release new data within twenty-four hours to GenBank, a public and publicly accessible database supported by the National Library of Medicine. Though it disagreed with this approach, Celera nonetheless took advantage of GenBank's data, allowing the company to reanalyze its results with greater accuracy. Celera then restricted its own data's availability, use, and redistribution (Butler, 2000). In the United States, the government has traditionally financed basic science research, and private industry has financed and privatized applied research for product development. However, in the case of Celera, the basic research sequencing of the genome directly overlaps with the company's proprietary interests.

One explanation for these conflicts is that, in contrast to earlier biomedical developments in which the path from basic research to a patentable product was long and complicated, the path from DNA sequencing to a product seems more direct. Also, a major change was made to patent law that allowed DNA to be patented much earlier in the product development process. Essentially, patenting now takes place at the basic research level of DNA sequencing. Therefore, the goals of basic researchers working to sequence the genome and identify the gene's functions became synonymous with many propriety goals (Weiner, 1986; Schmidtke, 1992; Etzkowitz and Webster, 1995; Eisenberg, 1996; Lin, 1996; Gilbert and Walter, 2001).

On the one hand, Celera's entry into the race for the DNA sequence quickened the HGP's pace so that the project was essentially completed several years before the anticipated date (Wade, 1999). In that sense, the public and the pharmaceutical companies benefitted from Celera's role in the project (Wade, 2000). On the other hand, Celera's policies regarding access to sequence information could retard progress in further research by imposing unacceptable restrictions or financial costs on some researchers. This stance challenges the long-held premise that basic research is not proprietary and belongs in the public domain.

Product Development

Case 2: Commercializing a Treatment for a Genetic Disease—an Orphan Drug for an Orphan Disease

The dynamics of the race for the human genome sequence reflect the tension between potential synergistic and antagonistic interactions involving public and private ventures. But there are other cases in which the government has effectively facilitated the private development of medical advances. Even here, the successes can be accompanied by consequences that may limit the benefits. An example is the development and marketing of a treatment for the genetic condition known as Gaucher disease.

Treatments for genetic diseases are still relatively few. One of the big success stories in the biotechnology industry, both financially and in terms of improving health, is Ceredase, a drug used to treat the symptoms of Gaucher disease. Gaucher disease is a condition affecting about fifteen thousand people in the United States who are missing an enzyme that breaks down certain body fats. The disease varies in its severity, and many sufferers die at an early age from debilitating effects on organs and bones.

In the early 1990s, Genzyme Corporation received permission from the Food and Drug Administration (FDA) to market a purified preparation of the missing enzyme that resulted in significant improvements in patients with Gaucher disease. The drug was developed and marketed under the Orphan Drug Act (ODA) of 1983 (PL-97–414). This act applies to drugs that alleviate conditions affecting fewer than 200,000 people in the United States or drugs whose sales are unlikely to recoup research and development costs. It gives companies various tax incentives and exclusive marketing rights for seven years. During this period, no other company can market a molecularly identical drug for the same FDA-approved use as the original orphan drug (Malinowski and Littlefield, 1999). The ODA was meant to encourage the development of treatments for diseases that might otherwise never be researched due to their lack of commercial attractiveness.

The biotechnology industry, realizing the potential financial benefits of the ODA's exclusivity clause, has tackled a number of orphan diseases. Today, there are more than 218 orphan products (National Organization of Rare Disorders, 2001) on the market benefitting more than 8 million Americans (Reider, 2000). Although the ODA was designed in anticipation of new drugs that would have low profitability, Ceredase has been very profitable for Genzyme, becoming a major source of revenue for the company. In 1999, sales for this drug represented 70 percent of the company's total product revenue (Genzyme Corporation, 2000). In the early years of Ceredase treatment, the estimated cost per year to the patient ranged from almost $100,000 to over $500,000. Genzyme agreed to provide the drug free to anyone who had exhausted their health insurance or did not have health insurance (Schwartz and Friday, 1992; U.S. Congress, Office of Technology Assessment, 1992), but in 1994 only about thirty-two people received the drug at no cost (Knox, 1994). The government repeatedly criticized Genzyme for pricing the drug too high (Leary, 1995), and the events led to questions about the government's role in fostering drug development. It appeared that the majority of the research and development had been done by government researchers, but there was very little if any governmental input into the pricing structure of the drug (U.S. Congress, Office of Technology Assessment, 1992).

Drug pricing is only one example of how the ODA has been exploited in the name of profits, abuses that were certainly not in the minds of the writers of the act. One critic of the existing ODA stated, "A drug company can drive a Brinks truck though the loopholes in the Orphan Drug Act" (Love, 1992, p. 267). As a result, Congress has attempted to limit company profits through a congressionally approved bill that has the support of the National Organization of Rare Disorders and the Biotechnology Industry Association. In 1990, however, President George Bush Sr. vetoed the bill, which proposed curbing the seven-year exclusivity clause if costs were recovered through sales in less time.

Another potential loophole of the ODA relates to the demarcation and definition of an orphan disease. As genetic technologies progress and allow for a narrower definition of a disease or condition caused by a specific gene mutation, patient populations can be subdivided into smaller and smaller groups until their numbers are 200,000 or fewer, thus fitting the definition of an orphan disease. Cancer is just one example of how this is happening. While there are approximately 6.8 million Americans diagnosed with the disease called cancer, cancer can be subclassified into many disease types (e.g., ovarian, breast, or pancreatic cancer). Ovarian cancer is the fifth leading cause of death among women, affecting nearly 164,000—a number still well below the 200,000 limit (Love, 1992). This ability to narrowly define an orphan disease or condition requires that we reexamine what is meant by orphan diseases or conditions.

Genzyme's marketing practices for Ceredase also raise a specter for the future marketing of medical treatments or diagnostic tests such as screening kits for genetic diseases—namely, direct-to-consumer marketing of prescription drugs. To target potential Ceredase patients, company representatives obtained names through seminars sponsored by the National Gaucher Foundation, some of which were funded by Genzyme. The foundation claimed that their mailing lists were never made public (Knox, 1994). In addition to the potential informational bias and pressure on patients and physicians to use the product, some patients were concerned about potential loss of confidentiality owing to the tactics used to obtain mailing lists. Although improved patient and physician information is desired, the information needs to be unbiased.

While the ODA has benefitted large numbers of people, the defects in this legislation have caused problems for those people with limited health care resources. Is it in the public's best interest to provide companies with government assistance and incentives to develop and market such drugs and then allow those companies to recover their costs, and then some, with no limitation on the amount of profit to be made? Were other treatments available but not investigated because of the ODA's marketing exclusivity? Public policies need to be developed to guarantee affordable access and fair pricing for the company, the patient, and society.

Evaluating Products: Clinical Trials and Potential Conflicts of Interest

Case 3: Gene Therapy and the Death of Jesse Gelsinger

The case of Ceredase illustrates the complicated issues involved in government efforts to provide incentives for product development and some of the broader concerns surrounding the direct-to-consumer marketing of prescription drugs. Once developed, new therapies need to be evaluated. The recent death of a research subject at the University of Pennsylvania's Institute for

Human Gene Therapy raises numerous questions about the role of universities and their faculties in uniting financial ventures with clinical research.

The field of molecular biology began as a purely academic, basic science. However, with the development of new DNA technologies in the 1970s, molecular biology turned to more and more practical applications. Many researchers entered the corporate sphere as they found they could potentially apply their science to solving societal problems such as human disease. In addition, they could add to their income by founding new companies, sitting on scientific advisory boards, or acting as scientific consultants (Natowicz and Ard, 1997). Biotechnology companies initially multiplied as collaborations formed among a variety of players: academics, entrepreneurs, venture capitalists, for-profit and not-for-profit institutions, governmental agencies, and large multinational pharmaceutical companies (Malinowksi and O'Rourke, 1996, p. 167).

In the meantime, more and more industrial funds were supporting university-based research (Krimsky, Ennis, and Weissman, 1991; Clemmit, 1993; Blumenthal, Causino, and Campbell, 1997). Restricted federal funding for biology in the 1970s and 1980s also caused many academic biomedical researchers to turn to industry for research support. They performed research in their own laboratories designed to aid in the development of commercial products. By the 1990s, numerous academic institutions were closing deals with pharmaceutical and biotechnology companies who sought access to the scientific expertise found in university settings. All of these factors have led to a blurring of the lines between government, industry, and the university, the consequences of which often reach the public. This was the case when efforts to treat a genetic disease with gene therapy at the University of Pennsylvania made newspaper headlines.

Gene therapy refers to the attempt to cure genetic diseases that are the result of an absent or malfunctioning single gene by restoring a normally functioning gene to the patient's cells. Even before the establishment of the HGP, numerous laboratories were working on gene therapy. But with the advent of the HGP, public promises for rapid benefits from genetic research were ratcheted up a notch. In the process of promoting the HGP, scientific leaders such as Frances Collins spoke of the medical revolution that would result (Guyer and Collins, 1993). Among the benefits would be the development of gene therapy techniques. Frequent reports appeared in the media, heralding supposedly successful uses of gene therapy for treating such diseases as cystic fibrosis, but actual gene therapy successes were not as anticipated (Orkin and Motulsky, 1995; Thompson, 2000). Researchers in the field expressed increasing frustration with the failures. In the meantime, a number of biotechnology companies began to explore the potential of gene therapy. Given the promises, the financial connections, and the many years of research, the stakes for those pursuing this research were very high.

During this period, the University of Pennsylvania established its Institute for Human Gene Therapy, headed by Dr. James Wilson. Dr. Wilson also founded a company that contributed millions of dollars to the university's institute in exchange for exclusive patent rights to develop the institute's discoveries. As a university dean, Dr. Kelly, as well as the university itself, stood to benefit from patent royalties if the gene replacement techniques succeeded (Stolberg, 1999; *New York Times*, 2000).

In April 1997, researchers at the institute initiated a Phase 1 (safety assessment) clinical trial to assess a gene therapy for the inherited disorder ornithine transcarbamoylase (OTC) deficiency. Mr. Jesse Gelsinger, an 18-year-old male with mild OTC deficiency symptoms, was the eighteenth subject enrolled in the OTC gene therapy trial. Four days after receiving infusion of the gene therapy material, he died. Investigations by the university, the FDA, and other agencies identified several irregularities in the researchers' adherence to procedures for the protection of human research subjects (Food and Drug Administration, 2000; Institute for Human Gene Therapy, 1999). The University of Pennsylvania researchers, like many others in the field, had used virus vectors to carry copies of the desired gene into patients' cells. The viruses, after entering the cells, would insert themselves into the cell's chromosomes, along with the needed gene. However, when a monkey given a viral vector (though not the identical vector) died, it had raised questions about the safety of this approach for human testing. It was also determined that two other patients enrolled before Mr. Gelsinger in the trial had experienced significant side effects. Furthermore, initial testing of Mr. Gelsinger had revealed increased levels of ammonia in his blood, which, according to the initial approved study protocol, should have made him an inappropriate candidate for the study. Mr. Gelsinger's parents accused the doctors of failing to properly inform their son of these risks of participating in the trial. They charged that he had not been given the opportunity to give his truly informed consent (*New York Times*, 2000).

Research carried out at academic institutions such as the University of

Pennsylvania has always been regarded as objective and not tainted by commercial interests. Academic institutions are expected to oversee the conduct of research and assess the potential conflicts of interests of individual investigators, according to federal guidelines (National Institutes of Health, 1989). The original guidelines prohibited investigator-industry relationships that might result in conflicts of interest. However, with the increasing prevalence of such relationships, the original guidelines were weakened to require merely the disclosure and peer review of the relationships (*Federal Register*, 1995). Of note, these regulations apply only to federally funded research; they do not apply to non–government-funded private research. As a result of the increased use of private funding and corporate connections at U.S. medical schools and research institutions (as was the case at the University of Pennsylvania), institutional conflict-of-interest policies show a wide variability in the types of practices permitted (Cho et al., 2000; McCrary et al., 2000; Lo, Wolf, and Berkeley, 2000). In addition, the institutions themselves, as well as the individual researchers, may benefit economically from their research through royalties and patent rights. Consequently, it may be very difficult for the institution to act as an objective overseer of the research.

The commercial connections now common in university settings raise concerns, whether founded or not, that biases and interests of investigators and sponsors for timely completion of the clinical protocol or desired outcomes might unduly influence subject participation and protections. As a result, the Gelsinger case has became a watershed for improvements in human research subject's protection and for increased public debate on industry-university connections (Korn, 2000; National Institutes of Health, 2000; Shalala, 2000).

Many of the issues raised by this case relate more generally to the protection of human research subjects and the ethical conduct of researchers. But the problems of the Gelsinger case are particularly pertinent to genetic research, as they highlight the convergence of three factors: (1) the extraordinary public attention that has been directed toward genetics as a solution to health problems in general; (2) the rapid expansion of the biotechnology industry; and (3) the remarkable increase in direct involvement of universities in promoting potentially lucrative biotechnological and clinical research in genetics. The potential conflicts of interest may have colored views of those monitoring the safety of genetic technologies and the potential effects of commercialization on the ethics of clinical research and scientific integrity.

Case 4: Genetic Tests for Susceptibility to Breast Cancer:
Conflicting Interests in Test Development, Marketing, and Use

The Gelsinger gene therapy case at the University of Pennsylvania involved the development and testing of a biotechnology therapy. Such research was subject to government regulation. The problems arose, in part, because of limitations in the implementation of the regulations. The development of tests that are able to detect mutations in a single gene is probably the most concrete and widespread achievement to date of human genome research. Unlike the activities involved in the Gelsinger case, the marketing of DNA tests for genetic diseases by private biotechnology corporations is subject to only limited regulation. There is still no consensus on what kinds of mechanisms are most appropriate for overseeing the rapid development of genetic testing—specifically predictive tests. Yet, the marketing and use of these tests are proceeding, and many problems are surfacing. The topic of genetic and predictive testing is extensive, and we refer you to other publications for additional discussions (Holtzman and Watson, 1997; Welch and Burke, 1998; U.S. Department of Health and Human Services, 2000; Evans, Skrzynia, and Burke, 2001; U.S. Department of Energy and the National Institutes of Health, 2001). In this case study, we focus on the problematic commercial aspects of the genetic tests for the so-called breast cancer genes, BRCA1 and BRCA2.

Breast cancer is the most prevalent cancer in women worldwide, and about 5 to 10 percent of cases are thought to be hereditary. The remaining 90 to 95 percent of cases, termed *sporadic,* are thought to result from complex interactions between an individual and the environment. Studies of certain families with histories of early onset breast and ovarian cancers helped researchers in 1994 to identify a region of human chromosome 17, termed the BRCA1 gene, that plays a role in the development of this cancer (Futreal et al., 1994; Miki et al., 1994). Shortly thereafter, another gene, located on chromosome 13 and called BRCA2, was also found to contribute to susceptibility to these malignancies in different sets of families (Wooster et al., 1994; Tavtigian et al., 1996). Identification of BRCA1 and BRCA2 allowed researchers to determine which specific mutations in these genes were associated with these cancers in high-risk families. While this research continued, private companies began to develop, patent, and market genetic tests for these mutations, to be used in clinical evaluations of breast cancer risk.

On the surface, this sounds like a success story for patients, researchers, and venture capitalists alike, all of whom benefit from the commercialization of breast cancer tests. However, while companies hoped for a profitable market and pushed to make these breast cancer tests available, groups such as the American Society of Human Genetics and the National Advisory Council for Human Genome Research questioned whether these tests were ready for widespread clinical use (Weiss, 1996). Several reasons for this caution can be cited:

1. Tests for specific sequences of DNA can be developed before their relevance, interpretation, or potential clinical utility is fully understood. The actual functions of the BRCA genes and the extent to which they will likely increase cancer risk in any one individual is not fully understood. Researchers have determined the frequencies of these mutations in broader populations of patients both with and without significant family histories or diagnoses of breast and ovarian cancers (Shattuck-Eidens et al., 1995; Durocher et al., 1996; Serova et al., 1997; Whittemore, Gong, and Itnyre, 1997). In one study, blood samples were collected from Ashkenazi Jewish women for testing not related to breast cancer. Specific BRCA1 and BRCA2 gene mutations previously identified in Ashkenazi Jewish women with familial early onset breast cancer (e.g., BRCA1:85delAG) were found to be present in increased frequency in this broader Ashkenazi Jewish population. Those women in this broader population with the BRCA1 and BRCA2 mutations but without a strong family history of breast and ovarian cancer showed a much lower breast cancer rate than those women with the mutations who came from high-risk families (Struewing et al., 1997). This result exemplifies a methodological problem in genetic analyses. Researchers looking to find a disease-associated gene initially seek mutations associated with the disease in those families that show a strong family history of that disease. However, these special cases may represent a unique subset. For example, the high frequency with which the BRCA1 mutation correlates with breast cancer in these families may be influenced by other genes that these families tend to carry or by environmental factors that they are all exposed to. To conclude that the mutations will confer the same degree of susceptibility to breast cancer in another family is unfounded. Owing to the resulting uncertain predictive value of the genetic tests, many researchers are therefore dubious about their utility for widespread clinical practice.

2. Offering predictive tests make little sense if no effective intervention

follows a positive predictive test result. What are the options following a positive test for BRCA1 or BRCA2? In order to decrease the risk of developing breast cancer, some clinicians suggest behavioral and life-style changes as well as more frequent mammographies. The only current preventive therapy involves radical mastectomy, clearly not a benign intervention. Breast cancer is a serious disease, but the predictive accuracy value of the genetic test in low-risk populations is limited and the surgical intervention is drastic. It is evident that a positive genetic test result puts both patients and their physicians in very difficult decision-making positions (Schrag et al., 1997; Fasouliotis and Schenker, 2000; Unic et al., 2000). For some women, the costs resulting from lack of appropriate response options to a positive test result can outweigh the benefits of the test's availability.

3. Predictive genetic tests provide information not only about the individuals tested but also about their family members and possible broader populations (e.g., a specific ethnic group). Who should receive these results? What is the responsibility of the tested member in providing that information to other family members at potential risk? Someone being tested for a condition may not wish to reveal that information to his or her family, yet it may be important to the health of other family members. Results of one member's test may suggest a need for testing others in the family. Assume, for a moment, that a parent in a high-risk family tests positive for a mutation in BRCA1 that is linked to familial cancer. Should the children be tested for this mutation? Or should the children have the option when they become of age to make that decision themselves? Again, one needs to weigh the risks and benefits of having the knowledge and the treatment options. Do we have preventive techniques that are adequately effective to warrant obtaining that test without the child's true informed consent?

4. Predictive tests raise the problem of genetic discrimination in such areas as health insurance and employment (see Chapter 12). Women found to carry a BRCA1 or BRCA2 mutation who are perfectly healthy may be denied health benefits or a job because of the probability that they will develop breast cancer.

To a commercial organization, successfully developing a diagnostic medical test depends upon feasibility, production, and profitability. Its profitability is clearly tied to the number of tests sold in the marketplace, which in turn depends upon clinical use. For the breast cancer tests, their clinical utility depends on how well the test measures what it is supposed to measure (e.g., how accurately it determines presence of a mutation); how well the test correlates with the clinical condition (e.g., how well the identification of a BRCA1 mutation correlates with the development of breast cancer in the future for the individual being tested); whether the results of the test will be useful (e.g., are there effective interventions to prevent breast cancer in a person with a BRCA1 mutation); and, finally, whether the test is appropriate for the patient (medically appropriate, feasible, and desired by the patient). The issues surrounding judicious use of these genetic predictive tests is at the heart of many of the challenges this genetic technology poses to individuals and society (Collins, 1996; Healy, 1997).

Many of the difficulties that have arisen with the breast cancer tests derive from this gap in knowledge regarding the tests' predictive capabilities and from the lack of clear clinical criteria for their use. A number of factors impact whether or not patients obtain medical tests appropriately. Clinicians need to assess whether or not the test is medically indicated. Unfortunately, there is a significant need for improvement in the education of clinicians with regard to medical genetics (Hofman et al., 1993; Stephenson, 1997; Caulfield, 1999). In addition, much of the information available to practitioners about specific genetic tests comes from the companies producing those tests and, therefore, may be biased in favor of test use. The number of genetic counselors who are aware of many of the issues involved in genetic testing is still far too small to handle the recent rapid expansion of the availability of such tests. Recognizing this, some companies have developed mechanisms to try to ensure appropriate test use. OncorMed, one of the companies developing the breast cancer tests, has been held up as the gold standard because they set requirements for using their genetic tests. They required a physician's referral, pre- and post-test counseling, that results are to be given in person by the doctor, and that there be a three month follow-up by the doctor. Unfortunately, not all companies hold to the same standards for patient care (Malinowski and Blatt, 1997).

In a study that looked at psychological responses to predictive genetic testing, the number of patients that actually choose to obtain genetic testing was actually low. As the accuracy of the predictive test was lowered, so, too, was the interest in undergoing the testing. If companies marketing genetic tests are required to provide pre- and post-test counseling, some are concerned about how "independent" that counseling would be. Such counseling can affect patients' decisions to take the test—in other words, help determine whether they purchase the product (Marteau and Croyle, 1998).

Because all of these problems are specific to the utilization of predictive genetic tests, there has been considerable discussion about how to best regulate the use of these tests. While biotechnology companies and private clinics are eager to widely market their products, many observers fear widespread problems—medical, psychological, and financial—if their introduction is not carefully monitored. Task forces have been convened to look at these issues and assess current applicable regulations. The development of genetic tests is regulated by the Code of Federal Regulations to protect human subjects and their identifiable DNA (45 CFR 46, 21 CFR 50, and 21 CFR 56) (U.S. Department of Health and Human Services, 2000). However, genetic test development that is not federally funded or in the FDA marketing-approval stage is not subject to these policies, and so their regulation remains in question (Huang, 1998). The Secretary's Advisory Committee on Genetic Testing (SACGT) is currently addressing some of these concerns. This committee was formed to advise the Department of Health and Human Services on the medical, scientific, ethical, legal, and social issues raised by the development and use of genetic tests and assess, in consultation with the public, the adequacy of current oversight of genetic tests. Presumably, the recommendations of this committee will affect the ongoing development of public policy at both the federal and state levels.

Conclusion

As the opportunities increase for individuals to have genetic tests and for researchers to gather DNA data, and as biotechnology and medicine collide with profit, social issues for many different communities are affected. In this chapter we have explored different groups and the various stages of commercialization. The HGP-Celera case examined basic research conducted or sponsored by the federal government and showed the blurring boundaries between public and private efforts. The Ceredase case involved early research and development conducted by public ventures and the transfer of that knowledge to industry, with the assistance of government regulations, to create a product. The gene therapy case emphasized the need for the protection of human subjects and the potential conflicts of interest in clinical research. We argue that because of the field's rapid development, genetic technologies still in the research stage are being offered prematurely to the public. Even though genetic tests or diagnostic devices that find their way to the marketplace are regulated by the federal government, that does not mean that their appropriate uses are clear. The breast cancer example showcases the dilemmas resulting from the combination of industry's need for profit, society's interest in improving medical dianostics, and the need for remaining research to clarify the tests' optimal use. Moreover, individuals are faced with the dilemma of whether to be tested or not. All four cases confront the difficulty in finding a balance between government involvement, active public involvement, and the commercial sector—particularly when technological capability outpaces policy making. Resolution is all the more pressing now that when millions of consumers have greater and quicker access to newer, riskier drugs, diagnostics, and treatments.

Society's hopes for biotechnology are tempered by considering how genetics and genetic technologies might bring about discrimination and psychosocial harms. Just as important are the issues of potential erosion of public trust with regard to scientific research and the public's continued commitment to the development of science in the name of societal advancement. Therefore, it is critical to ensure an appropriate balance as the growth of such technology continues. The increasing influence of the biotechnology and pharmaceutical industries, within both the U.S. economy and the delivery of health care, requires increased vigilance and oversight, not just by the government but also by the public.

REFERENCES

Blumenthal, D., N. Causino, and E. G. Campbell. 1997. "Academic-Industry Research Relationships in Genetics: A Field Apart." *Nature Genetics* 16:104–8.

Butler, D. 2000. "US/UK Statement on Genome Data Prompts Debate on 'Free Access.'" *Nature* 404:324–25.

Caulfield, T. 1999. "Gene Testing in the Biotech Century: Are Physicians Ready?" *Canadian Medical Association Journal* 161 (9):1122–24.

Clemmit, M. 1993. "US Drug Industry's Research Support." *Nature* 361:757–60.

Cho, M. K., R. Shohara, A. Schissel, and D. Rennie. 2000. "Policies on Faculty Conflicts of Interest at US Universities." *Journal of the American Medical Association* 284 (17):2203–8.

Collins, F. S. 1996. "BRCA1—Lots of Mutations, Lots of Dilemmas." *New England Journal of Medicine* 334 (3):186–88.

Durocher, F., D. Shattuck-Eidens, M. McClure, F. Labrie, M. H. Skolnick, D. E. Goldgar, and J. Simard. 1996. "Comparison of BRCA1 Polymorphisms, Rare Sequence

Variants and/or Messense Mutations in Unaffected and Breast/Ovarian Cancer Populations." *Human Molecular Genetics* 5 (6):835–42.

Eisenberg R. 1996. "Patents: Help or Hindrance to Technology Transfer?" Pp. 161–74 in *Biotechnology: Science, Engineering, and Ethical Challenges for the Twenty-First Century*, ed. F. B. Rudolph and L. V. McIntire. Washington, D.C.: Joseph Henry Press.

Etzkowitz H., and A. Webster. 1995. "Science as Intellectual Property." Pp. 480–505 in *Handbook of Science and Technology Studies*, ed. S. Jasanoff. Thousand Oaks, Calif.: Sage Publications.

Evans, J. P., C. Skrzynia, and W. Burke. 2001. "The Complexities of Predictive Genetic Testing." *British Medical Journal* 322 (7293):1052–56.

Fasouliotis, S. J., and J. G. Schenker. 2000. "BRCA1 and BRCA2 Gene Mutations: Decision-Making Dilemmas Concerning Testing and Management." *Obstetrical and Gynecological Survey* 55 (6):373–84.

Federal Register. 1995. "Objectivity in Research." FR Doc:95–16799 July 11, Vol. 60, No. 132.

Food and Drug Administration. 2000. "Food and Drug Warning Letter of March 3, 2000, to Dr. James M. Wilson." http://www.fda.gov/foi/warning.htm.

Futreal, P. A., et al. 1994. "BRCA1 Mutations in Primary Breast and Ovarian Carcinomas." *Science* 266 (5182):120–22.

Genzyme Corporation. 2000. *Genzyme General 2000 Annual Report*. Cambridge, Mass.

Gilbert, P., and C. Walter. 2001. "Patents and the Human Genome Project: New Claims for Old?" *Trends in Biotechnology* 19 (2):49–52.

Guyer, M. S., and F. S. Collins. 1993. "The Human Genome Project and the Future of Medicine." *American Journal of Diseases of Children* 147 (11):1145–52.

Healy, B. 1997. "BRCA Genes: Bookmaking, Fortunetelling, and Medical Care." *New England Journal of Medicine* 336 (20):1448–49.

Hofman, K. J., E. S. Tambor, G. A. Chase, G. Geller, R. R. Faden, and N. A. Holtzman. 1993. "Physicians' Knowledge of Genetics and Genetic Tests." *Academic Medicine* 68 (8):625–32.

Holtzman, N. A., and M. S. Watson, eds. 1997. "Promoting Safe and Effective Genetic Testing in the United States." Final Report of the Task Force on Genetic Testing: NIH-DOE Working Group on Ethical, Legal, and Social Implications of Human Genome Research. http://www.nhgri.nih.gov/ELSI/TFGT__final/.

Huang, A. 1998. "FDA Regulation of Genetic Testing: Institutional Reluctance and Public Guardianship." *Food Drug Law Journal* 53 (3):555–91.

Institute for Human Gene Therapy. 1999. "Preliminary Findings Reported on the Death of Jesse Gelsinger." http://www.med.upenn.edu/ihgt/findings.html.

Knox, R. A. 1994. "Drug Makers' Aggressive Marketing Questioned." *Boston Globe*, May 11, pp. 1, 14.

Kolata, G. 1994. "Selling Growth Drug for Children: The Legal and Ethical Question." *New York Times*, August 15, pp.1, A13.

Korn, D. 2000. "Conflicts of Interest in Biomedical Research." *Journal of the American Medical Association* 284 (17):2234–37.

Krimsky, S., J. G. Ennis, and R. Weissman. 1991. "Academic-Corporate Ties in Biotechnology: A Quantitative Study." *Science, Technology and Human Values* 16 (3):275–87.

Leary, W. E. 1995. "A Partial Cure for Drug Bills for a $370,000-a-Year Ailment." *New York Times*, March 8, p. C12.

Lin, M. 1996. "Conferring a Federal Property Right in Genetic Material: Stepping into the Future with the Genetic Privacy Act." *American Journal of Law and Medicine* 22 (1):109–34.

Lo, B., L. E. Wolf, and A. Berkeley. 2000. "Conflict of Interest Policies for Investigators in Clinical Trials." *New England Journal of Medicine* 343 (22):1616–20.

Love, J. 1992. "Comments on the Orphan Drug Act and Government Sponsored Monopolies for Marketing Pharmaceutical Drugs." U.S. Senate, Committee on the Judiciary, Subcommittee on Antitrust, Monopolies and Business Rights, Anticompetitive Abuse of the Orphan Drug Act: Invitation to High Prices. January 21, J-102–48, pp. 259–83.

Malinowski, M. J., and R. J. R. Blatt. 1997. "Commercialization of Genetic Testing Services: The FDA, Market Forces, and Biological Tarot Cards." *Tulane Law Review* 71:1211–1311.

Malinowski, M. J., and N. Littlefield. 1999. "Transformation of a Research Platform into Commercial Products: The Impact of United States Federal Policy on Biotechnology." Pp. 29–54 in *The Commercialization of Genetic Research: Ethical, Legal, and Policy Issues*, ed. Caulfield, T. A. and B. Williams-Jones. New York: Kluwer Academic/Plenum Publishers.

Malinowksi, M. J., and M. A. O'Rourke. 1996. "A False Start? The Impact of Federal Policy on the Genotechnology Industry." *Yale Journal on Regulation* 13 (163):167.

Marteau, T. M., and R.T. Croyle. 1998. "The New Genetics: Psychological Responses to Genetic Testing." *British Medical Journal* 316 (7132):693–96.

McCrary, S. V., C. B. Anderson, J. Jakovljevic, T. Khan, L. B. McCullough, N. P. Wray, and B. A. Brody. 2000. "A National Survey of Policies on Disclosure of Conflict of Interest in Biomedical Research." *New England Journal of Medicine* 343 (22):1621–26.

Miki, Y., et al. 1994. "A Strong Candidate for the Breast and Ovarian Cancer Susceptibility Gene BRCA1." *Science* 266 (5182):66–71.

National Institutes of Health. 1989. "National Institutes of Health Guide, 1989: Proposed Guidelines for Policies on Conflict of Interest." NIH Grants and Contracts, Vol. 18, No. 32. Bethesda, Md. September 15.

———. 2000. "Financial Conflicts of Interest and Research Objectivity: Issues for Investigators and Institutional Review Boards." NIH Guide Notice: OD-00–040 Bethesda, Md. June 5, 2000

National Organization for Rare Disorders. 2001. "Testimony Submitted regarding FY 2002 Funding for the Orphan Product Research Grants Program." April. http://www.rarediseases.org/new/senate402.htm.

Natowicz, M. R., and Ard, C. F. 1997. "The Commercialization of Clinical Genetics: An Analysis of Interrelations between Academic Medical Centers and For-Profit Clinical Genetics Diagnostic Companies." *Journal of Genetic Counseling* 6 (3):337–55.

New York Times. 2000. "Suit Filed over Death in Gene Therapy Test." September 19, p. A23.

Orkin, S. H., and A. G. Motulsky, Co-chairs. 1995. "Report and Recommendations of the Panel to Assess the NIH Investment in Research on Gene Therapy." National Institutes of Health, Bethesda, Md. December 7.

Orsengio, L. 1989. *The Emergence of Biotechnology: Institutions and Markets in Industrial Innovations.* New York: St. Martin's Press.

Reider, C. R. 2000. "The Orphan Drug Act: Provisions and Considerations." *Drug Information Journal* 34:295–300.

Schmidtke, J. 1992. "Who Owns the Human Genome? Ethical and Legal Aspects." *Journal of Pharmacy and Pharmacology* 44 (Suppl. 1): 205–10.

Schrag, D., K. M. Kuntz, J. E. Garber, and J. C. Weeks. 1997. "Decision Analysis: Effects of Prophylactic Mastectomy and Oophorectomy on Life Expectancy among Women with BRCA1 or BRCA2 mutations." *New England Journal of Medicine* 336 (20):1465–71.

Schwartz, J., and C. Friday. 1992. "Beating the Odds in Biotech: Boston's Genzyme Puts Business before Science." *Newsweek*, 12 October, p. 63.

Serova, O. M., S. Mazoyer, N. Puget, V. Dubois, P. Tonin, Y. Y. Shugart, D. Goldgar, S. A. Narod, H. T. Lynch, and G. M. Lenoir. 1997. "Mutations in BRCA1 and BRCA2 in Breast Cancer Families: Are There More Breast Cancer-Susceptibility Genes?" *American Journal of Human Genetics* 60 (3):486–95.

Shalala, D. 2000. "Protecting Research Subjects: What Must Be Done." *New England Journal of Medicine* 343 (11):808–10.

Shattuck-Eidens, D., et al. 1995. "A Collaborative Survey of 80 Mutations in the BRCA1 Breast and Ovarian Cancer Susceptibility Gene: Implications for Presymptomatic Testing and Screening." *Journal of the American Medical Association* 273 (7):535–41.

Specter, M. 1999. "Decoding Iceland." *New Yorker*, 18 January, pp. 40, 42–46, 48–51.

Stephenson, J. 1997. "As Discoveries Unfold, a New Urgency to Bring Genetic Literacy to Physicians." *Journal of the American Medical Association* 278 (15):1225–26.

Stolberg, S. G. 1999. "F.D.A Officials Fault Penn Team in Gene Therapy Death." *New York Times*, December 9, p. A1.

Struewing, J. P., P. Hartge, S. Wacholder, S. M. Baker, M. Berlin, M. McAdams, M. M. Timmerman. 1997. "The Risk of Cancer Associated with Specific Mutations of BRCA1 and BRCA2 among Ashkenazi Jews." *New England Journal of Medicine* 336:1401–18.

Tavtigian S. V., et al. 1996. "The Complete BRCA2 Gene and Mutations in Chromosome 13q-Linked Kindreds." *Nature Genetics* 12:333–37.

Thompson, L. 2000 "Human Gene Therapy: Harsh Lessons, High Hopes." *FDA Consumer Magazine* 34 (5). http://www.fda.gov/fdac/features/2000/500_gene.html.

U.S. Congress, House Committee on Science, Subcommittee on Energy and Environment. 1998. "The Human Genome Project: How Private Sector Developments Affect the Government Program." Washington, D.C.: U.S. Government Printing Office, June 17.

U.S. Congress, Office of Technology Assessment. 1992. "Federal and Private Roles in the Development and Provision of Alglucerase Therapy for Gaucher Disease." OTA-BP-H-104. Washington, D.C.: U.S. Government Printing Office, October.

U.S. Congress, Senate. 1992. "Orphan Drug Amendments of 1992." Senate Report 102–358. Washington, D.C.: U.S. Government Printing Office, August.

U.S. Department of Energy and the National Institutes of Health. 2001. "Human Genome Project Information Website." http://www.ornl.gov/hgmis/medicine/genetest.html.

U.S. Department of Health and Human Services, Secretary's Advisory Committee on Genetic Testing (SACGT). 2000. *A Public Consultation on Oversight of Genetic Tests.* http://www4.od.nih.gov/oba/sacgt/reports/Public_Consultation_document.htm.

Unic, I., L. C. Verhoef, P. F. Stalmeier, and W. A. J. van Daal. 2000. "Prophylactic Mastectomy or Screening in Women Suspected to Have the BRCA1/2 Mutation: A Prospective Pilot Study of Women's Treatment Choices and Medical and Decision-Analytic Recommendations." *Medical Decision Making* 20 (3):251–62.

Wade, N. 1999. "Talk of Collaboration in Decoding of the Genome." *New York Times,* November 14, p. 22.

———. 2000. "Rivals on Offensive as They Near Wire in Genome Race." *New York Times,* May 7, p. 26.

Weiner, C. 1986. "Universities, Professors, and Patents: A Continuing Controversy." *Technology Review* (February–March): 33–43.

Weiss, R. 1996. "Tests' Availability Tangles Ethical and Genetic Codes." *Washington Post,* May 26, p. A1.

Welch, H. G., and W. Burke. 1998. "Uncertainties in Genetic Testing for Chronic Disease." *Journal of the American Medical Association* 280 (17):1525–27.

Whittemore, A. S., G. Gong, and J. Itnyre. 1997. "Prevalence and Contribution of BRCA1 Mutations in Breast Cancer and Ovarian Cancer: Results from Three U.S. Population-Based Case-Control Studies of Ovarian Cancer." *American Journal of Human Genetics* 60 (3):496–504.

Wooster, R., et al. 1994. "Localization of a Breast Cancer Susceptibility Gene, BRCA2, to Chromosome 13q12–13." *Science* 265 (5181):2088–90.

Individual, Family, and Societal Dimensions of Genetic Discrimination

A Case Study Analysis

Lisa N. Geller, Joseph S. Alper, Paul R. Billings,
Carol I. Barash, Jon Beckwith, and Marvin R. Natowicz

The growing knowledge of human genetics, stimulated in part by the Human Genome Project, has engendered a societal need to understand potential hazards as well as benefits of this knowledge. With our increased ability to identify genetic differences, it is important to elucidate appropriate uses of genetic information from the perspectives of both individuals and the public. At the same time, safeguards must be developed to minimize inappropriate uses of this information (Holtzman, 1989; Wilford and Nolan, 1993; Andrews et al., 1994; Nelkin and Tancredi, 1994). One area of concern is genetic discrimination.

An earlier version of this chapter appeared as "Individual, Family, and Societal Dimensions of Genetic Discrimination: A Case Study Analysis," in *Science and Engineering Ethics* 2, no. 1 (1996): 71–88. The authors are grateful to many individuals who were generous in their cooperation with this study and to the Huntington Disease Society of America, the Hemochromatosis Research Foundation, the National MPS Foundation, and the PKU Clinic at Children's Hospital, Boston, Massachusetts. We also wish to thank all members of the Genetic Screening Study Group for helpful discussions. In addition, we thank Professors Dorothy Nelkin and Dorothy Wertz for consultations and Jane Alper, J.D., and Vicki Laden, J.D. for discussions of the legal issues. The study was supported by a grant from the U.S. Department of Energy and funding from the Department of Mental Retardation of the Common-Wealth of Massachusetts.

All authors contributed equally to this work.

The term "genetic discrimination" has been used to describe the differential treatment of individuals or their relatives based on actual or presumed genetic differences, as opposed to discrimination based on phenotype (Billings et al., 1992; Natowicz, Alper, and Alper, 1992a; Gostin, 1991). Sources of genetic information that enable such discrimination include genetic and sometimes nongenetic medical tests, family histories, and information obtained from clinical examinations. Each of these sources has important limitations in terms of its reliability in predicting whether a particular genetic condition will occur and, if so, the clinical course of the associated disease. These limitations include but are not restricted to the sensitivity and specificity of genetic tests, the intrinsic clinical variability of many hereditary conditions, and the importance of environmental factors.

A pilot study of genetic discrimination showed this problem to involve more disorders than was previously revealed by isolated reports. The reported incidents involved a variety of social institutions, such as life and health insurance organizations, and suggested that genetic discrimination may become a significant social policy problem. Based on this work and reports of genetic discrimination by others, many are seriously concerned about this problem (Billings et al., 1992; Dewar, 1992; U.S. Congress, Office of Technology Assessment, 1992; NIH/DOE Working Group on Ethical, Legal, and Social Implications of Human Genome Research, 1993; Alper et al., 1994; Andrews et al., 1994; Nelkin and Tancredi, 1994). This concern is intensified by the proliferation and increasing utilization of genetic tests, made possible in part by technological advances resulting from the Human Genome Project and by the application of these technologies by commercial interests (Holtzman, 1992; Caskey, 1993; Nowak, 1994).

Previous reports of genetic discrimination involved studies of relatively small numbers of individuals and, consequently, would not be expected to reveal a full range of the discriminatory experiences faced by affected individuals and their families. Here we report on case studies obtained in 1992–1993 of individuals living throughout the United States at risk for or related to people at risk for the following disorders: hemochromatosis, phenylketonuria (PKU), mucopolysaccharidoses (MPS), and Huntington disease. We describe the spectrum of discrimination reported by some of these individuals and discuss its implications through analysis of selected informative cases.

Methods

Study Design

Individuals at risk for genetic discrimination were sent questionnaires during 1992–1993. The definition of genetic discrimination presented above distinguishes genetic discrimination from discrimination based on phenotype (Alper and Natowicz, 1993). Consequently, only those cases in which individuals appeared to have no symptoms (i.e., no apparent phenotype at the time of the reported discrimination) were included in this study.

Questionnaires and Interviews

Two questionnaires and an interview instrument were developed based on findings from our pilot study. They were reviewed by consultants experienced in qualitative research methods and questionnaire design and were approved by the Shriver Center's Institutional Review Board. Two questionnaires were distributed through the mailing lists of genetic disease organizations selected according to the criteria described below, and were accompanied by a letter describing the research group and the goals of the study. One questionnaire was directed at individuals who had or were at risk of developing a genetic condition. The other questionnaire was directed at parents who had a child with a genetic condition. Both were designed to acquire information about whether an individual believed that she or he, or a relative, had experienced discrimination because of a genetic diagnosis or assumption of genetic predisposition to the disorder. The questionnaire also requested a brief description of the alleged discriminatory event(s) (Table 12.1). These descriptions were used to screen the returned questionnaires for cases that appeared to fit the definition of genetic discrimination used in this study. That is, the person alleging discrimination was not symptomatic for a genetic disorder (or any other disease that might confound the claim of discrimination), nor did the complaint appear to involve legitimate actions by companies or individuals that were simply construed as "unfair" by the individual claiming discrimination. Some cases were included in which an apparent conflict between the perception of the individual and the point of view of an institution illustrate areas of ambiguity concerning the "fairness" of the situation.

Telephone interviews were conducted with individuals who, from their responses to the questionnaire, appeared to have experienced genetic discrimination as described above. An attempt was made to interview all individuals whose questionnaire answers met the above criteria and who had indicated that they were willing to be contacted by telephone. The script (available by request) used to conduct the interviews was designed to obtain more detailed information about the perceived discriminatory event(s) (Table 12.2). For example, in cases of alleged discrimination by an insurance company, the interviewee was asked about how the company found out about their genetic status, correspondence and conversations held with individuals at the company, reasons given by the company for actions taken, whether outside support or counsel had been sought, whether the case was reconsidered after communication with the company, the length of time of response, who within the company handled the case, whether alternative policies were offered, and so on. In addition, general information was elicited regarding the economic and educational status of the individual, as well as pertinent medical information including whether the individual was asymptomatic. We also sought to determine the origin of the genetic diagnosis or supposed genetic risk factor, perceived ability to redress a grievance, the extent to which an individual challenged adverse decisions, and the impact of personal genetic information on the individual and her or his family. After conducting a number of interviews, it became apparent that the respondents differed widely in their knowledge concerning avenues for seeking redress for complaints involving insurance. Consequently, questions concerning whether the individual knew of the Medical Information Bureau, Inc. (MIB), and state insurance commissions—institutions that are useful to individuals seeking redress from insurance companies—were added to subsequent interviews. Consenting interviewees were tape recorded anonymously to aid in the transcription of information. In addition, documentation of discriminatory events, such as letters from insurance companies and medical and personal notes, was sought.

Study Groups

The specific disorders targeted for this study were chosen because they met the following criteria: (1) the genetic basis of the condition is known and unambiguous; (2) discrimination directed against individuals with these conditions would most likely be due to the genetic bases of these conditions, rather than due to physical symptoms; and (3) support groups for persons with these conditions exist so that individuals could be contacted easily. These conditions were also selected because they cover a spectrum of situations including dominant and recessive disorders, treatable and untreatable disorders, relatively common disorders for which screening programs exist, and rare disorders for which screening programs are not indicated. Note that the individuals with recessive disorders included both those with the genotype for the disorder and those who are simply carriers.

By these criteria, the diseases chosen for study were Huntington disease, hemochromatosis, phenylketonuria (PKU), and mucopolysaccharide disorders (MPS). Huntington disease is a fatal, untreatable, autosomal dominant disorder with symptoms typically appearing during middle age. There is currently a molecular genetic test available to diagnose this condition. Hemochromatosis is an autosomal recessive iron storage disorder with a variable phenotype; some individuals are completely asymptomatic. This disorder is treatable with phlebotomy (blood-drawing). PKU is an autosomal recessive disorder for which all newborns in the United States are tested. If left untreated the disorder results in mental retardation. However, PKU is successfully treated by placing the child on a special diet. MPS disorders are usually associated with mental retardation and organomegally (enlarged organs).

A total of 27,790 questionnaires were mailed by the following groups to their members: the Huntington Disease Society of America, the Hemochromatosis Research Foundation, the National M.P.S. Foundation, and the PKU Clinic at Children's Hospital, Boston, Massachusetts. Mailing lists for these groups included donors and interested individuals who were not appropriate respondents to the questionnaire, leading us to expect a low response rate. However, contacting individuals through a national organization was more likely to get a broader response than that obtained by contacting individuals through a few clinics. Respondents to the questionnaire included individuals who were at risk to develop a genetic disorder but who had not been informed of their genotype, individuals who were presymptomatic for a specific genetic condition, and individuals who either were asymptomatic because of therapy or were heterozygotes and thus only "carriers" for an autosomal recessive condition.

Results

Of the 917 returned questionnaires, 455 respondents asserted that they had experienced genetic discrimination and 437 that they had not. The remainder gave ambiguous answers that could not be specifically classified. Some respondents reported experiencing genetic discrimination in more than one setting. After screening the questionnaires for cases that appeared to fit the definition of genetic discrimination used in this study, we were able to set up interviews for 206 individuals who reported that they experienced genetic discrimination. Detailed breakdowns of the respondents, categorized by disease group, are given in Table 12.3.

A variety of different institutions allegedly discriminated against the respondents. The majority of cases involved discrimination by health and life insurance companies; the remainder involved clinical professionals, adoption ser-'vices, the armed services, employers, educational institutions, and blood banks. The cases reported below are grouped according to agents or institutions allegedly engaged in the genetic discrimination, followed by results of the impact of genetic discrimination on individuals and family members, responses and countermeasures taken to mitigate the effects of genetic discrimination, and information pertinent to the underlying bases of this phenomenon.

Agents or Institutions Engaging in Discriminatory Practices
Health and Life Insurance Corporations

Four aspects of discrimination are illustrated by the cases involving health and life insurance: (1) discrimination against individuals who were asymptomatic; (2) differential treatment of asymptomatic individuals or families once a genetic diagnosis was established, thus treating the genetic diagnosis as a pre-existing condition; (3) the failure of some group insurance plans to provide coverage for qualified individuals with a genetic diagnosis; and (4) the loss of insurability suffered by relatives of an individual with a presumed genetic disease.

Case 1. An HMO had covered the medical expenses of a child since birth but refused to pay for occupational therapy after she was diagnosed with MPS-I, claiming that the condition was pre-existing. All bills relevant to the condition had been paid up to the time of diagnosis, and the occupational therapy had been pre-approved by the managed care corporation. The situation was remedied after the family complained to a customer service representative of the HMO.

Case 2. A private insurer in Colorado notified the parents of a 3-year-old recently diagnosed with an MPS syndrome that the child's policy had been terminated, although the family had been on the policy for nine months before the diagnosis. After an extended negotiation that included retention of a lawyer and the threat of a lawsuit, the insurance policy was reinstated. However, a rider was added to the policy excluding coverage for two common MPS-related complications.

Case 3. A 24-year-old woman was denied life insurance due to her "strong family history of Huntington's Chorea" and the fact that she has never been tested to determine if she is "currently a carrier." The rejection letter stated that if she "should be tested and if found to be negative," the company would issue a standard contract.

Case 4. A mother submitted applications for employment-based life insurance policies simultaneously for her two children, one of whom had Hurler syndrome, a form of MPS. Both were rejected. The rejection letter indicated that the child with Hurler syndrome was denied a policy because the condition is fatal; no reason was given for the denial of a policy to the other child. She was later able to obtain coverage for the healthy child through a different employer.

Clinical Professionals

In several cases, medical professionals reportedly pressured patients or clients at risk for having children with serious genetic conditions to undergo prenatal diagnostic testing or to forsake having children.

Case 1. A PKU gene carrier reported that during a routine pediatric visit, her child's doctor advised her that it would be unwise to have more children and that she should consult a genetic counselor to understand "the implications of PKU."

Case 2. A couple in which one member was at risk for Huntington disease reported that physicians tried to compel them to undergo prenatal genetic testing and coerced them to sign a document agreeing to abort an affected pregnancy. They also reported being required by a health care provider to undergo genetic counseling despite their belief that they had comprehensive knowledge about the genetic risks and their decision to continue any pregnancy irrespective of Huntington disease status.

Adoption

Three issues are illustrated by the cases of alleged discrimination by adoption agencies. They are: (1) a misunderstanding of the nature of the presumed genetic condition with consequent unfair treatment of the prospective parents; (2) the requirement that individuals "pass" a genetic test before being allowed to adopt a child; and (3) the assumption that individuals with genetic diagnoses should adopt only children at risk of having a disability.

Case 1. One respondent, a carrier for MPS, was required by an adoption agency to repeat the blood and urine tests routinely required of prospective parents. It was reported that agency personnel found it "inexplicable" that the original test results were normal in someone who was a carrier for a genetic disorder.

Case 2. A married woman learned that she was at risk for Huntington disease when she was 25 years old. A year later, on the advice of her physician, she and her husband decided to adopt a child. The physician had told her it would be better for her not to have her own children and that she could easily adopt. She therefore underwent a tubal ligation and the couple began the adoption process. The adoption agency application asked why the couple was not able to have children biologically, inquiried about the presence of hereditary disorders, and required certification from a doctor that the couple was sterile. Shortly after filing the application, the couple received a letter from the adoption agency refusing them the opportunity to adopt, based on the woman's risk of Huntington disease.

Case 3. A birth mother with Huntington disease was refused the opportunity to place her child up for adoption through a state adoption agency, but the child was accepted by a private agency. A couple with one member at risk for Huntington disease had been unsuccessful in trying to adopt a child who was assumed to be genotypically normal. However, that at-risk couple was permitted to adopt the at-risk infant.

Armed Services

The case described below involving the armed services shows that even institutions as structured as the military may not have a consistent policy with regard to people at risk for genetic conditions.

Case 1. An individual enlisted in the Air Force and revealed his (approximately 50%) risk status for developing Huntington disease. When applying for reenlistment, he was discharged due to his risk status, although he was asymptomatic. The brother of this individual served in the Marines (who were aware of his risk status) until he became symptomatic for Huntington disease at which time he received a medical discharge and treatment at a V.A. hospital.

Employers

In many of the cases involving employment, individuals believed that they were not hired or were fired because they were at risk for genetic conditions. In other cases, individuals who were employed reported that they were reluctant to seek either a more desirable job or a job in a different location because they feared that they would be unable to obtain health insurance in their new position.

Case 1. A 24-year-old woman was fired from her job as a social worker shortly after her employers learned that she was at risk to develop Huntington disease. In the eight-month period prior to her termination, she had received three promotions and outstanding performance reviews. However, while conducting an in-service training on admitting and caring for Huntington disease patients, she revealed that she had a family member with Huntington disease. Shortly afterward, she was given a poor performance review, though her employers declined to give examples of poor performance. She was soon fired and told by a coworker that the employer was concerned about her risk to develop Huntington disease.

Case 2. A 53-year-old man was interviewed for a job with an insurance company. During his first interview, he revealed that he had hemochromatosis but was asymptomatic. During the second interview, the company representative told him that the company would be interested in hiring him but would not be able to offer him health insurance because of his hemochromatosis. He agreed to this condition. During the third interview he was told that although they would like to hire him, they were unable to do so because of his hemochromatosis.

Educational Institutions

Our study elicited a few reports of genetic discrimination occurring in educational institutions. As in the cases described above, the examples of genetic discrimination by educational institutions involved the denial of opportunities to apparently qualified individuals because of a perceived (genetic) abnormality in those individuals.

Case 1. In a small town, two healthy children attended the same school as their disabled brother. That brother had MPS II and attended a special-education class. In second grade, one of the healthy children was judged to have poor penmanship. A teacher decided that this indicated the onset of MPS II and sent the child back to first grade without consulting the parents or a physician. The parents protested and the child was placed in the appropriate grade.

Blood Banks

Twenty-two respondents with hemochromatosis reported that they were not able to donate blood. The American Red Cross has a policy of rejecting blood donations from all individuals with hemochromatosis, arguing that the donations are treatments, not gifts (Grindon, 1993). A significant number of respondents stated that they donated blood because their health insurance would not pay for phlebotomy treatments. In some cases, blood banks were willing to perform phlebotomies as treatment for a fee. Several of these cases have been previously discussed (Alper et al., 1994). In the case below, prejudice or ignorance of a medical condition apparently played a role in inappropriately denying potential donors the opportunity to give blood.

Case 1. A man who had regularly donated blood for a number of years was deemed ineligible to donate blood by a nurse who learned that he had been diagnosed with Huntington disease. Donating blood was important to this man as a way of making a contribution to society. His neurologic findings, if any, were apparently not an issue since the director of the blood bank invited him to resume his blood donations once that particular nurse retired.

Personal Reactions among People at Risk for Genetic Discrimination

Not unexpectedly, experiencing one or more episodes of genetic discrimination engenders a gamut of personal and psychological reactions for both the affected individual and, often, for other family members. These involve loss of self-esteem, alienation from family members and others, and alterations in family dynamics. For example, some individuals reported that they felt stigmatized and unworthy of marriage or believed that they should only marry disabled individuals. Others behaved as if they had a genetic condition even though they had not been diagnosed. In some instances, family members blamed each other for problems caused by a genetic diagnosis. The cases excerpted below illustrate some of these complex feelings and interpersonal dynamics.

Case 1. A woman at risk for Huntington disease chose her profession (school teacher) because it provided good benefits, especially disability benefits. Although some of her friends know of her risk, she keeps her genetic information from her employers because, in her words, she "doesn't trust" them.

Case 2. A woman at risk for Huntington disease reported that friends and co-workers continually pressure her to undergo genetic testing arguing that if information can be obtained, she should not remain ignorant. As a result, she feels less free to discuss her risk status with friends and is resentful of the intrusion.

Case 3. A woman learned of her risk of Huntington disease in adolescence. She reported feeling that she could not have a "normal" life, had no interest in marriage or children, and chose a career that had good disability benefits available. Later, genetic testing revealed that she was at low risk to develop Huntington disease. Since then she has actively pursued a career change and marriage.

Strategies to Avoid Genetic Discrimination

Many individuals used strategies to prevent themselves from experiencing genetic discrimination. These strategies included purchasing insurance policies before genetic testing, being tested anonymously, paying out-of-pocket for tests so that insurance companies would not obtain the results, providing partial disclosure of relevant information and, sometimes, providing incorrect information (see also Smith, 1995).

Individuals reported avoiding genetic testing and/or avoiding situations where genetic information could be used against them. For example, several of these respondents reported that they had never been rejected for insurance because they had not applied for it: they stated the belief (true in the case of Huntington disease) that their applications would necessarily be denied.

Case 1. The parent of an individual died of Huntington disease. Fearing adverse consequences at work if the diagnosis became known, the individual arranged for the diagnosis of "asphyxiation" to be reported as the cause of death so as to avoid mention of the disease in an obituary.

Case 2. An 18-year-old man, at risk for Huntington disease, wished to enlist in the Marines in order to serve in the Persian Gulf War. He believed it unlikely that he would become symptomatic during his tour of duty but worried that his risk status would disqualify him from service. He therefore answered "no" to questions regarding hereditary disorders on his application and did not include Huntington disease in his family medical history.

Knowledge of the Medical Information Bureau

The Medical Information Bureau, Inc. (MIB), is a private, nonprofit corporation that provides insurance companies with medical and certain nonmedical information about potential insurees (Ostrer et al., 1993). Member organizations (mostly insurance companies) have access to its computerized data bank of information about individuals. Thus, genetic information provided by the MIB could result in inappropriate discrimination in obtaining health or life insurance, particularly if recorded data are incorrect or misleading (Norton, 1989; Ostrer et al., 1993). The MIB does offer individuals the opportunity to examine their MIB records and request corrections. However, doing so requires knowledge of the existence and function of the MIB. We therefore questioned individuals concerning their awareness of the MIB. Only 10 of the 55 (18%) respondents asked about the MIB knew of its existence and none had asked for access to their MIB records.

Knowledge and Use of State Insurance Commissions

State insurance commissions are charged with regulating the insurance industries in their states. Consequently, appeal to a state insurance commission is one mechanism for challenging a perceived discriminatory decision regarding procurement of insurance. Therefore, study participants were sampled regarding their knowledge of state insurance commissions. Nineteen out of 58 respondents (33%) knew of the existence of state insurance commissions, and many of the nineteen thought the purview of these commissions was limited to automobile insurance.

Discussion

The purpose of this study was to determine the varieties and impact of genetic discrimination using the case studies of individuals who have, or who are at risk of having, abnormal genotypes. The results extend the findings of the pilot study: genetic discrimination exists and has significant impacts on individuals and their families. The pilot study provided evidence of genetic discrimination in several social arenas: health insurance, life insurance, and adoption. This study confirmed these findings, providing many more instances of genetic discrimination in each of these areas and identifying additional institutions engaged in discrimination.

This study also revealed several additional ramifications of genetic discrimination. First, some cases were reported in which clinical professionals appeared to give judgmental and possibly coercive counsel to persons who were at risk for abnormal genotypes or having offspring with abnormal genotypes. While all individuals, professional or otherwise, have personal positions on ethical issues, the imposition of a clinician's values with respect to reproductive decisions is regarded as inappropriate (President's Commission for the Study of Ethical Problems in Medicine and Biomedical and Behavioral Research, 1983). It is not possible to determine whether the alleged incidents occurred exactly as they were related to us. Nonetheless, even if some of these cases reflect a misunderstanding between the health care provider and patient, they suggest that poor communication can give rise to the perception of discrimination.

Second, while this study was not designed to evaluate the psychological effects of genetic discrimination, the pervasiveness and importance of these effects became apparent. The cases that we have summarized illustrate typical feelings expressed by respondents. Individuals reported stigmatization by relatives, friends, coworkers, and other members of their communities. Some respondents reported that a genetic diagnosis resulted in feeling a loss of self-worth; others reported feeling powerless to challenge adverse decisions. These responses were common and indicate the significant impact that genetic discrimination can have on people's lives.

Third, although many of the individuals reported that they had not experienced genetic discrimination, comments on their questionnaires revealed that many of them had adopted strategies to ensure that others would not learn of their genetic backgrounds. Apparently they perceived the possibility of genetic discrimination and took action to avoid it.

Fourth, most respondents lacked either the information or the inclination to deal with the discrimination they encountered. For example, although state insurance commissions might appear to be the appropriate avenues for redress of grievances against insurance companies, only 33 percent of individuals who reported experiencing discrimination knew these commissions existed. A recently published study found that state insurance commissioners were unaware of incidents of genetic discrimination (McEwen, McCarty, and Reilly, 1992). Our results indicate that this lack of awareness arises not because genetic discrimination does not exist as was suggested by that study, but rather because affected consumers did not appeal to the insurance commissions.

Even individuals who were aware of regulatory agencies often did not avail themselves of opportunities to redress their grievances. Some felt they had little hope of successfully challenging discrimination. In one case, an attorney who had been denied health insurance because of diagnosis of (asymptomatic) hemochromatosis did not reapply or fight the denial because she "didn't want to be reminded" that she had a genetic diagnosis.

To increase our understanding of the causes of genetic discrimination and suggest strategies for minimizing discriminatory incidents, we attempted to determine whether instances of genetic discrimination occurred as a result of ignorance on the part of the discriminating institution or as a result of institutional policy. Our study revealed instances of both causes of discrimination and, in some instances, these two causes were difficult to distinguish. For example, in several reported cases involving a few specific companies, life insurance agents in a branch office were unaware of company policy that individuals with asymptomatic hemochromatosis should not be denied an insurance policy. This pattern suggests not only ignorance on the part of the agents but also that the company is not troubled by and may even condone such ignorance.

Other cases provide additional examples of ignorance giving rise to genetic discrimination. Representatives of an adoption agency reportedly thought that parents of children with MPS could not be healthy. Some teachers and school officials apparently believed that unaffected siblings of affected relatives must themselves be at risk for MPS and in need of special treatment.

The single clear example of genetic discrimination due to institutional policy is that of the American Red Cross's refusal to accept blood donations from people with hemochromatosis. Because the standard treatment for hemochromatosis, phlebotomy, is not covered by many health insurers, some individuals donate blood as an alternative to treatment. There is no apparent medical reason to restrict the use of this blood; instead, the policy of the American Red Cross is based on the nonaltruistic nature of the donation (Grindon, 1993).

The instances of differential treatment based on genetic tests described in this paper raise questions concerning the legality of this discrimination. Under what circumstances is it legal to limit an individual's opportunities for employment, insurance, education, or for adopting a child on the basis of genetic information? Existing federal legislation such as the Rehabilitation Act of 1973 and the Americans with Disabilities Act of 1990 (ADA) provides that much differential treatment against those with disabilities is unlawful. The question of whether the ADA provides protective coverage for individuals who have abnormal genes but are asymptomatic or presymptomatic has been the subject of considerable debate (Holtzman and Rothstein, 1992; Natowicz et al., 1992b). Recent guidelines from the EEOC (Equal Employment Opportunity Commission) regarding the definition of "disability" under the ADA specifically address the issue of genotypically abnormal individuals who are asymptomatic or presymptomatic, stating that those individuals are covered under the definition of "disability" in the ADA if they are regarded as disabled (Equal Employment Opportunity Commission, 1995).

Although the ADA provides broad legal protections against genetic discrimination, it is apparent that, for the most part, its provisions do not apply to insurance underwriting (Gostin, 1991; Natowicz, Alper, and Alper, 1992a; Ostrer et al., 1993; Equal Employment Opportunity Commission, 1995). There is growing concern that insurance companies are abandoning the practice of community rating, in which all people in a given geographical area pay the same premiums, in favor of underwriting, that is, setting premiums on the basis of an individual's risk. In principle, there is no need for underwriting since the rates set in community rating reflect the known incidence of morbidity and mortality in that geographical area. However, insurance companies are concerned that other companies will skim (i.e., insure only those individuals with the lowest risks). In addition, they fear that individuals who know that they are at risk for increased morbidity or mortality will buy an excessive amount of insurance (Ostrer et al., 1993). Our study showed that this possibility is real; several individuals who were at risk for Huntington disease reportedly attempted to buy life insurance or increase the amount of their coverage when they first learned of their at-risk status or when symptoms of the disease appeared. Given these pressures on insurance companies to resort to underwriting, it is likely that insurance companies will increasingly use genetic as well as other sophisticated medical tests.

Since federal regulation of insurance companies is extremely limited, any meaningful restrictions of the use of genetic tests by insurance companies will need to be mandated by state legislation. States vary widely in their regulation of genetic testing by insurance companies (McEwen and Reilly, 1992; Ostrer et al., 1993). Some states have already enacted legislation prohibiting or limiting the use of genetic information in insurance underwriting. Although at this time the prospect of a universal health care policy in the United States is uncertain, any such policy will have to deal with the increasing use of genetic tests by medical professionals and insurance companies.

This study of genetic discrimination is limited in several respects. The respondents are members of genetic disease support groups who do not represent the entire population of affected individuals. In addition, they are a self-selected subgroup of the membership of those groups. In many instances, documentation of discrimination was difficult to obtain. Some types of discrimination, such as employment discrimination, cannot be documented easily. In other instances, records of discrimination had not been kept, especially if the individuals believed that there was no recourse for appeal of an adverse decision. Thus, it is difficult to determine to what extent reports of genetic discrimination are of actual rather than perceived discrimination.

The low response rate to the questionnaires, even taking into account the actual incidence of genetic discrimination, is due to several factors. No follow-up mailings of the questionnaire were sent, a practice that greatly increases response rates. Further, some questionnaires were returned by people who noted that they were not appropriate respondents, indicating that the mailing lists of the disease organizations include many individuals who are not personally affected by the disorders and so would not respond to the questionnaire. It is also possible that the response rate reflects a real result—namely that genetic discrimination exists at this time but is not a widespread phenomenon.

Finally, we emphasize that this study is not a survey but rather an attempt to collect case studies in order to examine the varieties of genetic discrimination. Consequently, any statistical analysis of the cases would be both inappropriate and unnecessary.

This first extensive study of genetic discrimination extends and confirms the results of earlier ones. The cases from this study are consistent with the interpretation that although not systematic, genetic discrimination does occur in a wide variety of contexts and can cause hardship to affected individuals and their families. Many instances of genetic discrimination described in this study are similar to other types of discrimination. The distinctive nature of this type of discrimination lies in its effect on individuals who are asymptomatic and may never become symptomatic. Because the number and use of genetic tests are expanding rapidly and will continue to increase, it is vital that standards be developed in the near future to ensure that genetic information be used fairly. As our society struggles to become more equitable in its treatment of people regardless of race, age, or gender, it cannot ignore or justify inequities based on genotype.

REFERENCES

Alper, J., L. Geller, C. I. Barash, P. R. Billings, V. Laden, and M. R. Natowicz. 1994. "Genetic Discrimination and Screening for Hemochromatosis," *Journal of Public Health Policy* 15:345–58.

Alper, J. S., and M. R. Natowicz. 1993. "Genetic Discrimination and the Public Entities and Public Accommodations Titles of the Americans with Disabilities Act," *American Journal of Human Genetics* 53:26–32.

Andrews, L. B., J. E. Fullarton, N. A. Holtzman, and A. G. Motulsky, eds. 1994. *Assessing Genetic Risks: Implications for Health and Social Policy*. Washington, D.C.: National Academy Press.

Billings, P. R., M. A. Kohn, M. de Cuevas, J. Beckwith, J. S. Alper, and M. R. Natowicz. 1992. "Discrimination as a Consequence of Genetic Testing," *American Journal of Human Genetics* 50:476–82.

Caskey, C. T. 1993. "Molecular Medicine: A Spin-off from the Helix," *Journal of the American Medical Association* 269:1986–92.

Dewar, M. A., R. Moseley, H. Ostrer, L. Crandall, D. Nye, and B. Allen. 1992. "Genetic Screening by Insurance Carriers." *Journal of the American Medical Association* 267:1207–8.

Equal Employment Opportunity Commission. 1995. *Compliance Manual*. March 14, vol. 2: EEOC order 915.002, section 902. Washington, D.C.

Gostin, L. 1991. "Genetic Discrimination: The Use of Genetically Based Diagnostic and Prognostic Tests by Employers and Insurance," *American Journal of Law and Medicine* 17:109–44.

Grindon, A. J. 1993. "Blood Donation from Patients with Hemochromatosis," *Journal of the American Medical Association* 270:880.

Holtzman, N. A. 1989. *Proceed with Caution: Predicting Genetic Risks in the Recombinant DNA Era*. Baltimore: Johns Hopkins University Press.

———. 1992. "The Diffusion of New Genetic Tests for Predicting Disease," *FASEB Journal* 6:2806–12.

Holtzman, N. A., and M. A. Rothstein. 1992. "Eugenics and Genetic Discrimination," *American Journal of Human Genetics* 50:457–59.

McEwen, J. E., K. McCarty, and P. Reilly. 1992. "A Survey of State Insurance Commissioners Concerning Genetic Testing and Life Insurance," *American Journal of Human Genetics* 51:785–92.

McEwen, J. E., and P. R. Reilly. 1992. "State Legislative Efforts to Regulate Use and Potential Misuse of Genetic Information," *American Journal of Human Genetics* 51:637–47.

Natowicz, M. R., J. K. Alper, and J. S. Alper. 1992a. "Genetic Discrimination and the Law," *American Journal of Human Genetics* 50:465–75.

———. 1992b. "Genetic Discrimination and the Americans with Disabilities Act," *American Journal of Human Genetics* 51:895–97.

Nelkin, D., and L. Tancredi. 1994. *Dangerous Diagnostics: The Social Power of Biological Information*. Chicago: University of Chicago Press.

Nowak, R. 1994. "Genetic Testing Set for Takeoff," *Science* 265:464–67.

NIH/DOE Working Group on Ethical, Legal, and Social Implications of Human Genome Research. 1993. "Genetic Information and Health Insurance: Report of the Task Force on Genetic Information and Insurance." *Human Gene Therapy* 4:789–808.

Norton, C. 1989. "Absolutely Not Confidential," *Hippocrates* (March–April): 53–59.

Ostrer, H., W. Allen, L. A. Crandall, R. E. Moseley, M. A. Dewar, D. Nye, and S. V. McCrary. 1993. "Insurance and Genetic Testing: Where Are We Now?" *American Journal of Human Genetics* 52:565–77.

President's Commission for the Study of Ethical Problems in Medicine and Biomedical and Behavioral Research. 1983. *Screening and Counseling for Genetic Conditions: A Report on the Ethical, Social, and Legal Implications of Genetic Screening, Counseling, and Education Programs.* Washington, D.C.

Smith, K. 1995. *Consequences of Genetic Discrimination.* Master's Thesis, School of Public Health, University of California, Berkeley.

U.S. Congress, Office of Technology Assessment. 1992. *Genetic Counseling and Cystic Fibrosis Carrier Screening: Results of a Survey.* Washington, D.C.: U.S. Government Printing Office.

Wilford, B. S., and K. Nolan. 1993. "National Policy Development for the Clinical Application of Genetic Diagnostic Technologies: Lessons from Cystic Fibrosis," *Journal of the American Medical Association* 270:2948–54.

APPENDIX: TABLES

Table 12.1. Questionnaire.

1.	What is your genetic diagnosis?
2a.	Do you think that you may have been refused social benefits or denied opportunities because of your diagnosed condition?
2b.	If no, do you have any concerns for the future, or other comments?
3.	In what year did the event(s) occur?
4.	Around what issue did you experience difficulties? (Health insurance, life insurance, adopting children, military, social services, church/synagogue, community/neighbors, other.) Please specify.
5.	Please describe your experiences, explaining why these are discriminatory.
6.	Are there any other comments that you would like to make?
7.	Please note which institution sent you this questionnaire.
8.	May we contact you for more information (name, address, telephone)?

Note: The above questions were distributed in a questionnaire to individuals associated with genetic disease support groups who were likely to have a genetic diagnosis (see Methods). In addition to the questions listed above, the questionnaire had a brief definition of genetic discrimination and an assurance of confidentiality. A nearly identical questionnaire was distributed to individuals likely to be carriers for a genetic disorder.

Table 12.2. Partial List of Questions from the Telephone Guide Used for
Interviews on Genetic Discrimination.

Number of children/family members affected by the condition
Pedigree
Presence or absence of confounding disabilities
Context of the occurrence or the event
   (Insurance, employment, public entities & accommodations/housing, education,
   government, community, other)
Insurance
   Type? (Health, life, disability, automobile, home/mortgage, commercial loan)
Obtaining, renewing, or switching insurance?
   Company name?
Employment
   (Hire, promotion, transfer, job responsibilities, compensation, eligibility for benefits,
   provision for disability, association with someone disabled, other)
   Company name?
   Employer/title?
   Probe about type of job and relevance of the condition to job performance
   Was physical accessibility to an activity curtailed in any way?
   Were reasonable accommodations requested? If so, were they provided?
   After the incident, where did you work?
   If you changed jobs, why?
   Describe educational background and qualifications for job
   Jobs held before and after (title/duties/length of time/why left)
Public entities and accommodation
   (Adoption agency, public housing, obtaining a loan, professional licensing, other
   licensing, transportation services, place of education, day care center, recreational
   facility, other)
Education
   (Admission, activity restriction, termination, health service, other)
Government
   (Military, benefits, social security entitlement, federal, state, local, other)
   Military
   (Entrance, transfer, job responsibilities, activity restrictions, termination, promotion,
   other)
   Army, Navy, Air Force, Marines, National Guard, other
Benefits
   (Type: eligibility criteria and dates)
Community
   (Neighborhood, religious community, recreational facilities)

How was information about your condition revealed?
Did the institution get information from the Medical Information Bureau? What
information did they get? How did you find out?
What did you request and why? (Describe all events, contacts/correspondence which
precede the institution's denial.)

Table 12.2. continued

Who did you first contact? (include job title)

Type of correspondence (letters, phone, person)

What if any additional medical information were you required to disclose? (May we receive a copy of their request?)

Were you given a reason why this information was required?

Did you voluntarily submit additional information or medical letters of support? (May we receive documentation?)

Did you seek help from an outside source, such as personnel or other people you know, a disease support group, etc.?

What was the nature of their reply?

 (Refusal to consider case, request for additional information—if so, what was requested? Were you or your physician requested to submit information? Other?)

Did the person making the decision explain to you what they thought and why? How was this communicated to you?

How long did the institution take to respond to your initial inquiry?

Was the response made in person? by phone? by letter? (personalized form or letter? May we obtain a copy? If not, why?)

Who replied? (job title)

Did this person continue to handle your case, or was it referred to a supervisor? If so, how high up within the organization did consideration of your case go? Did you ever request that a supervisor take charge?

Table 12.3. Tabulation of Questionnaires.

Disorder	Questionnaires (returned/sent)	Reporting Genetic Discrimination		
		Yes	No	Ambiguous
Huntington disease	623/25,924	276	329	18
Hemochromatosis	138/1,250	53	85	0
MPS	57/420	44	10	3
Phenylketonuria	22/200	12	8	2
Other*	77/none	70	5	2
Total	917/27,790	455†	437	25

*This category includes questionnaires with information regarding disorders other than those listed above or questionnaires for which it was not possible to ascertain the disorder the individual had. Questionnaires returned blank are not included.

†The 206 interviewees were from the 385 individuals in this category reporting an association with Huntington disease, hemochromatosis, MPS, or phenylketonuria. See Methods for a more detailed description of the selection of individuals interviewed.

CHAPTER THIRTEEN

Current Developments in Genetic Discrimination

Lisa N. Geller

Increased research in the field of molecular genetics has led to the development of genetic tests for a variety of disorders. The scientific discoveries leading to these tests, and in some cases the tests themselves, have been well publicized. Increasing numbers of people are now being tested for genetic disorders and predispositions to such disorders because of the increased availability of tests as well as increased public awareness of genetics. While the genetic information obtained from those tests is useful for diagnosis, for assessing predisposition to a genetic disorder, or for selecting a treatment regime (see Alper, Chapter 1 in this volume), many are concerned that such information will be used to discriminate against individuals. Furthermore, genetic testing of populations may lead to discrimination against groups based on the perception that people in those groups carry "faulty" genes (see Beckwith, Chapter 2 in this volume).

Discrimination based on an individual's genetic makeup (genotype) is termed *genetic discrimination.* Such discrimination can be based on knowledge of an individual's actual genotype or on a belief about his or her genotype. By the early 1990s, it had become clear that there were questions about the possible negative effects of genetic information. One important question was whether genetic discrimination would occur. To clarify this, the Genetic Screening Study Group undertook a preliminary study (Billings et al., 1992), which was followed by a more extensive survey (Geller et al., 1996, reprinted as Chapter 12 in this volume) investigating the experiences of people reporting genetic discrimination and the venues in which such discrimination occurred. The first contribution of these studies was demonstrating that genetic discrimination did occur. Respondents in these studies reported genetic discrimination in a number of settings including insurance (health and life insurance), the armed forces, adoption agencies, blood banks, educational institutions, interactions with clinical professionals, and employment.

It is now generally accepted that genetic discrimination occurs. This chapter focuses on how society has responded to the threat of genetic discrimination. Because government officials are regarded as representing their constituencies (i.e., the public), legislative and regulatory actions can serve as one measure of public reaction to genetic discrimination. Increased calls for education on genetic issues serve as another measure. Some of the responses to concerns about genetic discrimination have occurred in the venues previously reported in the Geller et al. study, while several additional venues have also shown a potential for genetic discrimination. In all of these cases, privacy and fairness are the main issues that underlie public concern about genetic discrimination and motivate the enactment of legislation. Such legislation is intended to prevent the use of genetic information for discriminatory purposes and create a tension between people's desire to know about their own genetic makeup and use it for their own purposes, at the same time limiting access to the information by others that may cause harm.

Agents and Institutions Engaging in Discriminatory Practices

Health and Life Insurance Corporations

Insurance, especially health insurance, is the most prominent venue in which genetic discrimination has been reported and about which individuals voice concerns. For example, there are major concerns over insurance companies' practice of creating high-risk pools. People who purchase insurance are assigned to such pools based on the perceived risk of their incurring high health care costs and are charged higher rates for insurance than those assigned to lower-risk pools. Genetic testing could provide insurers with another means of assessing people for assignment to risk pools.

In an effort to address these concerns, about forty states have enacted some type of legislation related to health insurance and genetic information. Most legislation prohibits the use of genetic information for restricting enrollment in insurance plans (at least in the absence of symptoms) and provides some kind of privacy protection of genetic information. In this legislation, the definition of *genetic test* (the mechanism by which genetic information is procured) varies. Many definitions include not only tests that provide information about genes and chromosomes but also those tests based on evaluation of gene products.

Fear of genetic discrimination among adults who are at risk for or have a disease with a genetic component has been found in several studies (e.g., Lynch et al., 1999; Williams et al., 1999; Phillips et al., 2000). Discrimination by health insurance companies was found to be of particular concern. It is difficult to say whether the fear expressed by participants in these studies truly reflects public knowledge of the risks associated with genetic information or whether the study participants were particularly sensitive to the issues by virtue of their specific interest in a genetic disease. Regardless of the cause for fear, these studies support the proposition that there is a perception of serious potential for genetic discrimination by insurers.

Another study found that, although there was little current evidence of discrimination by insurance companies and agents, it appeared likely that genetic information would be used in the future (Hall, 1999). For example, it was reported that:

> About half of insurers who responded to the general inquiry (eight of seventeen) and about two-thirds of those who responded to the breast cancer example (ten of fourteen) conceded that they might or probably would use such information in some fashion, if legally permitted to do so. Also, four of six insurer subjects said that in the future it is likely that so much more genetic information will exist and predictive data will be so much more precise that genetic test results probably will be much more relevant to medical underwriting. These subjects thought that, whether this information will be used is largely a cost-benefit business decision, in response to market forces. Agents gave similar responses. Ten of fifteen agents said insurers might or would use genetic information in some fashion if legal and it came to their attention, and two of

four said use of this information is likely some time in the future. (Hall, 1999, p. 112; footnotes omitted)

This finding is consistent with others who also found that at least some insurers are interested in using genetic information, if not now, then in the future (e.g., U.S. Congress, Office of Technology Assessment, 1992; Volpe, 1998).

An additional finding of the Hall study was that insurers and agents were not well informed about laws designed to prevent genetic discrimination by their industry. The main point of such laws is to deter the misuse of genetic information as well as to provide legal recourse for those injured by misuse. Therefore, it is important that the insurance industry provide its members with increased education about laws and regulations related to genetic information.

Clinical Professionals

Health care professionals are the providers of most genetic information to individuals, and so they are the logical focus of concern about genetic discrimination. Studies have found that these professionals may themselves discriminate. For example, a health care provider may try to influence a patient to terminate a fetus that has a genetic anomaly even though ethical standards require that they remain nonjudgmental when counseling patients.

Although health care providers may discriminate, especially by trying to influence a patient's health care decisions, they are also the first line for educating patients about the potential for genetic discrimination. Many genetic tests, current and potential, fall into the fields of oncology or reproductive services. Therefore, more attention has been given to the attitudes and knowledge of the professionals in these fields regarding their attitudes and knowledge about genetics. One survey of cancer genetics specialists found that the majority would pursue genetic testing if they had a 50 percent risk of carrying a gene that predisposed them to a hereditary form of cancer. However, the majority of those electing testing would not bill their insurance companies for fear of discrimination, and some would even use an alias (Matloff et al., 2000). In a 1998 study it was reported that "eighteen percent of physicians underestimated the importance of informed consent for [genetic] testing and 34% of discussing the risk of insurance discrimination" (Geller et al., 1998). This presumably means that 66% of physicians were conscious of the importance of discussing genetic discrimination with their patients. Obstetricians/gynecologists were also found to be sensitive to the potential for genetic discrimination, at least with respect to breast cancer (Rowley and Loader, 1996). This may tell a somewhat different story than an earlier survey that found physicians training in these fields (residents) were underinformed about genetics.

Legislation that protects genetic information often imposes a burden on the patient and health care provider by requiring "informed consent." This means that the patient must understand medical procedures and their possible negative consequences before agreeing to such procedures. I maintain that such consent should include informing patients about the possibility of genetic discrimination. Informed consent is desirable in that, among other things, it represents an attempt to prevent paternalism by health care providers and to empower patients to maximize their control over health care decisions. Obtaining meaningful informed consent for a genetic test requires that the person administering the test be competent to provide sufficient education to the patient. Concepts associated with genetic information are complicated because information about an individual may also reveal information about genetically related family members.

A number of authorities have called for increased education about genetics for health care providers, including educating them about the risk of genetic discrimination. There is a developing literature designed to inform specialists and general practitioners about these issues (e.g., American Society of Clinical Oncology, 1996; Roth and Painter, 2000). Little is known about the effectiveness of such education, and it is not clear how practitioners are to incorporate educating their patients into their practices. There will be a clear need for the evaluation of such counseling to permit construction of effective education programs.

Although nonjudgmental counseling is a goal for health care professionals, it does not seem possible or even reasonable for those who perform genetic counseling to achieve this ideal. The mere offering of a genetic test to a pregnant woman or to a couple contemplating parenthood may be construed as pressure not only to have the test but to carry through with the implied "solution" (often an abortion) should a chromosomal or genetic abnormality be discovered.

Some legislation holds a health care provider responsible if they disclose genetic information without the consent of the individual. This is in addition to laws protecting general medical information. Presumably this additional legal threat adds incentive for health care providers to be especially careful about the disclosure of genetic information.

Adoption

Unlike most of the situations discussed above, adoption law permits, and often requires, collecting genetic information about adoptees as well as prospective adoptive parents. Such practices are recommended by professional organizations such as the American Society of Human Genetics and the Child Welfare League (Andrews and Elster, 1998) and are advocated by some in the legal system (e.g., Blair, 1996). There appears to be little concern about genetic discrimination against adoptees. In fact, genetic information about an adoptee can, in some states, be obtained before the adoption is finalized. This means that adoptive parents are able to reject a child if they believe the child is or may become "defective." Lawsuits for wrongful adoption, in which adoptive parents sue an adoption agency essentially for giving them a "defective" child, support the notion that some parents regard the adoption process as a commercial interaction.

The disregard for genetic privacy in the context of adoption also extends to policies regarding prospective parents, whose medical records are often subject to inspection by adoption agencies. States generally do not require medical testing of prospective parents, although their medical records may be inspected. Nevertheless, such testing is sometimes required (Geller et al., 1996).

The reasons for such an apparent lack of concern regarding the genetic privacy of prospective parents and adoptees deserves careful examination, especially since the trend in other contexts is toward increasing protection of genetic information. The reasons for this difference in attitudes toward genetic privacy in adoption are complex. It is likely that the transactional nature of adoption, especially when the adoption is particularly costly to prospective parents in time and money, could encourage the attitude that a child with a medical problem is a defective good. Misinformation or incomplete information about genetics—for example, the belief that genes are equivalent to "fate" and the blanket belief that it is advantageous for an individual's health to "know" about their genetic makeup—also contribute to the notion that it is necessary to gain information about an adoptive child's genetic information.

Much of the information sought in adoption is about the child's biological parents, information that may be anecdotal and irrelevant. This increases potential for adoptive parents to engage in assumptions about their adopted children and sets up a scenario for genetic discrimination. Such discrimination dovetails with the larger issues of how parents view genetic information, including the importance that many assign to being genetically related to their children.

Other recent developments in adoption law raise questions regarding genetic discrimination and privacy that arise years after an adoption is finalized. For example, Oregon law directs licensed adoption officials to inform the object of a confidential search by a blood relative that the reason for the inquiry is "a serious medical condition in the person's immediate family that is, or may be, an inheritable condition." (Oregon House Bill 2860, 1997). The object of the bill is to permit adoptees to obtain medical information from their birth families, opening files that the biological parents may have thought were to remain confidential.

On a related note, reproductive technologies entail privacy issues similar to those arising in adoption. The genetic information of those who participate in reproductive technologies should be protected. For example, sperm banks collect "genetic" information, and in some cases they are obligated by law to disclose genetic information about donors to those who make use of the specimens. In such cases there are issues, similar to those in adoption, of whether to make donors completely untraceable or whether to permit some mechanism by which they can be contacted, an action that would endanger their privacy.

Armed Services

Most discussion of genetic discrimination in the military has focused on a series of memoranda issued by the Department of Defense mandating that members of the armed services provide a sample that can be used for DNA analysis. The primary purpose of collecting such DNA samples is to aid the identification of remains in case of death. The terms and conditions of the military's DNA registry have evolved since the initial memorandum was published in 1991 (Deputy Secretary of Defense, 1991). The current policy is reflected in the March 2, 1993, Notice in the Federal Register (63 FR 10205) regarding the Armed Forces Repository of Specimen Samples for the Identification of Remains. Initially the military was apparently either unaware of or insensitive to the issues raised by keeping DNA samples obtained from members of the armed services and certain civilians associated with the Department of Defense. Several individuals who refused to provide samples were subject to court martial proceedings and, ultimately, convicted. In their testimony, these individuals expressed their concern about the potential misuse of their genetic information, both in the military and, in the case of the inappropriate release of their military genetic records, in civilian life.

A statement by an African American military officer, Air Force Technical Sergeant Warren J. Sinclair, illustrates not just a general fear of genetic discrimination but also a fear that it would be used to exacerbate the evils of our society (e.g., racism).

> Would we ask the Jews to give their genes to the Germans? No! But we think nothing of asking black people to give their complete genetic blueprint to a racist power structure. Until the issue of racism is resolved Afro-Americans should maintain possession of their genetic material. This is a unique opportunity for the armed forces to address a problem that will only intensify if we do not do something to bring healing to our nation. Surely you can understand why it is reasonable for us not to submit.
>
> I have mental scars because of my negative experiences with racist[s] and racism that will not allow me conform to this request at this time. Because the uniqueness of this requirement [to provide a DNA sample] touches the very essence of each individual, we should allow those who cannot conform to depart from the service or be given special status. (United States v. Sinclair, 1996)

Sinclair was sentenced to a reduction in grade to E-4 and to fourteen days of hard labor without confinement.

The present regulations regarding the military's DNA repository provide for early destruction of samples, the stipulation that such samples are to be treated with the same degree of privacy afforded medical samples, and that the samples will not be analyzed unless analysis is believed necessary for identification of human remains. There are a few exceptions, largely having to do with legitimate criminal cases. Presumably, the changes in regulations regarding the military's DNA repository are due in part to individual members of the military becoming aware of possible misuse of their genetic information and the increasing awareness of these issues among members of Congress. The basis for protecting the genetic privacy of military personnel stems from the Federal Privacy Act of 1974 (5 U.S.C. 552a).

Employers

Genetic discrimination in the workplace is addressed in state and federal legislation as well as in policy and administrative regulations. About half of the states have enacted some type of legislation related to genetic information and the workplace (for example, see Office for Human Genome Policy, 2000). This legislation can be divided into three areas, illustrating the major concerns about genetic discrimination and employment.

The first area addresses the concern that genetic information will be used as a criterion for hiring. For example, a person may not be hired because of a possible susceptibility to a disorder that the employer believes will affect job performance. Legislation attempts to ameliorate this scenario by prohibiting requirements that a potential employee undergo a genetic test as part of the hiring process.

A second area of concern is that genetic information could be used to justify firing an employee. Although laws can be enacted to prohibit such uses of genetic information, the efficacy of the legislation would be limited. This is because, as with most genetic discrimination, it is unlikely that any company would document the fact that genetic discrimination was used in a firing decision. This makes it difficult for employees to prevail in lawsuits alleging genetic discrimination.

Finally, there is concern that employers who provide group health or disability insurance will use genetic information as a basis for hiring decisions. An employer might not question an individual's ability to perform a job but still believe, based on real or perceived genetic information, that the individual will become ill and require so much medical care that providing health care benefits for that individual will drive up the cost of the group health plan. This is a particular concern of small employers.

The Equal Employment Opportunity Commission (EEOC) has interpreted the Americans with Disabilities Act of 1990 (ADA) to apply to cases of genetic information (see also Natowicz, Alper, and Alper, 1992). The EEOC ruled that the ADA should apply even when an individual is not actually disabled but discriminated against because of a belief (accurate or not) about their genetic makeup. Some state legislation also adopts this position. For example, legislation passed in 1998 in Maine (S.P. 384) prohibits the use of genetic information in decisions concerning hiring, firing, compensation, terms, or conditions of employment. Under this law, employers are not permitted to consider the information that a genetic test was requested by an applicant or an employee, nor are they permitted to consider the fact that an employee or potential employee refuses to provide results from a genetic test. As in most legislation involving genetic information and the workplace, employers are, however, permitted to use genetic information if it is related to a genuine "occupational qualification."

In April 2001, the EEOC filed its first legal case challenging workplace genetic discrimination by an employer. Burlington Northern Santa Fe Railway was allegedly testing employees who filed claims for work-related carpel tunnel syndrome injuries for a genetic marker, without the knowledge or consent of the employees. The railway settled the case before going to trial and agreed to halt the testing program (U.S. EEOC, 2001). This case represents promise that the ADA may indeed be an effective weapon to combat genetic discrimination in the workplace.

The federal government has also attempted to play a role in providing protection from genetic discrimination in the workplace. The Health Insurance Portability and Accountability Act of 1996 (HIPAA) prohibits the use of genetic test for a preexisting condition if the person is not actually ill. The HIPAA also prevents group health insurance plans from using genetic information as an exclusionary criterion for eligibility, though it does not place limits on the cost of such insurance. As discussed above, although the ADA is not a federal law specifically designed to address genetic discrimination, it has been interpreted by the EEOC, including in those cases where the individual is not actually ill.

On February 2, 2000, President Clinton issued an "Executive Order on Discrimination in Federal Employment," whose stated purpose is "to prohibit discrimination in federal employment based on genetic information." This administrative order prohibits the use of genetic information regarding an individual or their family members with respect to hiring, discharge, or other employment decisions. There are certain exceptions, such as information relating to a condition that may prevent the individual "from performing the essential functions of the position held or desired" (Clinton, 2000, at 301 [a] [3]).

Legislation focused on genetic information may not be necessary to protect individuals if those individuals are already members of a class protected under Title VII of the Civil Rights Act. For example, in *Norman-Bloodsaw v. Lawrence Berkeley Laboratories,* the Ninth Circuit Court of Appeals ruled that pre-employment screening of African Americans for sickle cell trait was a violation of Title VII.

Changes in current legislation make it clear that there are widespread concerns about genetic discrimination in the workplace. This concern is shared by both the executive and legislative branches of the government and at the state and federal levels. The efficacy of governmental precautions against genetic discrimination has yet to be settled in the courts (Miller, 2000; Rachinsky, 2000). It is likely that any cases brought under these laws, even more so than in the case of insurance discrimination, will be difficult to prove since discrimination can be covert.

Educational Institutions

There is little information directly concerning the occurrence of genetic discrimination in education. Yet, as the tendency toward testing and categorizing schoolchildren continues, this is likely to become an area where there is an increase in genetic discrimination. Genetic information is the sort of data that educators may be tempted to use for the "benefit" of a child. For example, as many as 10 percent of school-age boys are being medicated to treat attention deficit hyperactivity disorder (ADHD) and similar disorders. Some who study ADHD have suggested that it has a genetic component. Furthermore, it has been suggested that identification of a gene or genes associated with the disorder (if it is, indeed, a single disorder) would provide a method, via genetic testing, of obtaining early treatment for these boys. Aside from the question of whether a "disorder" that purportedly affects such a large number of children should be considered abnormal, there are numerous reasons for alarm about this approach. For example, studies have shown that the best predictor of a child's classroom performance is a teachers' expectations of that child. A child who is expected to be a behavioral problem based on a predictive genetic test would likely be subject to unfair and adverse discrimination and could live up to that prediction because of the prediction itself.

In addition to being aware of a potential for discrimination based on supposed genetic contributions to behavior, we must be concerned that, despite the repeated failure of researchers to find good evidence of genes for "intelligence," schools may attempt to use such tests to evaluate a child's intellectual potential.

Blood Banks

Alper and his colleagues (1994) and I and my coauthors (Chapter 12) have reported that the American Red Cross discriminates against those with a genetic condition called hemochromatosis. This disorder affects about 1 in 200 people in the United States and about 1 in 100 in the Scottish-Irish and African-American communities, making it the most common Mendelian genetic disorder. The Red Cross does not accept blood donations from individuals who have been diagnosed with hemochromatosis because their disorder is generally treatable with regular bloodletting. Most experts assert that there is no medical reason to discard blood from these individuals.

The FDA permits the use of blood removed by phlebotomy from a hemochromatosis patient (subject to other safeguards) as donor blood as long as it is labeled (21 CFR Ch. 1 [4–1, 93 Edition]). However, the American Red Cross and the American Association of Blood Banks continue to refuse to use blood from hemochromatosis patients as donor blood, citing safety and the fact that blood received this way is not altruistically donated. An underlying reason for this refusal may be economic. The American Red Cross will draw blood from hemochromatosis patients, but to do so it charges for phlebotomies. A *U.S. News and World Report* article (Hawkins, 1997) estimated that phlebotomies for hemochromatosis patients are worth $200 million per year to blood banks, thus raising questions regarding the real motives behind the Red Cross's refusal to accept blood donations from these patients. It should also be noted that some locations *do* accept donated blood from hemochromatosis patients.

The position of the American Red Cross supports fears that increased genetic information may be used for purposes other than the benefit of an individual, even when experts believe there is no reason for such behavior.

Personal Reactions and Strategies to Avoid Genetic Discrimination

Studies report that individuals who are at risk for or who have genetic disorders are often concerned that they will experience genetic discrimination, primarily in obtaining or keeping insurance (e.g., Chapter 12; Lapham, Kozma, and Weiss, 1996). In some cases, concerns about genetic discrimination affected whether individuals decided to be tested for a genetic condition.

There is a particular need to attend to cultural differences when doing genetic counseling, as illustrated by the work of Diane Beeson (reported in this volume) within the African American community and that of H. T. Lynch and colleagues (1996) in the Navajo community. A study of Canadian Jewish women considering testing for a genetic form of breast cancer (Phillips et al., 2000) found that the decision to undergo testing was strongly influenced by altruistic factors and the belief that there would be a psychological benefit (primarily associated with a negative test result). However, the decision to undergo testing was balanced with a perception of associated risks, including insurance discrimination, impact on marriage prospects, and the focus placed by testing on the Jewish community.

As in earlier studies, it has been found that the main methods used for avoiding genetic discrimination are anonymous testing or avoidance of testing altogether. It should also be noted that, in general, people appear to conceal information that may lead to inferences about their genetic makeup, at least with respect to disease.

Genetic testing that is not necessarily associated with disease may also have great import to various communities in ways that cannot be predicted by the dominant community. The chapter by C. Phoebe Lostroh and Amanda Udis-Kessler in this volume illustrates that there is great diversity and controversy within gay/lesbian/bisexual/transsexual/transgender communities involving research related to "gay genes." Jon Beckwith and Joseph Alper, in Chapter 8 of this volume, point out some of the issues related to genetic discrimination that arise from studying minority populations under the auspices of the Human Genome Diversity Project.

Research Subjects

Individuals who participate in research studies are generally considered vulnerable to coercion, discrimination, or other dangers. For research subjects who participate in studies that require genetic information be collected, there is the possibility of an increased risk of discrimination against them or their families. Mere participation in a research study can suggest to an outsider (e.g., an insurer) that a study participant might be predisposed to a genetic disorder.

In general, there has been an increase in the protection of research subjects. National Institutes of Health guidelines stipulate a subject's medical privacy, including privacy regarding genetic information. Despite these guidelines, there have been reports that individuals were subjected to discrimination because of their participation in medical research studies, including a few reports related to genetic information. Computer searches of the Office for Human Research Protections website, using the terms *gene* and *genetics*, in October 2000 had no hits in 271 documents.

Groups who have been discriminated against in the past feel particularly vulnerable to stigmatization and discrimination arising from genetic research. For example, a 1996 case presented to the GenEthics Consortium of the National Human Genome Research Institute describes a proposed study of (and presumption of) a genetic basis for alcoholism in a Native American tribe. In a memo addressed to the institutional review board (IRB) chair, a representative body of the tribe urged that the research proposal be rejected, stating not only that had the tribe not been consulted about the study but also that they feared that "both communities as a whole and individuals within these communities may be stigmatized by such research. We [the tribe] cite the history of discrimination and stigmatization that has followed Native Americans, particularly in relation to alcoholism, as proof of this concern" (GenEthics Consortium, 2000). This is also an issue of particular importance in the pursuit of the Human Genome Diversity Project, as discussed by Jon Beckwith and Joseph Alper in this volume.

There generally appears to be no federal requirement for researchers to inform subjects of the genetic discrimination that could result from participation in genetic research. Even the final report of the Task Force on Genetic Testing (Holtzman and Watson, 1997) does not specify that consent forms for genetic tests should include information about genetic discrimination. This means that responsibility for assuring that research subjects are informed about the risk of genetic discrimination by researchers lies primarily with institutional review boards (IRBs). These boards are the committees within individual institutions charged with responsibility for oversight of research involving human subjects. These committees are generally unpaid and over-burdened and may not have the expertise to advise researchers about protecting subjects from genetic discrimination or even to provide appropriate cautions. As with most consent procedures administered to research subjects, the researcher has a conflict of interest: they are concerned that subjects will not participate in studies if the information in consent forms is onerous. Although there is an increasing effort to keep research participants' data confidential, it should still be required that the possibility of genetic discrimination be discussed with subjects of genetic research.

Paternity Testing and Crime-Related Databanks

Paternity testing raises possible issues for genetic discrimination. Although the genetic tests used for paternity testing are not generally designed to detect mutations associated with diseases or traits, mere sample collection itself can lead to fears that the sample will be misused at some later date. All fifty states have laws related to databanking of DNA samples from convicted felons. In some cases, samples of accused felons are taken and the procedures for destruction of these samples in cases of acquittal may require an affirmative action by the accused. The loss of convicted criminals' rights may include a loss of privacy with respect to genetic information and so subject these individuals to discrimination based on this information.

Studies of Genetic Discrimination

There have been relatively few studies of genetic discrimination published since 1996 that present more than case reports (or anecdotes). The reason for this shortage of follow-up information is unclear: it could be a lack of interest in the topic by funding agencies, the difficulty of conducting such studies, or a perception that further investigation is not required.

While the evidence that has been published since 1996 is generally consistent with earlier data showing that there is genetic discrimination, ongoing research in this area is needed to determine which remedies for genetic discrimination are effective. This is particularly important to pursue with the general public since some experts expect that, in the near future, everyone in the United States will have at least a portion of their genetic code analyzed. Therefore, the potential for genetic discrimination affects everyone and should be given attention by the public, researchers, legislators, and those institutions that anticipate beneficial uses of genetic information.

A pervasive theme underlying issues related to genetic discrimination is that of privacy. The culture of the United States emphasizes privacy to an extent not generally seen in other countries. This is reflected in the emphasis on medical privacy (e.g., New Jersey's 1996 law prohibiting physicians from disclosing genetic information to relatives of a patient unless there is consent or the patient is dead) and the emphasis on privacy in general regarding genetic information. Some state legislation (e.g., in New Hampshire) prohibits not only the use of genetic information in certain contexts such as employment or insurance but also prohibits giving genetic information about an individual to a third party.

Federal legislative efforts have been particularly focused on privacy. Dorothy Wertz (1999) reported that 110 bills with the phrase "privacy of genetic information" were presented in the 105th Congress (although none of the bills were passed). As discussed above, both the legislative and executive branches of the federal government have also attempted to address genetic discrimination in insurance and the workplace.

Conclusion

It appears that the public believes genetic discrimination to be a genuine threat to their well-being. Legislators have reacted at both the state and federal levels to these public concerns by enacting legislation to prevent certain types of genetic discrimination. Similarly, government agencies have promulgated regulations designed to prevent genetic discrimination.

The main venue in which action has been taken to prevent genetic discrimination is legislative. But before the legislative efforts can be fully effective, it is important for health care providers and the general public to be educated about genetic discrimination. Education will help people recognize discrimination and aid the effort to prevent it.

How is this education to occur? One obvious place to start is educating those who are considering undergoing a genetic test. Cho and colleagues (1997) reported that the majority of the pamphlets distributed by companies providing genetic tests did not contain information about "confidentiality, voluntariness, or the possibility of genetic discrimination." Only 3.4 percent (1 out of 29) of pamphlets intended for physicians, 26 percent (10 out of 39) of those intended for patients, and 47 percent (22 out of 47) of those intended for both mentioned these concerns about genetic testing.

Although educating people to recognize genetic discrimination is important, it is not sufficient. People also must be given information about how to avoid genetic discrimination. This means providing individuals with information about how to protect their medical privacy and their rights with respect to that privacy. If this type of education is not provided, individuals considering genetic tests must decide whether to acquire information that they want or need or forgo that information entirely for fear of discrimination. It is important that we develop a system in which individuals can have genetic information that they consider to be important and, at the same time, be protected from unfair discrimination that may result from that information. It is incumbent upon all advocates for genetic technologies to actively seek out and promote measures that permit the beneficial uses of genetic information and eliminate or at least minimize the harms.

The underlying concerns about genetic information are related to the desire for privacy and fairness. There appears to be something special about genetic information that makes people want to keep it private to an even greater extent than they want to keep their general medical information private. The question of fairness raises two sides of the genetic discrimination issue: individuals may want genetic information, but they do not want others such as insurers and employers to have such information. On the other hand, employers and insurers, particularly, can believe that it is unfair for employees and policy holders to be able to keep information secret that can affect business by increasing costs. Ongoing discussion between all interested parties must take place so we can seek solutions to these questions, which reflect the values of our society.

Finally, there are those who will continue to question whether there is enough genetic discrimination to merit so much attention. It is unlikely that we will ever know the extent of genetic discrimination. One measure of the prevalence of genetic discrimination would be the number of related lawsuits, but a lawsuit is a very public (and expensive) undertaking. People who experience genetic discrimination are generally concerned about privacy, something that cannot generally be preserved by filing a lawsuit. Thus, although laws prohibiting genetic discrimination serve to inform society that such behavior is not to be tolerated, enforcement of those laws and resulting litigation is unlikely to reflect the true prevalence of genetic discrimination. Nevertheless, it is clear from studies that genetic discrimination does exist, and no amount of such discrimination is acceptable. We must continue to work, through legislation, education, and public discussion, toward building a society that does not judge or penalize people because of their genes.

REFERENCES

Alper, J. S., L. N. Geller, C. I. Barash, P. R. Billings, V. Laden, and M. R. Natowicz. 1994. "Genetic Discrimination and Screening for Hemochromatosis." *Journal of Public Health Policy* 15:345–58.
American Society of Clinical Oncology. 1996. "Statement of the American Society of Clinical Oncology: Genetic Testing for Cancer Susceptibility, Adopted on February 20, 1996." *Journal of Clinical Oncology* 14:1730–36.
Andrews, L. B., and N. Elster. 1998. "Adoption, Reproductive Technologies, and Genetic Information." *Health Matrix* 8:125–51.
Billings, P. R., M. A. Kohn, M. de Cuevas, J. Beckwith, J. S. Alper, and M. R. Natowicz.

1992. "Discrimination as a Consequence of Genetic Testing." *American Journal of Human Genetics* 50:476–82.

Blair, M. B. 1996. "The Uniform Adoption Acts Health Disclosure Provisions: A Model That Should Not Be Overlooked." *Family Law Quarterly* 30:427–78.

Cho, M. K., M. Arruda, and N. A. Holtzman. 1997. "Appendix IV: Informational Materials about Genetic Tests." In *Promoting Safe and Effective Genetic Testing in the United States,* ed. N. A. Holtzman and M. S. Watson, National Human Genome Research Institute. http://www.nhgri.gove/ELSI/TFGI__final/.

Clinton, W. J. 2000. "Executive Order on Discrimination in Federal Employment." WL 141088 (White House).

Deputy Secretary of Defense. 1991. "Memorandum #47803 and Policy Statement, Deputy Secretary of Defense, to Secretaries of the Military Departments, Subject: Establishment of a Repository of Specimen Samples to Aid in Remains Identification Using Genetic Deoxyribonucleic Acid (DNA) Analysis (16 Dec. 1991)."

Geller, L. N., J. S. Alper, P. R. Billings, C. J. Barash, J. Beckwith, and M. R. Natowicz. 1996. "Individual, Family, and Societal Dimensions of Genetic Discrimination: A Case Study Analysis." *Science and Engineering Ethics* 2:71–88. Reprinted as Chapter 12 in this volume.

Geller, G., B. A. Bernhardt, T. Doksum, K. J. Helzlsouer, P. Wilcox, and N. A. Holtzman. 1998. "Decision-Making about Breast Cancer Susceptibility Testing: How Similar Are the Attitudes of Physicians, Nurse Practitioners, and At-Risk Women?" *Clinical Oncology* 16:2868–76.

GenEthics Consortium of the National Human Genome Research Institute. 2000. http://www.nhgri.nih.gov/About__NHGRI/Dir/Ethics/case__rev.html.

Hall, M. A. 1999. "Legal Rules and Industry Norms: The Impact of Laws Restricting Health Insurers Use of Genetic Information." *Jurimetrics Journal* 40:93–122.

Hawkins, D. 1997. "Throwing Out Good Blood." *U.S. News and World Report,* September 1. http://www.usnews.com/usnews/issue/970901/1bloo.htm.

Holtzman, N. A., and M. S. Watson, eds. 1997. *Promoting Safe and Effective Genetic Testing in the United States.* Bethesda, Md.: National Human Genome Research Institute.

Lapham, E. V., C. Kozma, and J. O. Weiss. 1996. "Genetic Discrimination: Perspectives of Consumers." *Science* 274:621–24.

Lynch, H. T., T. Drouhard, H. F. Vasen, J. Cavalieri, J. Lynch, S. Nord, T. Smyrk, S. Lanspa, P. Murphy, K. L. Whelan, J. Peters, and A. de la Chapelle. 1996. "Genetic Counseling in a Navajo Hereditary Nonpolyposis Colorectal Cancer Kindred," *Cancer* 77:30–35.

Lynch H. T., P. Watson, T. G. Shaw, J. F. Lynch, A. E. Harty, B. A. Franklin, C. R. Kapler, S. T. Tinley, B. Liu, and C. Lerman. 1999. "Clinical Impact of Molecular Genetic Diagnosis, Genetic Counseling, and Management of Hereditary Cancer. Part 2: Hereditary Nonpolyposis Colorectal Carcinoma as a Model." *Cancer* 86 (11 Suppl.): 2457–63.

Matloff, E. T., H. Shappell, K. Brierley, B. A. Bernhardt, W. McKinnon, and B. N. Peshkin. 2000. "What Would You Do? Specialists' Perspectives on Cancer Genetic Testing, Prophylactic Surgery, and Insurance Discrimination." *Journal of Clinical Oncology* 18:2484–92.

Miller, P. S. 2000. "Testing and Telling?: Implications for Genetic Privacy, Family Disclosure, and the Law." *Journal of Health Care Law and Policy* 3:225–65.

Natowicz, M. R., J. K. Alper, and J. S. Alper. 1992. "Genetic Discrimination and the Americans with Disabilities Act," *American Journal of Human Genetics* 51:895–97.

Norman-Bloodsaw v. Lawrence Berkeley Laboratories. 1998. 135 F.3d 1260 (9th Cir. 1998).

Office for Human Genome Policy. 2000. *Genetic Information and Workplace Legislation.* http://www.nhgri.nih.gov/policy__and__public__affairs/legislation/workplace .htm.

Oregon House Bill 2860. 1997. 69th Oregon Legislative Assembly, 1997 Regular Session.

Phillips, K. A., E. Warner, W. S. Meschino, J. Hunter, M. Abdolell, G. Glendon, I. L. Andrulis, and P. J. Goodwin. 2000. "Perceptions of Ashkenazi Jewish Breast Cancer Patients on Genetic Testing for Mutations in BRCA1 and BRCA2." *Clinical Genetics* 57:376–83.

Rachinsky, T. L. 2000. Genetic Testing: Toward a Comprehensive Policy to Prevent Genetic Discrimination in the Workplace." *University of Pennsylvania Journal of Laboratory and Employment Law* 2:575–98.

Roth, M. T., and R. B. Painter. 2000. "Genetic Discrimination in Health Insurance: An Overview and Analysis of the Issues." *Nursing Clinics of North America* 35:731–56.

Rowley, P. T., and S. Loader. 1996. "Attitudes of Obstetrician-Gynecologists toward DNA Testing for a Genetic Susceptibility to Breast Cancer." *Obstetrics and Gynecology* 88: 611–15.

United States v. Sinclair. 1996. Record of Trial at 105, *United States v. Sinclair* (Central Judicial Circuit, USAF Trial Judiciary, May 10, 1996). Warren J. Sinclair, Memorandum to Convening Authorities, Subject: Submission of Clemency Matters (June 27, 1996). As quoted in Gill, S. 1997. "The Military's DNA Registry: An Analysis of Current Law and a Proposal for Safeguards." *Naval Law Review* 44:175–222.

U.S. Congress, Office of Technology Assessment. 1992. *Genetic Tests and Health Insurance: Results of a Survey.*

U.S. Equal Employment Opportunity Commission (EEOC). 2001. "EEOC Settles ADA Suit against BNSF for Genetic Bias." Press release, April 18. http://www.eeoc.gov/ press/4-18-01.html.

Volpe, L. C. 1998. "Genetic Testing and Health Insurance Practices: An Industry Perspective." *Genetic Testing* 2:9–12.

Wertz, D. C. 1999. "Legislative Update: Genetic Privacy Bills." *Gene Letter* 3 (February): 2 http://www.geneletter.org/0299/legislativeupdate.htm. Cited in J. L. Dolgin, "Choice, Tradition, and the New Genetics: The Fragmentation of the Ideology of the Family," Connecticut Law Review 32 (2000): 523–66.

Williams J. K., D. L. Schutte, C. A. Evers, and C. Forcucci. 1999. "Adults Seeking Presymptomatic Gene Testing for Huntington Disease." *Image: The Journal of Nursing Scholarship* 31:109–14.

Index

reproductive issues, 15; adoption, 253–54, 272–
73; cost-benefit analysis in, 50; counseling
in, 48–50; eugenics and, 48–50; women's
role in decision making about, 102–22
research, genetic: benefits of, to sexual minorities, 205–9; dangers of, on sexual orientation, 209–11; famial studies in, 30–34, 180;
on gene therapy, 88–89; on homosexuality,
199–202; impact of, on women, 102–22; media reporting on, 9–10, 58–79; social/ethical
questions in, 4–5; subject protection in, 235–
36, 279–80; therapy vs. cure as goal of, 98–
99, 188; university-based, 233–36
responsibility, effect of genetic linkage on personal, 75–76
Risch, Neil, 27
Rist, Darrell Yates, 198
Roberts, Dorothy, 153–54
Rothman, Barbara Katz, 117
Roubertoux, Pierre, 52, 53
Rushton, J. Phillippe, 180

schizophrenia, 30–32. See also mental illness
science: GLBT mistrust of, 222–23; as neutral,
51, 72; news reporting on, 58–79
Science for the People, 3
Secretary's Advisory Committee on Genetic
Testing, 103, 241
Segal, Nancy, 47
self-help groups, 10. See also advocacy groups
sexual orientation, 12, 18; genetic influences in,
202–5; genetic research issues and, 205–11.
See also "gay gene"; homosexuality
Shaw, Margery, 49
Sheldon, William H., 179–80
Shockley, William, 180
sickle cell disease, 11, 152–74, 178; employment
discrimination and, 276; medical model vs.
family model of, 155–56; perception of, as irrelevant, 166–68; screening program for, 184–
85; study findings on, 159–69; study methods
on, 157–59; testing history of, 152–56
Sinclair, Warren J., 274
single-gene diseases, 20–21, 23–24, 24–26; behavior and, 29–30; cystic fibrosis, 24–25;
fragile X syndrome, 25–26; Huntington disease, 25–26

Skolnick, Mark, 67
social class: "gay gene" research and, 224–25;
prenatal testing and, 110–11
social policy, 42–43
sociobiology, 2–3
Sociobiology: The New Synthesis (Wilson), 2–3
Sociobiology Study Group, 3
species-typical functioning, 126–27
state insurance commissions, 258
Steinschneider, Alfred, 45
stereotypes, racial, 183
Stockdale, Alan, 10, 80–101
sudden infant death syndrome (SIDS), 45
support groups. See advocacy groups

Tacitus, 175
Tay-Sachs disease, 178, 183–84; reduction in, 153
Tentative Pregnancy, The (Rothman), 117
Terry, Patrick, 91–97
Terry, Sharon F., 10, 80–101
thalassemia, 23, 154, 178
therapeutic research, 98–99, 188
Tolin, Jonathan, 105
triplet repeats, 25–26
Tuskegee syphilis study, 162, 163
Twilight of the Golds, The (Tolin), 105, 106, 110
twin studies: behavior genetics and, 47; on
cancer, 26–27; on homosexuality, 200; on
intelligence, 181–82; on mental illness, 30–31

Udis-Kessler, Amanda, 12–13, 215–26
Ulrichs, Carl Heinrich, 199
ultrasound tests, 124
university-based research, collaboration of
commercial industry in, 233–36
University of Pennsylvania, Institute for Human Gene Therapy, 233–34, 235–36

values: conflicting, 5–6, 7; in genetic counseling, 49–50; geneticists' attitudes and, 51–54;
in science, 5; sickle cell disease and, 156; societal, 4–5
Venter, J. Craig, 229

Walker, Lynn, 137–38
Watson, James, 1, 18–19, 44, 48; on selective
abortion, 131

Printed in the United States
21395LVS00002B/97-99